Bottom Line's
HEALTH
BREAKTHROUGHS
2008

Bottom Line
Books
www.BottomLineSecrets.com

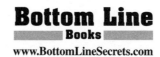

Health**Day**

Articles in this book were written by reporters for HealthDay, an award-winning international daily
consumer health news service, headquartered in Norwalk, Connecticut.

Bottom Line Books® publishes the opinions of expert authorities in many fields.

The use of this book is not a substitute for health or other professional service. Consult a physician
or other health-care practitioner for answers to your specific questions and before you make
any decision regarding your health.

Addresses, telephone numbers and Web sites listed in this book are accurate
at the time of publication, but they are subject to frequent change.

Bottom Line Books® is a registered trademark of Boardroom® Inc.

281 Tresser Boulevard, Stamford, CT 06901

Printed in the United States of America

Contents

1

Aging & Senior Health

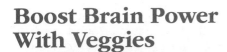

Boost Brain Power With Veggies

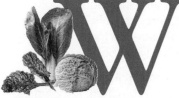ant to preserve your mental edge as you age? Vegetables—particularly green, leafy ones—will do the trick if you eat three servings a day, new research shows.

According to Martha Clare Morris, associate professor at Rush University Medical Center in Chicago, and lead author of the study, "People who consumed two or more vegetables a day had a 35% to 40% decrease in the decline in thinking ability over six years. That's the equivalent of being five years younger in age."

THE STUDY

Morris's team studied 3,718 men and women 65 years of age or older who live in Chicago. "We used a complete food questionnaire of 139 different food items," Morris said. "We asked about their usual intake and assessed the frequency of intake." During the six-year study, the participants received at least two cognitive tests that measured their memory and thinking speed.

"By far, the association with a slower rate of decline was found in the group that ate high amounts of green, leafy vegetables," Morris said. Such foods included lettuce and tossed salad, spinach, kale and collards.

EVERYDAY TASKS

Because the cognitive tests measured overall thinking ability, the benefits of eating vegetables may translate into an easier time with such everyday tasks as remembering phone numbers and names and balancing checkbooks, according to Morris.

Martha Clare Morris, ScD, associate professor, Rush University Medical Center, Rush Institute for Healthy Aging, Chicago.

Dallas W. Anderson, PhD, program director for population studies, Dementias of Aging Branch, Neuroscience and Neuropsychology of Aging Program, National Institute on Aging, Washington, DC.

Neurology, the scientific journal of the American Academy of Neurology.

1

THEORY

Morris suspects that vegetables may help protect memory and thinking speed because they contain high amounts of vitamin E, an antioxidant that can help reduce the damage caused by free radicals, unstable oxygen molecules that can damage neurons in the brain and contribute to dementia.

"We had found in previous studies that vitamin E in food protected against cognitive decline and the development of Alzheimer's disease," she said.

"When we eat vegetables, we tend to put the good fats on them, such as an oil-based salad dressing on salads, healthy-fat mayonnaise on coleslaw, and healthy-fat margarine on vegetables," Morris said. "Such fats help us to absorb the vitamin E, and perhaps are also beneficial to the brain. So that's one plausible explanation of why vegetables are good for you."

THE FINDINGS ON FRUIT

The research also suggests that fruit consumption does not have the same benefits as vegetable consumption.

Morris's study found that high consumption of fruit had no effect on thinking ability. It's possible that some fruit may contain compounds that counteract antioxidants. Further studies are still needed to determine whether fruit is brain-protective, she said.

Dallas Anderson is program director for population studies in the Dementias of Aging Branch of the National Institute on Aging's Neuroscience and Neuropsychology of Aging Program. "It may be premature to discount the role of fruit consumption in maintaining cognitive health," he said, citing recent research showing that weekly consumption of three or more servings of fruit and vegetable juices was associated with a reduced risk of Alzheimer's.

As for eating vegetables, Morris said it's too soon to say for sure that they actually preserve the brain from age-related decline. "But it's encouraging to see that it appears to slow the rate of decline," she said. "We know that eating vegetables is important for chronic diseases. So this might be one more reason why you should eat your vegetables."

MORE INFORMATION

info To learn more about the health benefits offered by vegetables, visit the US Department of Agriculture's Web site at *www.my pyramid.gov.*

■ ■ ■ ■

Relief for Leg Cramps

Many of my patients over age 50 tell me that they have recurrent lower leg cramps, usually in the evening. Their calf muscles seem to tighten up into a knot. Stretching does not alleviate the pain, though massaging the calves often helps.

The culprit is usually mineral deficiencies. This can happen even if you're taking a multivitamin. The three most common deficiencies, in order, are magnesium, calcium and potassium. All three are involved in nerve and muscle contraction. Blood tests can detect these deficiencies, but the tests often are not accurate.

The first thing to do is to consume foods rich in these minerals. Magnesium is found in whole grains, legumes and green, leafy vegetables. Good sources of calcium include broccoli, collard greens, kelp, yogurt and milk (unless you're dairy sensitive). Potassium-rich foods include apples, bananas, oranges, tomatoes and potatoes.

However, many of my patients get the best results by taking a combination supplement. Take a calcium (500 mg)/magnesium (250 mg) complex after dinner. For most people, this will resolve the problem within a day. If that doesn't help, a potassium deficiency may be the problem. Drink eight ounces of vegetable juice a day, such as low-sodium V8 juice.

Dr. Mark Stengler is a licensed naturopathic medical doctor and a leading authority on the practice of alternative and integrated medicine. An associate clinical professor at the National College of Naturopathic Medicine in Portland, OR, Dr. Stengler has served on a medical advisory committee for the Yale University Complementary Medicine Outcomes Research Project and is the author or coauthor of 16 books, including two best sellers—*The Natural Physician's Healing Therapies* and *Prescription for Natural Cures*. Dr. Stengler is the founder and director of the La Jolla Whole Health Clinic in La Jolla, CA. *www.DrStengler.com.*

■ ■ ■ ■

Almonds May Improve Memory

In a recent study, mice with a disease similar to Alzheimer's were fed an almond-rich diet and fared better on memory tests than mice fed a diet without almonds. Almonds contain substances similar to those found in drugs used to treat Alzheimer's.

Neelima Chauhan, PhD, assistant professor of anatomy and cell biology, University of Illinois, Chicago.

Low-Dose Aspirin Doesn't Help Memory

Jae Hee Kang, DSc, instructor of medicine, Brigham and Women's Hospital, Boston.

Gary J. Kennedy, MD, director, geriatric psychiatry, Montefiore Medical Center, New York City.

Sam Gandy, MD, PhD, chair, Medical and Scientific Advisory Council, Alzheimer's Association, and director, Farber Institute for Neurosciences, Thomas Jefferson University, Philadelphia.

British Medical Journal, on-line.

Despite earlier hopes, regular use of low-dose aspirin does not protect older, healthy women against cognitive decline, a major new study concludes.

The findings may lay to rest the notion that aspirin can prevent age-related shortfalls in memory and thinking.

"I certainly don't think that people should look at taking low-dose aspirin as a preventive measure for cognitive decline," said study author Jae Hee Kang, an instructor of medicine at Brigham and Women's Hospital in Boston. "I think that's pretty clear, especially among those women who are healthy."

Another expert, Dr. Gary J. Kennedy, director of geriatric psychiatry at Montefiore Medical Center in New York City, agreed. "It doesn't slam [the door] shut, but it does kind of close it," he said. "They had a large enough sample that, even for a short period of observation, they should have seen the effect."

Previous evidence had suggested that aspirin and other anti-inflammatory drugs might help protect aging brains from dementia. Larger randomized trials, such as this one, however, had been inconclusive.

Low-dose aspirin does have significant cardiovascular benefits. New expert guidelines recommend that women aged 65 and over consider taking low-dose aspirin on a routine basis, regardless of their cardiovascular risk, to help prevent both heart attacks and stroke. Women under 65 should not be taking aspirin routinely.

But this study focused on brain health. Kang and her colleagues looked at almost 6,400 women, aged 65 or over, who were all participating in the Women's Health Study between 1998 and 2004.

ABOUT THE STUDY

Participants were assessed cognitively every two years by phone. These tests tracked general cognition, verbal memory and category fluency (arranging things quickly by kind).

The women were randomly divided into two groups, one of which took a low-dose (100 milligrams) aspirin on alternate days and the other a placebo pill. The study lasted almost 10 years.

At the first assessment (after 5.6 years of treatment), cognitive performance was similar in the two groups, as it was at the second assessment (after 9.6 years of treatment). Risk of substantial decline in cognitive function was comparable between the two groups.

There was a hint that women taking aspirin performed better on the category fluency test than women in the placebo group, but the association was far from definitive.

The data also suggested that low-dose aspirin might be beneficial among people who are current smokers or who have elevated cholesterol. "However, these might be chance findings, as we could not find other studies that replicated this finding," Kang cautioned.

SOME LIMITATIONS

The data does have some limitations, namely that the population in question was generally "younger old" and white. "The risk of dementia really shoots up after age 85," Kang said. "Unfortunately, the trial had ended, so we can't follow these women when it really starts to go up. Whether or not aspirin may be beneficial in those who are older and in high-risk populations is really not known."

"I was not terribly surprised," Kennedy said. "I didn't have high hopes [that aspirin would prove effective], but it's a very useful study that was well-run with careful measures and a big sample. If there was a relationship, this study would have found it."

"This is a holdover from the flurry of older studies aimed at slowing Alzheimer's progression with cox-2 inhibitors and conventional anti-inflammatories," said Dr. Sam Gandy, chairman of the Medical and Scientific Advisory Council for the Alzheimer's Association. "Some of those studies were terminated prematurely due to risks or side effects, but the negative results from the low-dose aspirin study reinforces the notion that a positive outcome was unlikely, had those studies gone on to their intended endpoints."

info For more information on cognitive decline, contact the Alzheimer's Association at *www.alz.org*.

Simple Blood Test May Predict Memory Problems

American Psychological Association news release.

A simple blood test to measure uric acid levels may help predict cognitive problems associated with old age, according to researchers from Johns Hopkins and Yale University medical schools.

THE STUDY

For the study, researchers performed a blood test to measure the uric acid levels of 96 adults ages 60 to 92. The participants with uric acid levels in the high-normal range, defined as 5.8 to 7.6 milligrams per deciliter (mg/dL) in men and 4.8 to 7.1 mg/dL in women, had the lowest scores on tests of mental processing speed, verbal memory and working memory, regardless of age, sex, weight, race, education, diabetes, hypertension, smoking and alcohol abuse.

RECOMMENDATIONS

The findings suggest that uric acid testing may be a useful marker for the risk of cognitive impairment.

"It might be useful for primary-care physicians to ask elderly adults with high normal serum uric acid about problems they might be having with their thinking, and perhaps refer those who express concern, or whose family members express concern, for neuropsychological screening," said study author David Schretlen.

The authors said that further studies are needed to determine whether drugs that reduce uric acid, such as allopurinol, could help older people with high-normal uric acid avoid the cognitive decline that often precedes dementia.

Schretlen said that for reasons that are not entirely clear, uric acid levels increase with age. And higher levels of uric acid have been linked with high blood pressure, atherosclerosis, type 2 diabetes, and abdominal obesity and insulin resistance—all known risk factors for dementia.

Evidence of the connection between uric acid and cognitive function indicates that uric acid testing could be a valuable tool for detecting early cognitive problems in old age, according to the study.

info For more information about dementia, visit the Web site of the American Academy of Family Physicians at *http://familydoctor.org*.

Skin Test Could Detect Alzheimer's Disease Early

Daniel L. Alkon, MD, scientific director, Blanchette Rockefeller Neurosciences Institute, West Virginia University Health Sciences Center, Morgantown, WV.

Sam Gandy, MD, PhD, chair, Medical and Scientific Advisory Council, Alzheimer's Association, and director, Farber Institute for Neurosciences, Thomas Jefferson University, Philadelphia.

Proceedings of the National Academy of Sciences.

A simple skin test that would allow detection of Alzheimer's disease in its earliest stages is working its way to reality. The work "is based on the hypothesis that Alzheimer's disease doesn't just affect the brain, but affects the body systemically," said Dr. Daniel L. Alkon, a lead author of a report on the test.

HOW IT WORKS

The test zeroes in on two forms of an enzyme involved in the degradation of amyloid, the protein that accumulates in the brain of someone with Alzheimer's, said Alkon, scientific director of the Blanchette Rockefeller Neurosciences Institute at the West Virginia University Health Sciences Center.

The presence of Alzheimer's disease is indicated by a steep imbalance in the ratio of the two forms of the enzyme, MAP kinase Erk, in skin cells that are exposed to bradykinin, an inflammation-related molecule, Alkon said. That imbalance is not seen in cells of people without dementia or those with other forms of dementia, he said.

The test produced good results when run on 60 tissue samples: 30 from a tissue bank, 30 from autopsy samples of people diagnosed with Alzheimer's disease, Alkon said.

"We have seen a correlation with the duration of the disease," he said. "The earlier it is done in the course of the disease, the larger is the abnormality."

An as-yet unpublished study of the test done on 100 people showed equally good results, Alkon said. "We are ready to expand this to thousands," he added.

Such expanded testing is essential, said Dr. Sam Gandy, director of Thomas Jefferson University's Farber Institute for Neurosciences and chair of the Alzheimer's Association Medical and Scientific Advisory Council.

Technically, it looks perfectly sound, Gandy said of the published paper. But certainly nothing in science is accepted until it is replicated.

Having a test for early detection of Alzheimer's disease would be extremely valuable, both Alkon and Gandy said. "All the newest medications in clinical trials are aimed at the earliest stage of the disease," Gandy said.

"Drugs now are being tested on the basis of clinical diagnosis," Alkon said. "There is a major need for an early biomarker."

info To learn more about Alzheimer's disease, go to the Web site of the Alzheimer's Disease Education and Referral Center (ADEAR), *www.alzheimers.nia.nih.gov.*

How to Spot Early Signs of Alzheimer's Disease

Todd Feinberg, MD, chief of the Yarmon Neurobehavior and Alzheimer's Disease Center at Beth Israel Medical Center and professor of clinical neurology and psychiatry at Albert Einstein College of Medicine, both in New York City. He is coauthor of *What to Do When the Doctor Says It's Early-Stage Alzheimer's.* Fair Winds.

Alzheimer's disease was first identified 100 years ago, but only recently have significant breakthroughs been made in recognizing the sometimes subtle mental deficits caused by the condition.

Important development: With sophisticated new brain scans and neurological tests, doctors are now able to identify telltale signs of this dreaded disease in its early stages, when treatment is potentially most helpful. *What you need to know…*

HOW IT STARTS

With normal aging, our brains begin to shrink a few cells at a time, which slows brain functioning. In patients with early-stage Alzheimer's, however, a much more insidious process occurs. For reasons that are not well understood, abnormal accumulations of protein fragments and cellular material (plaques) that contain an insoluble protein called beta-amyloid develop, as do brain-damaging bundles of neurofibers known as neurofibrillary tangles.

When memory lapses occur as a result of normal aging, the information can almost always be retrieved at some point later. With early-stage Alzheimer's, however, memories of recent events— those that have taken place in past weeks, days or even hours—completely disappear.

Lesser-known symptoms that also characterize Alzheimer's in its early stages…

•**Loss of initiative.** The person may lose interest in what had been favorite activities, such as gardening or taking walks. He/she may become passive and spend more time sleeping or watching television.

•**Loss of smell.** One study has linked Alzheimer's to an inability to identify certain smells —specifically strawberry, smoke, soap, menthol, clove, pineapple, natural gas, lilac, lemon and leather.

•**Language problems.** Finding the perfect word or phrase becomes increasingly difficult, and vocabulary is diminished.

•**Difficulty reasoning.** This affects a person's ability to do things such as read and understand an instruction manual, balance a checkbook or follow a recipe.

People who have early-stage Alzheimer's also may have trouble making even simple decisions …take longer to perform routine tasks…or experience a change in personality (such as a person who is ordinarily very sociable becoming a recluse).

Important: Many early-stage Alzheimer's symptoms are similar to those caused by depression. Imaging tests, as well as a family history of either condition, can be used to distinguish the two.

During moderate-stage Alzheimer's disease, the patient may become less concerned with personal appearance…confuse the identities of family members (for example, thinking one's wife is one's sister)…hear, see or smell things that are not there…and/or need help with basic hygiene.

Late-stage Alzheimer's is typically characterized by loss of bladder and bowel control…an inability to recognize close family members… difficulties chewing and swallowing…and a need for total assistance with activities of daily living, such as eating, using the toilet, bathing and dressing.

MAKING THE DIAGNOSIS

People who are concerned about memory loss—or experience two or more of the symptoms listed above for early-stage Alzheimer's—should be evaluated by a neurologist, psychiatrist and/or psychologist to rule out treatable conditions that can mimic Alzheimer's. These include nutritional deficiencies (especially those involving vitamin B-12 and folate)…metabolic or hormonal disorders caused by diseases of the liver, pancreas or kidneys…lung problems that reduce oxygen flow, such as emphysema or pneumonia…and alcohol abuse. Certain drugs, such as tranquilizers and antidepressants, also can cause Alzheimer's-like symptoms.

A brain autopsy is the only definitive way to diagnose Alzheimer's disease, but doctors can now make a "probable diagnosis" that is accurate about 90% of the time by using high-tech brain scans and behavior and memory tests.

A computed tomography (CT) or magnetic resonance imaging (MRI) scan is typically used to identify loss of brain tissue and/or decreased brain activity. If results are inconclusive, three-dimensional imaging techniques known as positron emission tomography (PET) or single photon emission computed tomography (SPECT) are used.

EARLY TREATMENT

If a person is diagnosed with Alzheimer's, medication is usually started right away to help slow the progression of the disease as well as curb or stabilize the symptoms. Alzheimer's drugs include *donepezil* (Aricept), *rivastigmine* (Exelon) and *galantamine* (Razadyne). Side effects, such as diarrhea, nausea, appetite loss and insomnia, usually are mild and often diminish within a few months. More recently, *memantine* (Namenda) has been approved for the treatment of moderate and severe Alzheimer's.

PREVENTION

Certain health habits are believed to help protect against Alzheimer's…

•**Control weight,** blood pressure and cholesterol levels. A recent study of nearly 1,500 people in Finland confirmed that risk factors for Alzheimer's and cardiovascular disease are strikingly similar. Researchers found that people who were obese and had high blood pressure and elevated cholesterol levels were six times more likely to develop Alzheimer's than people without those health problems.

•**Eat the right foods.** A nutritious diet rich in brightly colored, antioxidant-rich fruits (blueberries, plums, strawberries, oranges, cherries, raspberries and cranberries) and vegetables (kale, spinach, broccoli, brussels sprouts, red peppers, eggplant and onions) helps curb the damage that brain cells undergo in response to disease-promoting molecules known as free radicals.

•**Stay physically active.** Any kind of physical activity is valuable. But cardiovascular exercise, including walking, is particularly good for overall circulation—and blood circulation to the brain.

'Fat' That May Lower Alzheimer's Risk

Ernst J. Schaefer, MD, senior scientist and director, Lipid Metabolism Laboratory, Jean Mayer US Department of Agriculture Human Nutrition Research Center on Aging at Tufts University, Boston.

Martha Clare Morris, ScD, epidemiologist, Rush University Medical Center, Chicago.

Archives of Neurology.

Adding further weight to the theory that fish may be brain food, new research found that people with diets rich in fish have a significantly lower risk of dementia and Alzheimer's disease.

The key may be docosahexaenoic acid (DHA), an omega-3 polyunsaturated fatty acid that appears to affect dementia risk and to be important for the proper functioning of the central nervous system.

"If you have a high level of DHA, a fatty acid found in fish, it reduced your risk of dementia by about half," said study lead researcher Dr. Ernst J. Schaefer, senior scientist and director of the Lipid Metabolism Laboratory at the Jean Mayer US Department of Agriculture Human Nutrition Research Center on Aging at Tufts University in Boston.

It's known that omega-3 fatty acids protect the heart and the circulatory system. "Just as fish is good for your heart, it's probably good for your brain as well," Schaefer said.

Fatty fish like mackerel, lake trout, herring, sardines, albacore tuna and salmon are high in DHA.

THE STUDY

In the study, Schaefer and his colleagues collected data on DHA levels and dementia in 899 men and women who were part of the Framingham Heart Study. Over nine years of follow-up, 99 people developed dementia, including 71 with Alzheimer's disease.

The researchers found that people with the highest blood levels of DHA had a 47 percent lower risk of developing dementia and a 39% lower risk of developing Alzheimer's, compared with those with lower DHA levels.

People with the highest blood levels of DHA said they ate an average of two to three servings of fish a week. People with lower DHA levels ate substantially less fish, the researchers reported.

REACTION

Schaefer thinks the same benefit can be realized by taking fish-oil supplements. "Everything that we know suggests that supplements would be as effective as eating fish," he said. "Since low fish intake appears to be a risk factor for developing dementia, either eat more fish or use one or two fish oil capsules a day."

However, Schaefer added that a randomized clinical trial is still needed to see if DHA really protects the brain from dementia.

Martha Clare Morris, an epidemiologist at Rush University Medical Center in Chicago, said, "This is the first study to link blood levels of DHA to protection against Alzheimer's disease." She added that recent animal studies have shown that DHA reduces amyloid plaques—a hallmark of Alzheimer's—in the brain and also improves memory.

"There is a lot of animal and biochemical evidence to support what this new study shows," Morris said.

But, she said, she's not sure there is enough data to suggest the value of fish oil supplements. "It looks like the protective benefits from omega-3 fatty acids are at a very low level. There is very little evidence that you get better protection from higher intake," she said. "Whether fish oil supplements are protective is yet to be seen."

info To learn more about dementia, visit the Web site of the Alzheimer's Foundation of America (AFA), *www.alzfdn.org.*

■ ■ ■ ■

Vaccine That Lowers Cause of Alzheimer's Nearly 40%

A new vaccine tested in animals reduced brain protein deposits, an underlying cause of Alzheimer's, by up to 38.5%. If further tests of the vaccine are promising, it could be tested in humans within three years.

The Wall Street Journal.

Dig into the Foods That May Cut Alzheimer's Risk

Nikolaos Scarmeas, MD, MSc, assistant professor of neurology, Columbia University Medical Center, New York City.

Sam Gandy, MD, PhD, chair, Medical and Scientific Advisory Council, Alzheimer's Association, and director, Farber Institute for Neurosciences, Thomas Jefferson University, Philadelphia.

Archives of Neurology.

People who eat a "Mediterranean" diet rich in fruits, vegetables, olive oil, legumes, cereals and fish have a lower risk of developing Alzheimer's disease, researchers report. "We have confirmed the association of a Mediterranean diet with Alzheimer's disease," said lead researcher Dr. Nikolaos Scarmeas, an assistant professor of neurology at Columbia University Medical Center.

This benefit does not appear to be due to the diet's effect on blood vessels, Scarmeas added. "The diet could be helping avoid Alzheimer's disease by protection from oxidative stress or by reducing inflammation in the brain," he said.

Another study finds that taking omega-3 fatty acid supplements slows cognitive decline in some patients with very mild Alzheimer's disease. However, supplements do not appear to affect people with more advanced cases of the disease, according to a team of Swedish researchers.

STUDY #1:
MEDITERRANEAN DIET

For the diet study, Scarmeas's team collected data on almost 2,000 people averaging 76 years of age. Of these, 194 had developed Alzheimer's. The researchers scored each person's diet based on how closely it followed what's known as the Mediterranean diet, which also includes mild-to-moderate drinking and little intake of red meat. Scores ranged from zero to 9. Higher scores were given for those closely following a Mediterranean diet.

People who closely followed that regimen had a significantly lower risk for Alzheimer's disease, the researchers found. For each additional point on the diet score, risk for Alzheimer's was reduced by 19% to 24%.

In fact, people in the top one-third of diet scores had 68% lower risk of developing Alzheimer's disease, compared with people in the bottom third. In addition, people in the middle third had a 53% lower risk of developing the disease.

"It seems that this diet is [health] protective," Scarmeas said. "Taking into account that this diet is protective for other conditions such as coronary heart disease, heart attack, high blood pressure, obesity and a series of cancers, it seems to make sense to follow this diet anyway, and the diet may also protect from Alzheimer's disease."

STUDY #2:
OMEGA-3 FATTY ACIDS

A team led by Dr. Yvonne Freund-Levi from the Karolinska Institutet in Stockholm, looked at the effects of omega-3 fatty acids supplements on 204 patients with Alzheimer's disease.

After six months, among the 174 people who completed the trial, the researchers found no difference in cognitive decline among people taking omega-3 fatty acids supplements at different doses or a placebo.

However, for a subgroup of 32 patients with very mild cognitive impairment at the beginning of the study, those taking the supplements experienced less cognitive decline compared with those who took a placebo, the researchers found.

And when patients who took a placebo during the first six months were given omega-3 fatty acids supplements, their cognitive decline decreased during the second six months of the trial.

REACTION

"The papers share a focus on the idea that diet plays a role in Alzheimer's, a consensus that has been building for the past five or six years," said Dr. Sam Gandy, the chair of the Medical and Scientific Advisory Council at the Alzheimer's Association and director of the Farber Institute for Neurosciences at Thomas Jefferson University.

"The common thread is that both papers point toward intervention at the earliest moment having a greater effect and the suggestion that prevention may have the greatest effect of all," Gandy said.

 To see more articles about Alzheimer's disease and diet, visit *www.medicinenet.com*.

■ ■ ■ ■

Mediterranean Diet Prevents Gallstones in Men

The diet, which includes lots of vegetable or olive oil, nuts and fish, already is believed to protect against heart disease and diabetes. New research shows it can cut gallstone risk in men by nearly 20%. The effect on gallstones in women is not clear.

Edward L. Giovannucci, MD, ScD, associate professor of nutrition and epidemiology, Harvard Medical School, Boston, and coauthor of a study of eating habits and medical histories of more than 45,000 men from 1986 to 2000, published in *Annals of Internal Medicine*.

■ ■ ■ ■

In Need of a Good Greek Salad Recipe? Try this…

1 bunch Romaine lettuce
1 small red onion
1 cucumber
4 Roma tomatoes
Kalamata olives
Feta cheese, crumbled

Dressing:

¼ cup good olive oil
3 to 4 tablespoons fresh lemon juice
1 or 2 cloves crushed garlic
1 teaspoon dried oregano

Whisk together dressing and let it sit while you prepare the vegetables.

Wash and spin-dry lettuce, tear into pieces. Slice onion, tomato and cucumber. Add olives and feta to taste. Whisk dressing before pouring on salad and toss.

Serves 4. Goes well with focaccia bread or pita and hummus.

 For more recipes, visit the Web site *www. recipegoldmine.com*.

Some Drugs No Better Than Placebo for Alzheimer's Patients

Dr. Thomas Insel, director, National Institute of Mental Health.
Dr. Gary J. Kennedy, director of geriatric psychiatry, Montefiore Medical Center, NY, and chairman of the Geriatric Mental Health Foundation, Bethesda, MD.
New England Journal of Medicine.

Antipsychotic drugs, which are commonly prescribed to treat psychosis, agitation and aggression in Alzheimer's patients, do benefit some patients, but the overall picture is bleak, new research suggests.

Two of the drugs studied in this multicenter national trial did seem to ease some symptoms, but the advantages were offset by the severity of the side effects.

MORE RESEARCH

"It's a call to arms to push the research forward much more quickly," conceded Dr. Thomas Insel, director of the National Institute of Mental Health, which sponsored the study.

Newer antipsychotic medications are used widely for Alzheimer's patients, despite an absence of solid evidence of their efficacy.

"I hope this will highlight behavioral interventions which are effective though not perfect," said Dr. Gary J. Kennedy, director of geriatric psychiatry at Montefiore Medical Center in New York City and chairman of the Geriatric Mental Health Foundation, in Bethesda, Maryland.

More than half of Alzheimer's patients experience delusions, hallucinations, aggression and agitation at some point in the progression of their disease. Traditional antipsychotics such as haloperidol have a lower risk of side effects than the newer agents, although both are thought to be equally effective.

SAFETY CONCERNS

Recently, however, new concerns about safety have emerged with the second-generation drugs. Namely, some studies have found an increased risk of cerebrovascular problems and even death.

This study involved 421 participants, all of whom had Alzheimer's disease along with psychosis, aggression or agitation. All participants also lived with a family member or caregiver or in an assisted-living facility, not a nursing home, to give the study more relevance to a real-world setting.

THE STUDY

In the first phase of the study, participants were randomized to receive one of three of the newer antipsychotic medications—*olanzapine* (Zyprexa), *quetiapine* (Seroquel), *risperidone* (Risperdal)—or a placebo.

The investigators were mainly interested in how long patients could take the drugs before discontinuing. Regardless of whether they were taking an actual drug or a placebo, patients discontinued their medication, on average, after about eight weeks.

There were some outliers who benefited from treatment, including 26% to 32% of those taking the active medications who improved, compared with 21% of those on the placebo. Zyprexa and Risperdal seemed to perform better than Seroquel.

Much of this benefit, however, was counterbalanced by side effects such as sedation, confusion and weight gain. Some 15% to 24% of those taking an active medication discontinued their use because of side effects vs. only 5% of those on the placebo.

Eight-two percent of participants discontinued their medications in Phase I. These individuals are now participating in Phase 2 of the trial, in which they are randomized to one of the medications not previously taken or to citalopram, an antidepressant. The results of this phase are not yet available.

MONITORING THE RESULTS

For now, some patients may still benefit from this class of medication. "Even if they don't look like they're effective in a whole population of people, there are some people who will respond and who will be able to tolerate them, so we will probably want to continue to use these drugs with great care and close monitoring of side effects," Kennedy said.

Insel advocates the development of new and better drugs.

"It's probably going to turn out that, in the future, treating psychosis [including schizophrenia] might be like treating hypertension," he said.

"One medication isn't going to be the magic bullet. We need more than one, particularly in those with severe cases."

MORE INFORMATION

info For more information on preventing Alzheimer's disease, visit the Geriatric Mental Health Foundation (GMHF) Web site, *www.gmhf online.org.*

New Ways to Improve Your Eyesight

Eleanor E. Faye, MD, an ophthalmologist in private practice and ophthalmic surgeon emeritus at the Manhattan Eye, Ear and Throat Hospital in New York City. She is medical director of Lighthouse International (*www. lighthouse.org*) and the author of *Clinical Low Vision.* Little, Brown.

Low vision, a permanent vision impairment that cannot be improved by standard eyeglasses, surgery or medical treatment, affects approximately 14 million Americans. Ninety percent of the eye diseases that lead to low vision—macular degeneration, diabetic retinopathy, glaucoma and cataracts accompanied by additional eye problems—occur in people over age 50.

Now: Vision aids—devices that provide magnification, light and/or contrast—can help people with low vision perform tasks that otherwise would be difficult or even impossible. Few doctors prescribe these aids for their patients—so only about 20% to 25% of people with low vision are using them.

GET A PROPER EVALUATION

If you have vision loss due to macular degeneration, diabetic retinopathy, glaucoma or cataracts, it is a good idea to consult an ophthalmologist (a medical doctor who diagnoses and treats eye diseases) or optometrist (a doctor who treats eye conditions not needing surgery) who specializes in low vision.

To find a low-vision specialist in your area, consult the free referral service sponsored by the American Academy of Ophthalmology, the

American Optometric Association and Lighthouse International, a not-for-profit organization that provides education, research, advocacy and rehabilitation services, 800-829-0500, *www.vision connection.org* (click on "Find Help Near You").

The doctor will perform a detailed evaluation of your visual function, including your contrast sensitivity and visual field. Based on his/her findings—and your lifestyle needs—the doctor will prescribe vision aids that best suit you. The products most widely used for low vision—including aids that do not require a prescription—are available at Maxi-Aids, 800-522-6294, *www. maxiaids.com*…and Independent Living Aids, 800-537-2118, *www.independentliving.com.*

Best vision aids for the following eye conditions…

MACULAR DEGENERATION

The most common cause of low vision, macular degeneration occurs when the macula (the central part of the retina, which is responsible for sharpness, color and daylight vision) is damaged by gradual degeneration of retinal cells or hemorrhaging of underlying blood cells into the retina.

Best vision aids: Macular degeneration destroys central vision, so magnification is necessary for most people who have this disease. Magnifiers can be handheld ($10 to $150)…placed on a stand ($20 to $150)…or even attached to your television or computer screen ($50 to $200). Tiny telescopes ($50 to $300) that magnify objects ranging from reading distance to far away can be held up to the eye or mounted on eyeglasses (by prescription only) to help you see better at the movies or the opera or while watching television.

Computer screen magnification is available with software such as BigShot ($99), which enlarges on-screen text up to two times its original size. The software can be purchased at Enable Mart, 888-640-1999, *www.enablemart.com.*

DIABETIC RETINOPATHY

A complication of advanced or long-term diabetes, diabetic retinopathy results in peripheral and central vision loss. It is caused by leaking blood vessels that damage the entire retina, including the macula.

Best vision aids: Diabetic retinopathy affects each individual differently, but most require a variety of aids, such as magnifiers and large-print books and periodicals.

Vision aids that help patients administer insulin are good for those with moderate vision loss from diabetic retinopathy. The Count-a-Dose syringe-filling device ($59.95) makes a clicking sound that can be heard for each dosage increment. The Magni-Guide Magnifier and Needle Guide ($12) magnifies syringe markings and helps guide the syringe needle into an insulin vial.

GLAUCOMA

Increased eye pressure, resulting from a buildup of fluid in the eyes that damages the optic nerves, often leads to the progressive eye disease known as glaucoma. In late-stage glaucoma, the optic nerve damage can cause an irreversible loss of peripheral vision.

Although glaucoma patients typically retain their central vision, it is impaired because their ability to see contrast is significantly reduced. This makes it difficult to distinguish edges, such as those on a curb or steps.

Best vision aids: Good lighting and contrast enhancement are crucial for people with glaucoma. They usually need double or triple the amount of light that a person with normal vision would use. For reading, good options are Verilux lamps (the Verilux Happy-Eyes Deluxe Desk Lamp is available at *www.egeneralmedi cal.com*, 866-844-9402, for $79.95) or an Ott-Lite table lamp (available at Ott-Lite Technology, 800-842-8848, *www.ottlite.com*, for $139.95). Both provide lighting that simulates the full spectrum of daylight, increasing clarity and reducing glare.

Warning: Regardless of whether you have low vision, never use halogen light for reading. Halogen is fine as an incidental light, but it is too intense as a direct reading light and can potentially damage the retina.

CATARACTS

Although cataracts can be surgically removed, some people must delay or even forgo surgery because of other health problems, such as stroke or a broken hip. For these cataract patients, low-vision aids can be helpful until surgery can be performed.

Best vision aids: Magnification makes reading easier, and polarized sunglasses ($12 to $35) eliminate glare and are helpful for people who have had cataract surgery.

Also helpful: To increase contrast on steps, sinks and bathtubs, mark the edges with brightly colored tape. Reduce glare by installing adjustable blinds on windows and covering shiny surfaces with dark tablecloths or towels.

■ ■ ■ ■

Exercise Cuts Risk of Eye Disease by 50%

Exercise helps reduce by half the odds of developing the wet form of macular degeneration, in which new blood vessels grow behind the eye, causing distorted vision and impaired sight. Even simple physical activity, such as walking three times a week or taking the stairs regularly, can help protect against the disease.

Michael Knudtson, MD, biostatistician, department of ophthalmology and visual sciences, University of Wisconsin School of Medicine and Public Health, Madison, and lead researcher of a 15-year study of 4,000 people, published in *British Journal of Ophthalmology*.

■ ■ ■ ■

How Complete Is Your Eye Exam?

Beginning at age 40, you should be screened annually for glaucoma symptoms. *See an ophthalmologist or optometrist, who should perform an exam that includes checking...*

- **Eye pressure.**
- **Optic nerve.**
- **Peripheral vision.**
- **The degree of angle opening.**

To find an ophthalmologist or optometrist in your area, contact the American Academy of Ophthalmology (415-561-8500, *www.aao.org*) or the American Academy of Optometry (301-984-1441, *www.aaopt.org*).

Sleep Apnea Increases Stroke Risk in Elderly

Thomas M. Hemmen, MD, PhD, assistant clinical professor of neurology, University of California, San Diego. *Stroke: Journal of the American Heart Association.*

Elderly people with severe sleep apnea, in which breathing repeatedly stops and starts during sleep, face more than twice the risk of stroke than people with mild sleep apnea or none, Spanish researchers report. Previous studies on stroke and sleep apnea have focused on middle-aged people, but it's older people who have the greatest incidence of stroke, according to study lead researcher Dr. Roberto Munoz, a neurologist at the Hospital de Navarra, in Pamplona, Spain.

THE STUDY

In the study, Munoz's team analyzed 394 people, ages 70 to 100. Over a six-year period, 20 of the study participants had strokes. Patients with severe sleep apnea had a 2.5-fold increased risk of stroke than patients with no apnea, mild apnea or moderate apnea, Munoz's team found.

WHAT TO DO

"Sleep apnea is two to three times more common in the elderly compared to middle-aged people," Munoz said. "However, typical symptoms of sleep apnea, such as loud snoring or excessive daytime sleepiness, are less prevalent in the elderly compared to middle-aged people. We should be aware of these symptoms, and specifically look for the presence of repetitive breathing pauses in our patients and relatives."

Apnea treatment should be started in patients who have a high rate of apnea episodes, particularly in patients with other cardiovascular risk factors, the researchers suggested.

"Snoring is the most important warning sign for sleep apnea," Munoz said. "People who live alone, which is common in the elderly, should be aware that excessive daytime sleepiness is another key risk factor."

One expert agrees that treating sleep apnea is important in reducing the risk of stroke.

Dr. Thomas M. Hemmen, an assistant clinical professor of neurology at the University of California, San Diego, noted that treatment for sleep apnea is becoming standard in reducing the risk of both heart attack and stroke. "People with sleep apnea are much more aggressively treated with respiratory aids during the night," he said.

Sleep apnea is typically treated with behavioral changes, such as losing weight or sleeping on your side. There are also oral devices that help keep the airway open.

info For more on sleep apnea and stroke, visit the Web site of the National Institute of Neurological Disorders and Stroke at *www. ninds.nih.gov/disorders*. Click on "Sleep Apnea."

■ ■ ■ ■

New Help for Common Sleep Problem

The FDA-approved *Pillar Palatal Implant* for sleep apnea—the sleep disorder that causes people to stop breathing intermittently—requires outpatient surgery, during which three pieces of polyester string are sewn into the soft palate. This causes the tissue to stiffen, which reduces sleep apnea and snoring. The procedure is comparable to somnoplasty, in which microwaves directed at the back of the throat stiffen tissue. Either operation is simpler and less painful than the standard surgery to remove excess throat and soft palate tissue.

Bruce Corser, MD, is medical director, Sleep Management Institute, Cincinnati.

Arm Workouts That Ease Leg Pain

American Heart Association news release.

Exercising the arms helps alleviate pain in the legs for people with peripheral arterial disease (PAD), in which narrowed arteries reduce blood flow to the limbs, a new study finds. Aerobic arm workouts can get patients up and walking better, too, researchers report.

In people with PAD, leg muscles can begin to hurt after walking just a short distance. The arteries have been narrowed by blockages, and not enough oxygen-rich blood makes it to the muscles, causing discomfort. The pain subsides after a few minutes of rest. Previous research found that treadmill training benefited PAD patients.

This study found that patients who used an arm ergometer—a tabletop device that has bicycle-like pedals that are operated by the arms—gained improved walking ability.

"This the first study showing that arm-only aerobics can provide results comparable to those seen with treadmill training," said study author Diane Treat-Jacobson, an assistant professor at the University of Minnesota School of Nursing.

THE STUDY

For the study, 35 PAD patients (average age 67) were randomly divided into four groups—no exercise, treadmill exercise, arm ergometer exercise or exercise with both arm ergometer and treadmill.

The patients in the exercise groups worked out for one hour three times a week. After 12 weeks, patients in all three groups showed improvements in the total distance they could walk and how far they could walk without pain.

"We were happy to discover that upper-body aerobics can help patients with PAD increase the distance they can walk without pain. We need additional studies to confirm the results, better understand why and how this works, and also identify the best training regimen for patients," Treat-Jacobson said.

"In the meantime, our results provide evidence that aerobic upper-body exercise is a pain-free alternative for patients with PAD who cannot or do not wish to perform treadmill exercises because of leg pain or some other disability," she said.

info To learn more about PAD, go to the Web site of the Society for Vascular Surgery at *www.vascularweb.org*.

■ ■ ■ ■

A Better Treadmill Workout

Gradually increase the treadmill incline as you run or walk at a brisk pace. To warm up, set the incline at an angle you can sustain comfortably—about a 2% incline for most people. After 10 to 15 minutes, increase the incline up to 3% to 5% over the course of one minute. Run or walk at that incline level for five to 10 minutes. Increase the incline as many as two to three times more, and run or walk for five to 10 minutes at each level.

Caution: Stay on the front of the belt. Running or walking at the back of the belt can result in injuries.

Also: Always check with your doctor before beginning an exercise program.

Derick Williamson, coach, Carmichael Training Systems, an endurance athlete training organization, Colorado Springs.

Why It's So Important to Prevent Shingles Now

Albert Lefkovits, MD, assistant clinical professor of dermatology and codirector of the cosmetic dermatological surgery training program at Mount Sinai School of Medicine in New York City. He also has a private practice in New York City and lectures widely at national and international medical conferences.

F ew people realize that a severe case of shingles—a viral infection characterized by a rash, blisters and sometimes excruciating pain—can lead to serious complications, such as blindness or hearing impairment.

That's why physicians are doggedly pursuing new ways to prevent shingles, and stressing the importance of early treatment to lessen its severity and duration.

Latest development: In 2006, the FDA approved a new vaccine, called Zostavax, that promises to reduce the risk of developing shingles in adults age 60 or older. However, the vaccine may not be appropriate for everyone who is at risk for the condition.

Here's what you need to know…

SIGNS AND SYMPTOMS

Shingles is caused by the varicella-zoster virus, the same virus that causes chicken pox. After an attack of chicken pox (usually in childhood), the virus remains dormant in nerve tissue until

it is reactivated by the onset of a serious illness, such as leukemia or lymphoma…weakened immunity, even from a bad cold…or normal aging.

Each year, approximately one million Americans develop shingles. The virus primarily attacks people over age 60, but it also can occur in children and teenagers. Half of all people age 80 or older can expect to develop shingles.

The first signs of shingles are easy to miss because they can mimic flu symptoms—chills, fever, nausea, headache, even difficulty urinating. Within a week, the virus spreads to the skin, causing the emergence of fluid-filled blisters in a band on one side of the body. The location of the blisters and pain correlates with the area of skin served by the infected nerve. While the rash and blisters usually appear on the trunk, they can appear on the face, near an eye, in the genital area or anywhere else on the body. The blisters usually dry and begin to scab about five days later. But the pain can continue for weeks, months or even years.

Shingles itself is not contagious. However, anyone who has never had chicken pox can develop chicken pox if he/she is exposed to the live virus in the skin of a shingles patient. The virus primarily is transmitted via direct contact with blisters that haven't completely dried. Airborne transmission, while rare, may occur.

Although the reason is unclear, doctors tend to see multiple patients with shingles at the same time—coinciding with a seasonal outbreak of chicken pox in grade-school children, typically in the fall or spring.

IF SHINGLES IS SUSPECTED

If you suspect that you may have shingles (based on the signs and symptoms already described), you should seek prompt medical attention (within 72 hours) either from your family doctor, a dermatologist or a neurologist.

Antiviral medication, which is generally taken for seven to 10 days, can be an extremely effective treatment for shingles. The antiviral agent *acyclovir* (Zovirax) is now available in a generic form, so it is the least expensive antiviral available. However, some people find acyclovir inconvenient to use because it must be taken five times a day. Both *famciclovir* (Famvir) and *valacyclovir* (Valtrex) can be taken three times a day. They are not available in generic forms and cost about $255 to $270 for a seven-day supply. If you start the medication right away, you'll decrease the odds of needing a painkiller later on. Side effects of antivirals may include nausea, headache and diarrhea.

When shingles pain does occur, sufferers describe it as itching, burning or cutting. At its extreme, the pain can be so severe that people contemplate suicide or are willing to undergo radical surgery (which entails cutting the infected nerve's roots) to relieve it. The standard painkillers used for shingles include topical and systemic steroids, the antidepressant *amitriptyline* (Elavil) and the antiseizure drug *gabapentin* (Neurontin).

A NEW VACCINE

As people grow older, their immunity tends to decrease. The new shingles vaccine contains a small dose of a live but weakened varicella-zoster virus. With exposure to the varicella-zoster virus, the recipient's immune system is stimulated to create antibodies against it. This helps protect people who receive the vaccine from developing shingles. The vaccine costs about $150 per dose, not including your physician's fee for the office visit.

Recent finding: In a study of almost 40,000 people age 60 or older, half of whom received a placebo, the vaccine reduced the occurrence of the virus by about 50%. The vaccine reduced postherpetic neuralgia (PHN), extreme nerve pain that can last for months or years after the rash is healed, by 66%. About 20% of shingles patients develop PHN, according to the Varicella-Zoster Virus (VZV) Research Foundation. However, in my experience, the incidence rate and the severity of PHN symptoms have decreased since the introduction of antiviral drugs to treat them.

Who should get the vaccine? That still hasn't been clearly established. The chance for a recurrence is low (about 5%), so people who have already had shingles do not need the shingles vaccine.

Because shingles responds well to treatment when it is initiated within the first 72 hours, I recommend using the new vaccine for adults over age 80 who are generally in good health but very frail. They are most likely to contract shingles and develop PHN.

The studies conducted thus far suggest that the vaccine has only mild side effects, such as redness, pain and tenderness, swelling at the site of the injection, itching and headache. However, many doctors—myself included—are prescribing cautiously because, like other live-virus vaccines used for other conditions, the live varicella-zoster virus can infect others.

Those who are at greatest risk of becoming infected after exposure to a person who has received the varicella-zoster virus vaccine include people with weakened immune systems due to cancer or AIDS and pregnant women, whose fetus could be harmed by a chicken pox infection. Anyone who gets the shingles vaccine should avoid the people mentioned above for about three months following vaccination.

Although doctors are optimistic about the potential of Zostavax, many of us are waiting to see whether widespread use results in yet-unreported adverse side effects.

■ **More from Dr. Lefkovits...**

Best Way to Relieve Shingles Pain

Shingles often causes severe pain. In a new survey conducted by the American Pain Foundation, 35% of 401 shingles sufferers reported "severe" pain...11% said it was "very severe"...and 6% called the pain "intolerable" during the first few weeks of the illness.

Suggested recommendations...

•**Take an over-the-counter (OTC) painkiller.** Some doctors recommend a *nonsteroidal anti-inflammatory drug* (NSAID), such as aspirin or *ibuprofen* (Advil), to help curb skin and nerve cell inflammation as well as pain. Because these medications are known to cause stomach problems, many shingles patients take *acetaminophen* (Tylenol). It has little effect on inflammation but is a very effective pain reliever.

To avoid possible liver damage: Do not exceed the maximum daily dose of 4 g (eight extra-strength tablets)—or 2 g daily if you're age 70 or older.

- **Use topical steroids.** Skin inflammation as well as burning and itching can be relieved with OTC creams and lotions that contain hydrocortisone (1%). These treatments can be used up to three times daily and do not cause side effects, such as weight gain, that are generally associated with oral steroids. If you must take oral steroids for an extended period, you should be closely supervised by your doctor.

- **Take warm baths.** Do this several times daily, if necessary. Warm baths are soothing and help relieve pain.

- **Go to a pain clinic.** People who cannot get adequate pain relief on their own should consider going to a pain clinic, where anesthesiologists, neurologists and other specialists will recommend different pain relief methods. Acupuncture also may be helpful.

info For more information, contact the Varicella-Zoster Virus (VZV) Research Foundation, *www.vzvfoundation.org*, 212-371-7280.

Uneven Leg Length May Boost Arthritis Risk

American College of Rheumatology news release.

People whose legs are of uneven lengths are at increased odds for knee and hip osteoarthritis, new research suggests. The study concluded that a difference of as little as two centimeters (about ⅘ of an inch) could raise the risk for osteoarthritis, the most common form of arthritis, characterized by the breakdown of joint cartilage.

THE STUDY

Researchers studied 3,161 people and found that 6.4% of them had legs of different lengths. Compared with people with legs of equal length, those with leg length differences of two centimeters or more were more likely to develop hip osteoarthritis (32.5% vs. 26.1%) and knee osteoarthritis (45.3% vs. 29%) and were more likely to have severe disease, the study found.

The actual location of osteoarthritis did not seem to be associated with either the longer or shorter limb, although right hip osteoarthritis was more common in people whose left leg was longer than in those with a longer right leg.

IMPLICATIONS

"Recognizing that leg length inequality has a significant association with hip and particularly knee osteoarthritis opens the door to more studies on whether leg length variances might cause the development and progression of the disease," said senior investigator Dr. Joanne M. Jordan, associate professor of medicine and orthopedics at the University of North Carolina, Chapel Hill.

"The findings from this study may help us predict who may develop osteoarthritis and who may have symptoms that worsen or have a potential risk of increased disability. Studies to test whether correction of leg length inequality with an orthotic or shoe lift can prevent the onset of osteoarthritis, or its progression, would be a logical next step," Jordan said.

info For more information about osteoarthritis, go to the Web site of the National Institute of Arthritis and Musculoskeletal and Skin Diseases at *www.niams.nih.gov*. Additional information can be found at *www.rheumatology.org*.

■ ■ ■ ■

Vitamin K Cuts Arthritis Risk

In a new study of 672 adults, those who had the highest vitamin K levels were less likely to have osteoarthritis of the hands and knees than people who had the lowest levels.

Theory: Insufficient vitamin K could affect proteins that build and maintain bone and cartilage.

Self-defense: Get the recommended daily intake of vitamin K—65 micrograms (mcg) for women and 80 mcg for men.

Good sources: Spinach, broccoli and olive oil.

Caution: If you take a blood thinner, vitamin K can reduce the drug's effectiveness.

Tuhina Neogi, MD, assistant professor of medicine, Boston University School of Medicine.

NSAID May Block Flu Vaccines

University of Rochester Medical Center news release.

Some nonsteroidal anti-inflammatory drug (NSAID) painkillers may react with the immune system in a way that reduces the effectiveness of flu shots and other types of vaccines, a University of Rochester study finds.

The researchers said this is an important finding because an estimated 50% to 70% of Americans use NSAIDs for relief from pain and inflammation.

BACKGROUND

"For years, we have known that elderly people are poor responders to the influenza vaccine and vaccines in general," said principal investigator Richard P. Phipps, a professor of environmental medicine and of microbiology and immunology at the University of Rochester.

According to Phipps, elderly people tend to be heavy users of NSAIDs such as Advil, aspirin, or Celebrex. "This study could help explain the immune system response problem," Phipps said.

THE STUDY

Phipps and his colleagues conducted studies on mice and also analyzed samples of blood from people who took part in early clinical trials of a new vaccine against human papillomavirus (HPV), which can cause cervical cancer.

They found that some NSAIDs hinder a vaccine's ability to prompt the immune system to produce antibodies against a specific illness or infection.

The researchers said their findings suggest that it may be wise for people to avoid taking an NSAID when they receive any vaccine.

info For more on vaccines, go to the Web site of the National Institute of Allergy and Infectious Diseases at *http://www.niaid. nih.gov/factsheets/evolution_vaccines.htm* and the Centers for Disease Control and Prevention at *www.cdc.gov*.

Testosterone May Keep Men Steady on Their Feet

JAMA/Archives, journals news release.

Higher testosterone levels may help protect elderly men from dangerous falls, a new study finds. Researchers found that older men with the lowest levels of testosterone in their blood were 40% more likely to fall and to have multiple falls than men with the highest levels of testosterone. Falls are a leading cause of bone fracture in older populations.

The association between falls and testosterone levels was strongest in men ages 65 to 69. The link was not apparent in men over age 80. Testosterone levels naturally decline as men age.

THE STUDY

A research team from Oregon Health & Science University in Portland studied nearly 2,600 men, ages 65 to 99.

The participants gave blood samples and filled out questionnaires on their medical history, medications, and lifestyle habits. The men also performed physical fitness tests.

At the end of the five-year study period, 56% of the men had fallen at least once. The link between falls and testosterone levels was apparent, even after the researchers factored in the men's scores on the physical performance tests.

That suggests that low testosterone levels may raise falling risk in other ways, including impairment of vision, thinking and coordination, the researchers said.

IMPLICATIONS

"These findings strengthen the link between testosterone and the health of older men," the team wrote. They added that testosterone measurements might be useful for identifying men at higher risk for adverse events.

"Moreover, these results provide additional justification for trials of testosterone supplementation in older men and should aid in the design of those studies," they said.

info For more information on low testosterone, go to the Medem Web site at *www. medem.com* and search for "low testosterone."

Amazing! Aspirin Shrinks Enlarged Prostate

Jenny St. Sauver, PhD, epidemiologist, Mayo Clinic, Rochester, MN.

Eric Jacobs, PhD, senior epidemiologist, American Cancer Society, Atlanta.

American Journal of Epidemiology.

Older men who regularly take aspirin or a similar medication may help keep prostate enlargement at bay, a new study finds. The common condition, called benign prostatic hyperplasia, typically affects one of every four men ages 40 to 50 and almost half of those over age 70, experts say. Enlarged prostate can lead to frequent urination and other bothersome effects.

However, men who regularly took a nonsteroidal anti-inflammatory drug (NSAID) "had a reduction of 50% in enlargement and a 35% reduction in moderate to severe urinary problems," said Jenny St. Sauver, a Mayo Clinic epidemiologist who led the study.

It didn't matter which NSAID a man was taking: aspirin, *ibuprofen* (Advil), *naproxen* (Aleve) or a more expensive cox-2 inhibitor such as *celecoxib* (Celebrex), St. Sauver said. "Eighty percent were taking daily aspirin," she said. "We did look at the other drugs, but the differences were not statistically significant."

This study included nearly 2,500 men living in the neighborhood of the Mayo Clinic in Minnesota. Data on NSAID use and prostate enlargement came from questionnaires the men completed every two years from 1990 to 2002.

EXPLANATION

There are several theories as to how NSAIDs might keep prostates from enlarging. According to St. Sauver, the drugs may reduce prostate cell growth or increase the natural death of these cells. Another theory credits the drugs' anti-inflammatory activity.

The findings should not be seen as a green light for men to rush out and start taking these painkillers without consulting a doctor first, the experts stressed. Men should always be cautious about taking NSAIDs, St. Sauver said, because the drugs raise risks for gastrointestinal bleeding and other side effects.

"We would like to see the results of our study replicated," she said. "If it can be, it would be important to figure out what kind of dose and what kind of timing would be proper."

Many of the men in the Mayo Clinic study were taking low-dose aspirin to protect against heart disease, said senior epidemiologist Eric Jacobs. "Currently, the decision about whether or not to take aspirin is based on balancing cardiovascular benefits with the risk of gastrointestinal bleeding," Jacobs said.

info For more information on prostate enlargement, visit the Web site of the National Kidney and Urologic Diseases Information Clearinghouse at *www.kidney.niddk.nih.gov.*

Ageless Fatherhood? Maybe Not

Harry Fisch, MD, professor of clinical urology and director of the Male Reproductive Center, Columbia University College of Physicians and Surgeons, New York City.

Avraham Reichenberg, PhD, assistant professor of psychiatry, Mount Sinai School of Medicine, New York City.

Archives of General Psychiatry.

Human Reproduction.

Journal of the American Medical Association.

Most women hoping to have a family are painfully aware of their biological clocks. They know their ability to bear children declines with age, even with all the innovation in fertility treatments.

Now, research is revealing that a man's potential for producing a child may not last forever, either—at least not without health consequences for the child. And, as men age, those who don't take care of their health may fall victim to a faster, louder clock.

"Men who are overweight, whose belly fat is very bad, have a higher chance of lower testosterone levels," reducing their ability to father a child, said Dr. Harry Fisch, director of the Male Reproductive Center and professor of clinical urology at Columbia University College of Physicians and Surgeons. Cigarette smoking can also adversely affect a man's fertility.

Fisch, author of *The Male Biological Clock*, doesn't believe there's a "cutoff" point for fatherhood. "But the sooner, the better," he said, citing recent research.

DOWN SYNDROME LINK

Several studies have found that older fathers risk having children with medical problems, including Down syndrome. Fisch and his colleagues evaluated more than 3,400 cases of Down syndrome, finding that if the woman and the man were both over age 35 at the time of conception, the father's age played a role in prevalence of the disorder. This effect was most pronounced when the woman was over 40, the researchers found. And, in those cases, the incidence of Down syndrome was about 50% attributable to the sperm, the researchers said.

AUTISM LINK

In another study, Dr. Avraham Reichenberg, of Mount Sinai School of Medicine in New York City, found that advanced age for fathers is associated with an increased risk for having a child with autism. His team gathered data on the age of fathers of more than 318,000 children born in Israel during the 1980s. The researchers found that the chances of having a child with autism or a related disorder were about six times greater if the father was 40 or older compared with men 29 or younger.

SCHIZOPHRENIA LINK

Still another study found that the risk for schizophrenia in children was tied to older age of the father. In the study, which included about 90,000 people, the researchers discovered that children whose fathers were 50 or older when they were born were nearly three times more likely to have the disorder than those born to younger fathers.

MISCARRIAGE AND OTHER LINKS

Another study found a higher risk for miscarriage in mothers 35 and older and fathers 40 and older. And, more research found that 20 different disorders in children—ranging from schizophrenia to skeletal disorders—have been linked to the advanced age of the father.

IMPLICATIONS

So, what's the next step for men who delayed becoming dads? "We need to know more about the 'biological clock' in men before making recommendations," said Reichenberg. "This is the first study to directly examine paternal age in autism in an entire population. There are other studies which, among other variables, also report that the age of fathers of children with autism is higher than those of normally developing children, but paternal age was not their main focus."

Other studies are needed to duplicate his finding, Reichenberg said.

Fisch believes "the sooner, the better" when it comes to having children—for both men and women. If parenthood must be delayed, men should try to stay in the best shape possible, paying attention to maintaining an ideal weight and not smoking, he said.

info For more on male fertility and infertility, visit the American Urological Association at *www.urologyhealth.org*.

How Your Brain Can Keep You Young

Gary Small, MD, Parlow-Solomon Professor on Aging and director of the University of California at Los Angeles Center on Aging and the Semel Institute Memory Center. He is the author of *The Longevity Bible: 8 Essential Strategies for Keeping Your Mind Sharp and Your Body Young*. Hyperion.

Today's American expects to live a long life. Those who make it to age 65 are likely to survive another 17 or more years. But will they be good years? To a great extent, that's up to the individual.

It's easy to say that a genetic roll of the dice determines how rapidly and gracefully we age, but studies have shown that only one-third of the factors that predict how well we age are controlled by genetics.

I've spent more than 20 years researching the lifestyle practices that lead to quality longevity. We all know that a healthful diet is the first step, followed by regular exercise. But there are other commonly overlooked, yet simple, steps that also can make a real difference in the way you age.

A HEALTHY BRAIN

Your brain is the "operating system" of your body. When you protect it, a ripple effect is created. With a sharp memory and positive outlook, you're more likely to take the actions that contribute to overall health and longer life, such as watching what you eat…exercising… and staying attentive to other people, which strengthens your relationships.

How to keep your brain healthy…

•**Brighten your outlook.** Optimists live longer. A Mayo Clinic study found that people who scored high on optimism in a personality test had fewer physical and emotional problems and were 50% more likely to survive another 30 years.

What to do: Practice mental habits that promote positive thinking—focus on your strengths and achievable goals, rather than what's wrong or missing in your life.

•**Do more than crossword puzzles.** Although research is not conclusive, mental workouts, such as those provided by crossword puzzles, have been touted as a key to maintaining brain health. However, crossword puzzles and other brain teasers, such as the number-logic game Sudoku, are of little value unless you really challenge yourself with difficult versions of these and other brain exercises.

What to do: Spend at least 10 minutes each day performing some form of challenging "brain activity." If you like crossword puzzles or Sudoku, choose ones that give your brain a rigorous workout, gradually progressing to even more difficult puzzles. They should be challenging but possible to complete. If you enroll in a class to learn a foreign language, put in the study hours it demands. If you join a book club, make sure you go beyond the best-seller list.

•**Be mindful.** Staying in the moment—aware of your thoughts and bodily sensations, and what's going on around you—promotes the health of both your brain and your body. If you stay in the moment, you're less likely to do things like overeating, tripping and hurting yourself or multitasking, which studies show can be stressful.

What to do: Keep your mind in the present to avoid worrying about the future and/or dwelling on past mistakes—it's a proven stress and anxiety reducer. To achieve mindfulness, sit down and meditate for five to 10 minutes, or simply take a few slow, deep breaths and tell yourself to focus on the present.

Also helpful: If you practice mindful awareness at mealtime, portion control—the key to weight control—will come naturally to you. Notice how your body feels before, during and after each meal. Eat when you're hungry, and stop just before you feel full.

STRONG RELATIONSHIPS

Spending pleasant time with other people can add years of good health. A Harvard study of about 3,000 men and women found that people who socialized most (attended sports events, played games, went to restaurants, etc.) had a 20% better chance of living long lives than loners. In addition, they had fewer disabilities and less cognitive decline.

Close, satisfying friendships and family connections are particularly helpful. The MacArthur Study of Successful Aging, conducted by researchers throughout the US, linked emotionally supportive relationships to lower levels of stress hormones. People with close relationships recover faster from surgery and need less pain medication.

Staying in the moment when talking with others—and being aware when your mind wanders—is the heart of true communication. The more attentive you are to another person's words, expressions and body language, the better you can feel what he/she is feeling. The capacity for empathy builds strong relationships.

What to do: Try this 15-minute exercise with a spouse, family member or friend: For three to five minutes, one partner talks about something that is going on in his/her life, such as a crisis, chronic issue or upcoming event. The listener should maintain eye contact and stay focused on what the other person is saying and should not interrupt. Switch roles for another three to five minutes, then discuss the experience.

COMBAT CLUTTER

A confusing, disorganized environment causes constant stress. When you can't find what you need, you face a constant reminder that you're not in control of your life.

What to do: Schedule 15 minutes a day to put things where they belong. Declutter one room—or one corner of the room—at a time. Put away rarely used items, such as clothes or sports equipment not needed until the next season. Consider donating or throwing away anything you haven't used in the last 12 months. Sort mail, groceries—anything—as soon as it comes into the house. Organize and store similar items together so they will be easy to find later.

Apply the same principle to your personal life. We often maintain friendships even when they become unfulfilling. "Declutter" your social world by staying away from people who make you feel unappreciated, guilty or who simply irritate you. Or at least see them less often. This will create time for healthy relationships.

Add Up to Ten Healthy Years to Your Life

Edward L. Schneider, MD, professor of gerontology and medicine at University of Southern California in Los Angeles and former deputy director of the National Institutes of Health's Institute on Aging. He is author of *What Your Doctor Hasn't Told You and the Health Store Clerk Doesn't Know: The Truth About Alternative Treatments and What Works.* Avery.

There are proven ways to lengthen our lives...or at least extend our "quality life span," when we can still take care of ourselves and enjoy the activities that make life worth living, according to gerontology expert Edward L. Schneider, MD.

Here are seven things you can do that really make a difference...

1. Cardiovascular exercise. Most people know exercise is good for you, but it's worth repeating here because it's the single best way to improve health. People who exercise 30 to 60 minutes per day can add five to 10 years to their quality life span. Exercise measurably reduces the risk of heart disease, stroke, obesity, diabetes, insomnia, depression and certain cancers.

Exercise need not be too strenuous. Walking briskly is sufficient.

Important: Don't exceed 60 minutes of strenuous exercise per day. After an hour, the damage your body absorbs from the prolonged strain outweighs the health benefits. Moderate exercise for more than 60 minutes is okay—for example, walking longer than an hour is fine.

2. Lifting weights for just five minutes each day will strengthen your bones and the surrounding muscles, making broken bones less likely. For seniors, broken bones can mean shorter lives—one of every four people who suffers a hip fracture after age 65 will die within 12 months. Building stronger muscles and bones also will keep you active and independent longer, so you can better enjoy the years you have.

Ask a physical therapist or personal trainer to design a low-impact weight-lifting regimen to tone the muscles of your arms, shoulders, abdomen, back and legs for a few minutes each day. Do not use the heaviest weights you can pick up—choose weights you can lift 20 to 30 times in a row. Increase the weight only when this becomes easy.

3. Mediterranean-style diet. Heart disease and cancer are two of the most imposing obstacles standing in the way of long life. The vitamins, antioxidants and monounsaturated fats found in a Mediterranean-style diet have been found to reduce these risks. The diet includes plenty of fruits, vegetables, whole grains, legumes, garlic, nuts, tomato sauce, berries and fish. You can also have one or two alcoholic drinks per day but no more—women have an increased risk of breast cancer if they have more than one drink a day. Multivitamins are not a suitable substitute for a healthful diet.

Minimize consumption of meat, saturated fats and fatty dairy products—these increase heart disease risk.

Important: Not all fat is bad. Olive oil is full of monounsaturated fats, which are wonderful for the heart. The residents of the Greek island of Crete consume more olive oil per capita than any other area in Europe. They have the lowest rate of heart disease and are 20% less likely to die of coronary artery disease than Americans.

4. Sufficient sleep. Your immune system is best able to fight off infection when it's armed with a good night's sleep. Sleep also keeps your mind sharp, reducing the odds that you'll die in an accident. Sleepy drivers are responsible for just as many fatal car crashes as drunk drivers.

How much sleep is enough? The answer is different for everyone. Some people need as little as five hours a night; others need as much as nine. If you're groggy during the day, try to add 15 minutes of sleep each night until you no longer feel sleepy during the day.

Don't use an over-the-counter sleep remedy even if you have chronic insomnia. These often have large doses of antihistamines that might make you groggy well into the following day. Instead, get more exercise…consume less caffeine…buy a more comfortable mattress and pillow…lightproof and soundproof your bedroom…and remove distractions, such as the TV and books, from the bedroom, so your mind associates the room with only sleep and sex.

Supplements such as valerian and melatonin work for some people but not for most people. Prescription sleeping pills should be used only to break cycles of insomnia. Try to avoid taking a nap during the day—this can wreak havoc with your internal clock.

5. A shared life. A good marriage and enjoyable social life truly do help you live longer. A 48-year-old man has a 65% chance of living to age 65 if unmarried, 90% if married. For a 48-year-old woman, marriage increases the odds of reaching 65 from 80% to 90%.

Friendships, too, contribute to living longer, making us feel better about ourselves and improving our lives.

6. Fish oil (omega-3 fatty acids). Fish oil pills are one of the few dietary supplements that actually can lengthen life. Research has confirmed that fish oil promotes heart and brain health.

Eat one to two servings of fatty fish, such as mackerel, herring or salmon, each week…or take a daily one-gram fish oil pill that contains equal amounts of eicosapentaenoic acid (EPA) and docosahexaenoic acid (DHA).

Caution: High intake of fish oil may cause excessive bleeding in some people.

Some people worry about toxins, such as mercury, in certain fish, including tuna. For most people, the benefits of eating one or two servings of fish a week outweigh potential risks. However, pregnant women, women who may become pregnant, nursing mothers and young children may want to avoid certain fish—talk with your doctor.

7. Sunlight and vitamin D. Studies suggest that vitamin D can help prevent breast, prostate and colon cancers, as well as arthritis. It also promotes the absorption of calcium, which is necessary for bone strength. Sunlight is the usual source of vitamin D. Spend three to five minutes in direct sunlight without sunscreen two to three times per week. (Put on sunscreen if you intend to stay in the sun longer, particularly if you're fair-skinned.)

If you live in the northern third of the US, it's impossible to get enough vitamin D from the sun between late November and the end of March, even if you spend all day outside. Multivitamins tend not to provide sufficient vitamin D, either. Take 1,000 international units (IU) per day of a vitamin D supplement during the winter.

A daily dose of sunlight also helps fight insomnia and depression, either of which could lead to a shorter life. However, vitamin D pills won't help here—you still need your three to five minutes of sun (winter sun is fine).

Boost Your Immunity With T'ai Chi

Michael Irwin, MD, director of the Cousins Center for Psychoneuroimmunology, University of California, Los Angeles, and professor of psychiatry, Semel Institute for Neuroscience and Human Behavior at UCLA.
Journal of the American Geriatrics Society.

T'ai chi, an ancient exercise that features slow martial arts-like movements and meditation, is one method used to prevent the pain and misery of shingles.

A new study finds that by itself, t'ai chi triggers an immune-boosting response in older people to fight the virus causing shingles that is on par with the standard vaccine.

When t'ai chi is coupled with a vaccine, immunity is strengthened even more—to levels normally seen in middle age, say researchers after studying the effects of both measures in 112 people ages 59 to 86.

VIRUS-SPECIFIC PROTECTION

"Since older adults often show blunted protective responses to vaccines, this study suggests that t'ai chi is an approach that might complement and augment the efficacy of other vaccines, such as influenza," notes study lead Dr. Michael Irwin, professor of psychiatry at the Semel Institute for Neuroscience and Human Behavior at the University of California, Los Angeles.

Shingles, which causes a painful and blistery rash, affects about one in three people after age 60. It is caused by the same virus as childhood chicken pox, often lying dormant for decades before reemerging in later years.

Explanation: Irwin says that t'ai chi—often recommended to help reduce stress and improve flexibility—strengthens specific immune-boosting cells that are especially useful at fighting recurrences of previously experienced infections that may lie dormant for decades. However, these cells typically die off as part of the natural aging process, explaining why previous infections (such as chicken pox) can return with a vengeance in older people (as shingles).

 The National Institute on Aging has more on shingles at *www.niapublications.org.*

2

Asthma & Allergies

How to Protect Against Killer Food Allergies

Many people with food allergies have mild symptoms, such as a rash, runny nose or itchy eyes, when they eat small amounts of a problem food. But they may still be at risk for a potentially deadly reaction.

In the US, food allergies cause up to 30,000 emergency room visits and 200 deaths annually due to anaphylaxis, an acute reaction that can cause respiratory distress and/or a heart arrhythmia (irregular heartbeat).

Recent development: The Food Allergen Labeling and Consumer Protection Act, which went into effect in 2006, requires food manufacturers to list eight major allergens on food labels to help people with food allergies identify and avoid problem foods.

IS IT REALLY AN ALLERGY?

Not all reactions to food are due to allergies. Tens of millions of Americans suffer from food intolerance. A food intolerance, such as a sensitivity to the lactose in milk, can begin in childhood. The most common symptom of lactose intolerance is gastrointestinal discomfort, including diarrhea, cramping and flatulence.

Food allergies affect about 11 million to 12 million Americans. With a food allergy, the immune system mistakenly identifies as harmful the various proteins—or even a single kind of protein—within one or more foods. This triggers a cascade of events that causes immune cells to respond to the "threat" by releasing large amounts of histamine and other chemicals that produce the allergic symptoms.

The most common food allergen is shellfish. Up to 2% of Americans are allergic to shrimp

Steve L. Taylor, PhD, professor of food science and codirector of the Food Allergy Research and Resource Program at the University of Nebraska, Lincoln. He is a leading expert on food allergies and serves on the editorial boards of the *Journal of Food Protection* and the *Journal of Natural Toxins*.

and/or other shellfish, such as lobster, crab and crayfish. This type of allergy often is ignored —primarily because most people tend to eat shellfish far less often than other allergenic foods, such as eggs, peanuts and fish.

TESTING FOR ALLERGIES

A food allergy usually can be diagnosed with a thorough medical history taken by an allergist.

The doctor will want to know…

•**When do symptoms occur?** Food allergies typically cause symptoms within a few minutes to several hours after exposure. Symptoms include stomach cramping, hives, lip swelling, runny nose, congestion and asthma. With a food intolerance, symptoms may not occur until the next day.

•**How much did you eat?** With food allergies, any exposure can trigger symptoms. For some patients, 1 mg—an amount that's almost impossible to see—will provoke an allergic response. A reaction can even be triggered by kissing—or sharing utensils with—someone who has eaten a substance to which you are allergic. A skin reaction can occur from touching the substance.

With a food intolerance, symptoms usually are linked to the amount consumed. Someone who's sensitive to milk, for example, can often drink a small amount without a reaction.

Two tests can identify most food allergies. *They are…*

•**Skin prick.** Extracts of suspected foods are pricked into the skin with a needle. The appearance of a rash within a few hours—or even a few minutes—indicates a food allergy.

Caution: The skin-prick test isn't advisable for patients with severe allergies. The tiny amounts of food used in the test could trigger a life-threatening reaction.

•**Radioallergosorbent test (RAST).** This blood test detects antibodies to specific food proteins. The test occasionally produces false positives—indicating an allergy where none is present. It's often combined with the skin-prick test for more accurate results.

TREATMENT

People with a history of serious food reactions must carry an EpiPen. Available by prescription,

it's a self-injector that delivers a dose of epinephrine. Epinephrine stimulates the heart and respiration and helps counteract deadly anaphylaxis.

Important: Use the EpiPen immediately if you experience difficulty breathing or throat constriction. Even if you take the shot promptly, get to an emergency room as soon as possible for follow-up treatments.

Also helpful: Take an antihistamine, such as Benadryl, according to label instructions. It can lessen the severity of symptoms while you get to an emergency room.

New development: *Omalizumab* (Xolair), a medication currently used for asthma, appears to significantly blunt reactions in food-allergy patients who receive a monthly injection of the drug. In an early study, patients who reacted to trace amounts of peanuts were able to eat eight to 10 nuts without experiencing problems. Further studies must be completed to determine whether the FDA deems it an effective—and safe—therapy for food allergies.

AVOIDING PROBLEM FOODS

Because there isn't a cure for food allergies —and even trace amounts of a protein can trigger reactions—strict avoidance is the best defense…

•**Always read food labels**—even if you've safely eaten that product in the past. Manufacturers frequently change or add ingredients.

•**Ask about "hidden" ingredients in medications.** Some prescription and over-the-counter (OTC) drugs, as well as vitamins and supplements, contain milk proteins or other common food allergens. This information should be on the label, but check with your doctor or pharmacist before taking any medication or supplement.

•**Talk to the chef or restaurant manager when eating out.** The waiter or waitress doesn't always have accurate information about food ingredients and preparation. Ask to speak to the chef or manager instead and tell him/her what you're allergic to. Explain that any contact with the offending food can be life-threatening.

If you're allergic to shellfish, for example, tell the chef or manager you can't eat a hamburger that was cooked on the same grill used to cook shrimp.

Other hidden sources of food allergens: Cooking oils that are used to cook different foods…knives and cutting boards that aren't washed clean between uses.

●**Wear a medical alert bracelet/necklace.** Anaphylaxis can potentially cause a loss of consciousness within minutes. A medical alert bracelet/necklace lets medical personnel know that you require urgent treatment for your allergy.

Astounding! Aspirin May Prevent Asthma

Tobias Kurth, MD, ScD, assistant professor, medicine, associate epidemiologist, division of aging, Brigham and Women's Hospital, Boston.

Rick Vinuya, MD, allergist/immunologist, Providence Hospital and Medical Center, Southfield, MI.

American Journal of Respiratory and Critical Care Medicine.

C an taking an aspirin each day stop asthma from developing in adults? Possibly, suggests new research that found adult-onset asthma risk was reduced by 22% in men who were already taking a daily aspirin for heart-disease prevention.

"Our findings suggest that low-dose aspirin may have beneficial effects on asthma," said study coauthor Dr. Tobias Kurth, an assistant professor of medicine and an associate epidemiologist in the division of aging at Brigham and Women's Hospital in Boston.

BACKGROUND

As many as 20 million Americans have asthma, according to the American Academy of Allergy, Asthma & Immunology (AAAAI). Despite advances in treatment, about 5,000 people die due to asthma every year in the US, the AAAAI reports.

The incidence of asthma has been rising in recent years. And that rise coincides with the decreased use of aspirin as people have switched to other over-the-counter pain relievers, or avoided aspirin use in children due to concerns about Reye's syndrome. That led researchers to wonder if the reduction in aspirin use was contributing to the rise of asthma.

THE STUDY

To test that hypothesis, Kurth and his colleagues reviewed data from 22,071 male physicians between the ages of 40 and 84 who were randomly assigned to receive either a daily dose of 325 milligrams of aspirin or a placebo. The original aim of the research was to study aspirin's role in heart-disease prevention.

During the five-year study period, 113 new cases of asthma were diagnosed in the aspirin group, compared with 145 in the placebo group. This represented a 22% decrease in the risk of developing asthma for those taking low-dose aspirin.

RECOMMENDATIONS

Kurth said the researchers weren't able to study the reasons why aspirin might have this preventive effect against asthma, but theorized that aspirin's anti-inflammatory effects might play a role.

He did caution, however, that for some people who already have asthma, aspirin could be an irritant that can actually trigger asthma symptoms. The question for researchers now, according to Kurth, is "for those at risk of getting asthma, should they be treated with aspirin or not?"

Dr. Rick Vinuya, an allergist and immunologist at Providence Hospital and Medical Center in Southfield, Michigan, echoed Kurth's comments.

"Any time you have an intervention to prevent the onset of disease, it's exciting, and a 22% reduction in risk is huge. This study needs to be followed up with a study specifically designed to answer whether aspirin really does have an affect and how does it work?"

Right now, Vinuya said, no one should start taking aspirin to prevent asthma. "This study adds on to the beneficial effects of aspirin. It's a healthy practice to take aspirin to prevent heart attacks and now it looks as if a secondary benefit is a possible decrease in the development of asthma. But, asthma prevention can't be the primary reason for taking daily aspirin," he said.

info To learn more about aspirin's role in heart attack and stroke prevention, visit the Web site of the American Heart Association at *www.americanheart.org*.

Sinusitis Could Start In the Stomach

Jordan S. Josephson, MD, director of the New York Nasal and Sinus Center, which treats people who suffer from sinus disease and related conditions, in New York City. He is the author of *Sinus Relief Now: The Groundbreaking 5-Step Program for Sinus, Allergy and Asthma Sufferers.* Penguin.

Chronic sinusitis is often part of a cluster of health problems that includes asthma and bronchitis as well as serious digestive problems, such as chronic heartburn. Sinusitis also is a cause of sleep apnea (temporary cessation of breathing while sleeping), which can indirectly lead to heart attack and stroke. Knowing that these conditions can be connected helps sinusitis sufferers to protect themselves from seemingly unrelated health problems.

SINUSITIS DANGERS

When the sinuses become inflamed by infection or allergy, the tissues swell, closing off the airflow and making it difficult to breathe through the nose. As a result of inflammation, mucus turns thick and sticky and can become yellow, green, brown or tan.

The inflammation and infection associated with sinusitis can spread to the respiratory tract and affect the digestive system as well, causing a broad set of health problems called chronic airway-digestive inflammatory disease, which results in...

•**Lung problems.** When the sinuses no longer cleanse the air properly, inflammation of the large and medium airways can result. This can lead to bronchitis, causing congestion, coughing and shortness of breath. Inflammation of the small airways can cause asthma.

•**Digestive disorders.** Infectious mucus dripping down the back of the throat may inflame the stomach, causing acid to back up into the esophagus, leading to chronic heartburn, a symptom of gastroesophageal reflux disease (GERD).

•**Sleep apnea.** Many people who snore also suffer from sleep apnea. Besides the stress of extreme fatigue caused by repeated awakenings, sleep apnea reduces oxygen levels in the blood, increasing heart attack and stroke risk.

BEST TREATMENT APPROACHES

Mild sinus symptoms should be treated the same way you would treat a cold—with lots of fluids to keep mucus thin and flowing, and plenty of rest (ideally, 12 or more hours each night). An over-the-counter decongestant, such as *pseudoephedrine* (Sudafed), can relieve stuffiness and pain. Decongestants have stimulant effects and should be used for no more than two days without the guidance of a physician. If used for longer than a few days, decongestants can have a rebound effect, leading to more congestion. Avoid antihistamines unless sinusitis is caused by an allergy.

If sinus symptoms last for more than 48 to 72 hours or are accompanied by even a mild fever or nausea, diarrhea, facial swelling or swollen neck glands, or if the pain is severe, see your doctor. You may have a bacterial infection and need to take an antibiotic.

Important: Some sinusitis symptoms are often overlooked—headache, typically around the eyes and forehead...persistent cough...hearing loss (caused by fluid buildup in the middle ear), resulting in ringing in the ears (tinnitus)...and toothache (the roots of some teeth are close to the sinuses).

To prevent sinusitis or if it recurs twice a month or more, or if symptoms linger despite treatment, follow a program of self-care that includes...

•**Irrigation.** Washing out the sinuses maintains healthy mucous membranes and keeps air passages open. When symptoms are acute, irrigate the sinuses twice a day. Daily irrigation will keep problems from returning, especially in the winter and during allergy attacks.

What to do: Use "normal saline"—a solution of salt water diluted to the same concentration as bodily fluids. Good sterile saline preparations, which are available at drugstores, include Ayr...Breathe-ease XL...or Goldberger's Ultra Saline Nasal Mist (available at 800-228-5382, *www.goldbergerspharmacy.com*).

•**Environmental control.** Airborne allergens...other irritants, including cleaning chemicals and smoke...and microorganisms, such as mold, trigger and exacerbate sinusitis. House-hold dust is a common allergen and irritant.

To minimize dust exposure: Wash bedding weekly in hot water, and place plastic covers or allergen-resistant fabric covers on the mattress and pillows…vacuum at least weekly, with a vacuum cleaner that has a high-efficiency particulate air (HEPA) filter…remove carpeting and shampoo area rugs once or twice a year…use sealed wood, plastic and metal furniture…and replace drapes with venetian blinds.

To prevent mold exposure: Clean mold-prone areas (in and around the shower, kitchen sink and washing machine) with a solution of bleach and water. Because mold thrives in damp places, don't let kitchen and bathroom walls and floors remain wet, and don't let water accumulate around the washer, sink or refrigerator. Leave the washer door open after use, to let it dry out inside. Repair roof and basement leaks promptly.

To keep sinus membranes from drying out, use a humidifier in the winter to add moisture to the air.

Important: Clean the humidifier at least weekly to prevent the growth of mold and other microorganisms.

SURGICAL OPTIONS

When sinusitis persists despite medical treatment and self-help, surgery may be necessary…

•**Debridement removes scar tissue,** scabs and infectious matter from the sinuses. It is usually performed in the doctor's office with a topical anesthetic.

•**Functional endoscopic sinus surgery (FESS)** involves opening passages and removing small growths and other blockages to promote free movement of air and drainage of mucus. FESS is usually outpatient surgery that is performed in a hospital under local or general anesthesia. Bleeding and postoperative pain are generally minimal.

■ **More from Dr. Josephson…**

What Are the Sinuses?

The sinuses are hollow spaces in the facial bones that surround the nose. Each sinus is lined with mucus to catch bacteria, viruses, fungi and other particles. Tiny hair-like cilia move most of these particles toward the back of the nose and down the throat into the stomach to be destroyed and excreted.

Easy Ways to Soothe Sinus Problems

Robert S. Ivker, DO, former assistant clinical professor of family medicine and clinical instructor of otolaryngology at the University of Colorado School of Medicine, past president of the American Holistic Medical Association (AHMA), cofounder and past president of the American Board of Holistic Medicine (ABHM), and author of *Sinus Survival: The Holistic Medical Treatment for Allergies, Asthma, Bronchitis, Colds and Sinusitis.* Tarcher.

Dry air is tough on sensitive mucous membranes, and closed windows and poor ventilation can lead to the build-up of noxious particles (including fumes from harsh cleaning products, paint, perfumes, etc.), the enemies of sinusitis and allergy sufferers.

Rob Ivker, DO, a family doctor for 35 years and past president of the American Holistic Medical Association, shares strategies to ease sinus suffering throughout the year.

KEEP AIR CLEAN AND MOIST

In every season, always have optimal air in your work and home, says Dr. Ivker. This means air that is clean (you can't see or smell it), moist (between 35% and 55% relative humidity), negative-ion- and oxygen-filled, and warm (between 65 and 75 degrees Fahrenheit).

•**Radiant heat/baseboard heating systems** are preferable to forced hot-air heating systems through ducts. Radiant heating keeps the hot dry air and dust particles from flying through the house.

•**If you have a forced hot-air heating system,** use an efficient furnace filter (such as Filtrete made by 3M) and change it monthly or more often during the winter months.

•**Have your home's air ducts cleaned every three years.**

•**Fill your home with high oxygen-producing and air-filtering plants** (such as spider plants, chrysanthemums, striped dracaena and Boston ferns), which can remove toxins from the air and generate oxygen.

•**Place a warm-mist humidifier in your bedroom** to keep air moist and to prevent sinuses from becoming dry and irritated. In Dr. Ivker's opinion, two leading brands are Slant/Fin (*www.slantfin.com/consumer*) and Bionaire (*www.bionaire.com*).

•**Invest in a negative-ion generator.** These devices efficiently clean air. Studies have shown that ionized air has improved the lung capacity of asthmatics. Ionizers that do not emit ozone are best (ozone is an irritant to the mucous membrane), says Dr. Ivker. He recommends the Sinus Survival Air Vitalizer (*www.sinussurvival.com*).

•**Consider a HEPA (high-efficiency particulate arrestor) air cleaner.** According to Dr. Ivker, these are also highly efficient in their ability to purify air. However, they have none of the other beneficial effects of negative ions.

•**Avoid air pollutants, strong odors and fumes.** Secondhand smoke is the single most harmful indoor air pollutant, warns Dr. Ivker. Others include radon, mold, dust, harsh cleaning products and air fresheners. Whenever possible keep chemical products out of your home, and instead use environment-friendly "green" cleaning products (baking soda, vinegar, borax, etc.), which are less irritating to the sinuses.

If allergies act as a trigger of your sinus problems, as they do with nearly half of all sinus sufferers, it's important to keep them under control. *To make your environment sinus-friendly and inhospitable to allergies and sinusitis, Dr. Ivker recommends...*

•**Identify your triggers**—foods (most common trigger) and food additives, mold, dust mites, animal dander, chemicals, etc.—and reduce your exposure to them.

•**Keep your home and workspace clean and dust-free.**

•**Stay on top of mold.** For example, wash your humidifier's tank once a week with vinegar and water. Otherwise it becomes home to mold and bacteria that are recirculated through the air.

•**Change pillow and mattress covers frequently,** and wash bedding and clothing in hot water.

•**Remove wall-to-wall carpeting and heavy drapes,** and invest in a vacuum cleaner with a HEPA filter.

■ ■ ■ ■

Are Fruits and Veggies Aggravating Your Allergies?

Does your mouth get itchy after you eat fresh fruits or vegetables? You may have oral allergy syndrome, say experts at the American Academy of Allergy, Asthma & Immunology (AAAAI). OAS, also called pollen-food syndrome, is caused by allergens such as ragweed, which begins to bloom in mid-August.

"In addition to sneezing and itchy, water eyes, and symptoms of OAS, ragweed allergies can take a heavy toll on the allergy sufferer's quality of life," said Dr. Suzanne S. Teuber, chair of the AAAAI's Adverse Reactions to Foods Committee.

OAS symptoms are the result of a "cross-reactivity reaction" between allergy antibodies directed toward target pollen proteins with similar proteins found in other parts of plants. Common symptoms of OAS included an itchy mouth and throat with mild swelling immediately after eating fresh fruits or vegetables.

People with ragweed allergies can experience OAS symptoms when they consume bananas, cucumbers, melon, zucchini, sunflower seeds, chamomile tea or echinacea.

OAS can also occur in people with birch tree allergy symptoms when they eat peaches, apples, pears, cherries, carrots, hazelnuts, kiwis, and almonds, the AAAAI said.

Generally, cooking foods will eliminate an OAS reaction, according to the AAAAI.

MORE INFORMATION

info For more information about allergies, visit the Web site of the American Academy of Family Physicians at *http://familydoctor.org.*

American Academy of Allergy, Asthma & Immunology news release.

Low Vitamin E in Pregnancy May Raise Asthma Risk

Graham Devereux, MD, PhD, department of environmental and occupational medicine, University of Aberdeen, Scotland.

Arun Jeyabalan, MD, assistant professor, division of maternal fetal medicine, department of obstetrics, gynecology and reproductive sciences, Magee Women's Hospital, University of Pittsburgh, PA.

American Journal of Respiratory and Critical Care Medicine.

C hildren of mothers who take in too little vitamin E during pregnancy may be at higher risk for asthma by age five, a new study suggests. The finding expands on previous research conducted by the same team that found that two-year-old children whose moms had relatively low vitamin E intake during pregnancy were more prone to wheezing—even when they were otherwise healthy.

THE STUDY

In the study of more than 1,250 pregnant women, maternal dietary intake was assessed dating back to conception, as were medical histories related to asthma, wheezing and related respiratory issues. The same information was gathered for the children of these women up until the age of five.

Maternal intake of nutrients such as vitamin C, beta-carotene, magnesium, copper, and iron during pregnancy did not seem to be correlated with an increased risk for wheezing or asthma, the team found.

However, low intake of vitamin E supplements, both dietary and supplemental, during pregnancy was associated with a higher risk among offspring for developing persistent asthma, beginning during the first two years of life and continuing until at least age five.

In fact, children born to mothers rated in the bottom 20% for prenatal vitamin E intake were more than five times more prone to asthma as children born to mothers in the top 20%.

Youngsters born to mothers with relatively poor vitamin E intake during pregnancy were also at higher risk for developing persistent wheezing in their first five years of life, the Scottish researchers reported.

The researchers stressed that a child's diet at age five appears to have no impact on their asthma risk.

They pointed out that fetal airways are fully developed 16 weeks following conception. That suggests that certain dietary deficiencies during pregnancy—particularly early pregnancy—may heighten risks for childhood asthma.

RECOMMENDATIONS

More research is needed to confirm that low prenatal vitamin E helps cause childhood asthma, said study lead author Dr. Graham Devereux, of the department of environmental and occupational medicine at the University of Aberdeen in Scotland.

For that reason, Devereux said, it is premature for women to take vitamin E supplements, at any dosage, to help ward off asthma in their offspring.

Vitamin E is abundant in many foods, such as green leafy vegetables, whole grain cereals, vegetable oils, meat and fish. The average adult's daily vitamin E needs could be fully met if these foods were included in a balanced and healthy diet, Devereux said.

Dr. Arun Jeyabalan, an assistant professor in the division of maternal fetal medicine at the University of Pittsburgh's Magee Women's Hospital, agreed.

"This is an important study because it is important to look at associations between nutrient intake, deficiencies, and potential pregnancy outcomes," she said. "However, women should be very careful about supplementation. Not all vitamins in high doses are good for anybody, and further study is needed before advocating any kind of vitamin E supplementation."

info For more information on pregnancy and nutrition, visit the Web site of the US Department of Health and Human Services at *http://www.4woman.gov/pregnancy/.*

■ ■ ■ ■

How to Beat Egg Allergies

E gg allergy is one of the most common food allergies among children in the United States. But according to new research, children who were allergic to eggs were able to overcome it by gradually increasing the amount of egg they ate, researchers say.

"Participants who took a daily dose of egg product over the two-year study period were able to build up their bodies' resistance to the point where most of them could eat two scrambled eggs without a reaction," said researcher Dr. A. Wesley Burks, chief of the division of allergy and immunology at Duke University Medical Center.

THE STUDY

For the study, seven children, ages one to seven, consumed small daily doses of powdered egg mixed with food. At the start of the study, the doses were the equivalent of less than one-thousandth of an egg. That was gradually increased to the equivalent of one-tenth of an egg, which was maintained as a "maintenance dose" for the remainder of the study.

RESEARCH ON OTHER ALLERGIES

This study was the first in a series of food allergy desensitization studies being conducted by researchers at Duke and the University of Arkansas. One of the studies is examining whether the desensitization method is effective in children with peanut allergies.

Duke University news release.

Six Shots Ease Allergies Full Season

Peter Socrates Creticos, MD, medical director, Johns Hopkins Asthma and Allergy Center, Johns Hopkins University School of Medicine, Baltimore.
Rick Vinuya, MD, allergist/immunologist, Providence Hospital and Medical Center, Southfield, MI.
New England Journal of Medicine.

If you're one of the millions of Americans who suffers every fall with ragweed allergies, long-term relief may be near. Researchers report that a new ragweed vaccine was effective for a year or longer in early trials. Even better, relief came from just six once-a-week injections, rather than the several years of weekly injections required for current allergy shots.

"We can provide relief, very effective relief that lasts for at least a couple of years with a very short treatment regimen," said study author Dr. Peter Socrates Creticos, medical director of the Johns Hopkins Asthma and Allergy Center at the Johns Hopkins University School of Medicine in Baltimore.

"You won't have to take several medicines every day of ragweed season. You won't need shots every week for years. We can turn this disease off for years with a concise six-injection regimen," he added.

"This study is very exciting, but I have to temper my excitement because it's a pilot study that has to be repeated on many more people. I'm optimistic about the future of these new immunomodulating (changing the body's immune system) agents," explained Dr. Rick Vinuya, an allergist at Providence Hospital in Southfield, Michigan.

HOW THE VACCINE WORKS

Vinuya said current allergy medications that suppress the immune system are like big guns that shoot down everything. That can lead to unwanted side effects because many immune system functions are vital.

"[The new vaccine] is a smart bomb. It hones in on a specific target. The end effect is that the agent allows the treatment to be more effective with fewer side effects," said Vinuya.

THE STUDY

For the current study, the Johns Hopkins' researchers recruited 25 people between the ages of 23 and 60 with documented ragweed allergies. During the first year of the study, 14 people received six weekly injections of the new vaccine before the ragweed season began. The remaining 11 received six weekly injections of a placebo. The participants kept close track of their allergy symptoms, recording when their noses ran and each time they sneezed or had watery eyes.

The vaccine group experienced a 60% drop in allergy symptoms during ragweed season when compared with the placebo group. In the year after the study, those in the vaccine group were still experiencing symptom relief, even though no additional vaccine was given.

THE NEXT STEP

Creticos said that because the vaccine is so specific, only targeting the ragweed allergy, there likely wouldn't be any long-term adverse effects. In fact, he pointed out that the vaccine is so specific that people who were vaccinated and who also have grass allergies in the spring still experienced symptoms from that particular allergy.

He said that after further clinical trials the vaccine could receive government approval. It could potentially become commercially available a few years down the road, said Creticos.

Creticos and his team are also planning trials of the vaccine for people with ragweed allergy-induced asthma.

info To learn more about ragweed and other allergens, visit the Web site of the American Academy of Allergy, Asthma & Immunology at *http://www.aaaai.org.*

Warning: Allergy Drug with Life-Threatening Allergic Reaction

David Weldon, MD, assistant professor, internal medicine, Texas A&M Health Science Center College of Medicine, and director, Allergy and Pulmonary Lab Services, Scott & White Clinic, College Station, TX.

Yucynthia Jean-Louis, president, Asthma and Allergy Foundation of America.

The US Food and Drug Administration (FDA) is calling for the strongest warning possible to be added to an asthma drug's label, due to the potential for a life-threatening allergic reaction. The new alert for *omalizumab* (Xolair), marketed by Genentech Inc., draws attention to anaphylaxis as a possible side effect of the medication.

Anaphylaxis is a sudden, potentially life-threatening allergic reaction that can include trouble breathing, tightness in the chest, dizziness, fainting, itching and hives and swelling of the mouth and throat.

BACKGROUND

Xolair was approved in 2003 to treat adults and adolescents 12 years and older with moderate to severe persistent allergic asthma whose symptoms can't be fully controlled with inhaled steroids.

According to one study, adding Xolair to a patient's medication regimen helps cut emergency medical visits. It also decreases the rate of asthma exacerbations.

RISK FOR ALLERGIC REACTION

Anaphylaxis due to an injection of Xolair has occurred at a rate of about one in 1,000 patients, the FDA said.

The new warning discusses the possibility of patients developing anaphylaxis after any dose of Xolair, even if there was no reaction to the first dose. Also, the reaction may occur up to 24 hours after administration of the drug.

RECOMMENDATIONS

"I think more allergists are going to equip patients with EpiPens [anaphylaxis remedies] to be able to utilize them, based upon the black box warning. It would be prudent that anybody who's on Xolair make sure they get one of the commercially available epinephrine sources like an EpiPen," said Dr. David Weldon, director of Allergy and Pulmonary Lab Services at Scott & White Clinic, in College Station, Texas

And Yucynthia Jean-Louis, president of the Asthma and Allergy Foundation of America (AAFA), said the group recognizes the importance of new treatments such as Xolair in fighting moderate to severe asthma. "AAFA encourages the companies and the FDA to continue to work together to assure a product label that is in the best interest of patients," she said.

info For more details about the new warning on Xolair, visit the US Food and Drug Administration's Web site at *www.fda.gov/cder/drug/infopage/omalizumab/.*

■ ■ ■ ■

Fish Oil May Fight Asthma?

Athletes who took 5.4 grams of omega-3 fatty acids daily had an 80% improvement in lung capacity, a benefit for athletes with exercise-induced asthma.

Theory: Omega-3s, found in fish oil, may reduce inflammation, so lungs dilate more easily.

Timothy Mickleborough, PhD, professor, department of kinesiology, University of Indiana–Bloomington, and leader of a study of 20 athletes, reported in *American Journal of Respiratory and Critical Care Medicine.*

■ ■ ■ ■

Smoking Quadruples Teens' Asthma Risk

Adolescents who smoke are about four times more likely to develop asthma during their teen years than those who don't smoke, researchers warn. "The results of our study provide clear evidence that regular smoking increases the risk for asthma and that important chronic adverse consequences of smoking are not restricted to individuals who have smoked for many years," said Dr. Frank D. Gilliland, of the Keck School of Medicine at the University of Southern California.

THE STUDY

Gilliland's group collected five to eight years of data on more than 2,600 grade school children with no prior history of wheezing or asthma. The team uncovered 255 cases of new-onset asthma. Children who smoked 300 or more cigarettes a year were nearly four times more likely to develop asthma than nonsmokers.

Surprisingly, the researchers found that this increased asthma risk in smokers was stronger in children with no history of allergies than in those who had allergies.

"The clinical and public health implications of our findings are far-reaching. Effective tobacco control efforts focusing on the prevention of smoking in children, adolescents and women of childbearing age are urgently needed to reduce the number of these preventable cases of asthma," Gilliland said.

info For more information on smoking and asthma, go to the Nemours Foundation Web site at *http://www.kidshealth.org/teen.* Type "smoking and asthma" into the search box.

American Journal of Respiratory and Critical Care Medicine.

Asthma Could Be Wrong Diagnosis in Overweight People

Chirag Mehta, MD, pulmonary critical care fellow, Newark Beth Israel Medical Center, NJ.
Bohdan Pichurko, MD, chief, pulmonology, Providence Hospital, Southfield, MI, and associate professor, medicine, Wayne State University, Detroit.
American College of Chest Physicians annual meeting.

Being overweight increases the odds you'll be misdiagnosed with asthma when other problems are actually to blame for shortness of breath or wheezing.

That's the conclusion of a study that determined that about 60% of overweight people diagnosed with asthma actually didn't have the lung disease.

Study author Dr. Chirag Mehta, a pulmonary critical care fellow at Newark Beth Israel Medical Center in New Jersey, explained that people who are overweight or obese can have other conditions that produce symptoms similar to asthma, such as shortness of breath from being out of shape or wheezing from acid reflux disease.

The bottom line, he cautioned other physicians, is that "we should be looking for other diagnoses with a patient with increased BMI." Body mass index (BMI) is a ratio of height to weight.

BACKGROUND

"It's the old question: Which came first, the chicken or the egg?" said Mehta, who explained that it's not clear whether obesity or asthma comes first. People with asthma may have to take oral steroids, which causes them to gain weight, which causes their asthma to worsen, he said.

Other research has shown that when morbidly obese patients undergo bariatric (weight loss) surgery and lose weight, their asthma symptoms are relieved. Such findings made the researchers behind the new study wonder if the original asthma diagnosis was correct.

THE STUDY

To assess the accuracy of asthma diagnoses in the overweight or obese, Mehta and his colleagues recruited 20 people who had been diagnosed with asthma but whose lung-function tests suggested they might not have the disease.

Ninety percent of the group was overweight, with 60% meeting the criteria for obesity.

The researchers performed lung-function tests and a test known as bronchoprovocation. In this test, the airways of a person with asthma will overreact or become hyper-responsive when provoked with methacholine, a substance that is a known irritant.

Only 39% of those overweight or obese individuals tested positive on this test, which meant that nearly two out of every three study participants had been misdiagnosed with asthma.

OTHER CAUSES

Dr. Bohdan Pichurko, chief of pulmonology at Providence Hospital in Southfield, Michigan, added that when someone is overweight, it's a matter of simple mechanics. The increased body mass stiffens the lungs and doesn't allow them to expand fully.

"You can't expel a full breath. It's like someone laying a bag of buckshot on your chest," said Pichurko. He said certain forms of high blood pressure or untreated heart disease can also cause wheezing.

Pichurko said this study provides important information to both doctors and their patients. "In overweight individuals, lung-function testing isn't something we can bank on," he said.

RECOMMENDATIONS

Pichurko recommended that anyone who is overweight and has symptoms of asthma see an asthma specialist, preferably at a specialized breathing lab. However, he said, in many areas of the country, breathing labs aren't accessible.

If a breathing lab or an asthma specialist isn't available, you can work with your doctor and keep track of your peak flow readings (a measurement of your ability to push air out of your lungs) three or four times a day. If they remain fairly constant, not varying by more than 10% or so, you may not have asthma. If, on the other hand, they're varying from reading to reading by 50% or 60%, you're likely to have asthma.

Getting the proper diagnosis is important. "With an incorrect diagnosis, patients aren't treated for what they do have, and they're taking costly medications that don't help and can cause side effects," said Pichurko.

info The Centers for Disease Control and Prevention has more information about obesity and suggestions for reducing your weight, at *http://www.cdc.gov/nccdphp/dnpa/obesity/.*

Experts' Favorite Ways to Allergy-Proof Your Home

Jeffrey C. May, principal scientist with May Indoor Air Investigations, LLC, an air-quality assessment company in Cambridge, MA. *www.mayindoorair.com.* He is author of three books on indoor environments, including his most recent, *My Office Is Killing Me! The Sick Building Survival Guide.* Johns Hopkins University.

Jeffrey May solves home air-quality and allergen problems for a living. He's also a lifelong allergy sufferer himself, as are his now-grown children. *Here's what he uses to improve the air quality in his own home...*

•**High-quality vacuum.** Most vacuums—even some expensive ones with high-efficiency particulate air (HEPA) filters—leak air while in use. Rather than collect dust and other allergens, these leaky vacuums actually churn up allergens and recirculate them throughout the home, reducing indoor air quality. Miele's HEPA Sealed System vacuums use high-quality filters and gaskets to dramatically reduce this problem.

Cost: $450 to $1,250, depending on the model. 800-843-7231, *www.miele.com.*

•**Dust mite covers.** Dust mites are microscopic organisms that thrive in warm, humid environments, such as bedding. A dust mite cover prevents mites from taking hold in your mattress—and kills dust mites that are already there by cutting off moisture. There are several varieties of covers on the market. The type I use—and the only type that works reliably—is a plastic mattress cover. My choice is Allergy Control Products' Economy Mattress Encasing.

Cost: $45.95 to $69.95, depending on mattress size. A standard-size Economy pillow cover costs $9.95. 800-ALLERGY, *www.allergycontrol.com.*

If you don't like the feeling of sleeping on plastic, place a mattress pad over the dust mite cover. Wash and thoroughly dry this mattress pad every week or two to kill new dust mites. We also wash our blankets and quilts monthly and run them through the dryer on the regular setting every two weeks. Twenty minutes of drying should kill any dust mites living inside.

•**Leather couches and chairs.** Dust mites can infest fabric-covered couches and chairs, but they can't penetrate leather. All the chairs and couches in our home that we use regularly are leather. In less frequently used rooms, we have futon-style fabric couches, but we have encased the mattress portion of the futons in plastic dust mite covers, with the fabric futon covers over the plastic covers.

We also change our clothes immediately upon returning from places where we might have been exposed to pet dander, pollen or other allergens so that we don't contaminate our couches, chairs or beds.

•**Hot-water radiators rather than a forced-air duct system.** When you have a forced-air ventilation system, there's no way to know what's inside your ducts. Mold could be growing and spreading throughout the home whenever the system is used. Even professional duct cleaning is no guarantee that all allergens will be removed.

The only air-quality challenge presented by hot-water heat is dust building up on and behind radiators and/or baseboard units. We use a vacuum attachment called a flat crevice tool to remove dust from tight spots, such as behind radiators and refrigerators. Mid America Vacuum's 36-inch Exten-Vac Crevice Tool fits most vacuums.

Cost: $17.49, plus shipping. 800-649-7996, *www.vacuumstore.com.*

If you live in a home with a duct system, have the ducts cleaned at least once every five years. (Make sure the person you hire to do this cleans your coil and blower as well as the ducts.) In the summer, we use portable air conditioners, which we clean with a solution of one-third bleach and two-thirds water yearly. We also replace the filters every year. Use high-quality air-conditioner and furnace filters with a Minimum Efficiency Reporting Value (MERV) no lower than eight. If you have serious allergy issues, use filters rated at least 11.

•**Hardwood floors.** Carpets collect dust and other allergens, and not even the best vacuum can remove them all. For people like me who suffer from severe allergies, switching from carpets to wood or tile floors can be like flipping a switch from chronic bad health to good. That's particularly true in the winter, when we spend more time inside with the windows closed.

We do have a few small rugs in our home. They are synthetic, not wool or cotton, and I subjected each of them to a sniff test at the store before I brought them into my home. I put my face close to the carpet and inhaled deeply. If I didn't experience any allergic reaction, I purchased the rug.

•**Dehumidifier in the basement.** The relative humidity in our basement was above 50%, creating the risk of mold and mildew growth. I measured the humidity with a humidity meter. Extech (781-890-7440, *www.extech.com*) makes good ones, ranging from $30 to $200. Don't buy a cheap one—it won't be reliable. I then purchased a Therma-Stor Santa Fe dehumidifier, and we keep it set to lower our basement's relative humidity level below 50%. Therma-Stor makes the most powerful and reliable dehumidifiers on the residential market.

Cost: $975 to $1,375, depending on the model. 800-533-7533, *www.thermastor.com.*

I attached the dehumidifier to a condensate pump, a device available in hardware and home-goods stores for around $50. The condensate pump automatically transfers water collected by my dehumidifier to a sink in the basement.

•**Face mask when I travel.** I carry a face mask with me so that when I start to feel allergy symptoms, I can put it on. I use an N95 mask made by 3M, available in hardware stores.

Cost: About $20 for a box of 20.

■ ■ ■ ■

Don't Count on Vitamin B-12 To Relieve Allergies

One recent clinical trial did show some improvement in allergy symptoms—after participants got 2,500 times the recommended daily allowance of three to four micrograms of B-12 for up to six weeks. But one trial is not conclusive—more research is necessary.

Good news: Even if vitamin B-12 does not help relieve allergies, it helps keep you healthy. But don't take huge doses of B-12 or any vitamin without consulting your doctor first.

Martha V. White, MD, director of research, Institute for Allergy and Asthma, 11160 Veirs Mill Rd., Wheaton, MD 20902.

Breathe Easy!
New Ways to Treat
Asthma—Naturally

Richard N. Firshein, DO, medical director of the Firshein Center for Comprehensive Medicine in New York City. Board-certified in family medicine and a certified medical acupuncturist, he is the author of *Reversing Asthma* (Warner), *Your Asthma-Free Child* (Avery) and *The Nutraceutical Revolution* (Riverhead).

Anyone who suffers from the wheezing, coughing and chest tightness caused by asthma knows all too well that conventional doctors typically treat these troublesome symptoms with prescription medication, such as steroids and bronchodilators (both available in inhalers and pills).

Problem: Long-term use of prescription drugs does nothing to solve the underlying causes of asthma (a disease of the lungs in which the airways become narrowed or blocked, resulting in breathing difficulties).

What's more, research shows that asthma medications can lead to dangerous side effects, including osteoporosis (from steroids) and heart damage (from bronchodilators, which accelerate the asthma sufferer's heart rate).

Latest development: Exciting new research confirms that asthma can be controlled with nondrug treatments, thereby reducing—or even eliminating—the need for medication.* *Here's how...*

*Consult your doctor before trying any nondrug therapies for asthma.

NUTRITIONAL SUPPLEMENTS

•**Omega-3 fatty acids.** This component of dietary fat—found abundantly in cold-water fish, such as salmon, herring and mackerel, as well as in flaxseeds and walnuts—may act as a natural anti-inflammatory for asthma sufferers.

Scientific evidence: In a three-week study, researchers at Indiana University followed 16 adults who had exercise-induced asthma (narrowing of the airways during and after vigorous exercise). Participants were given either a daily placebo capsule or fish oil capsules containing two types of omega-3 fatty acids—*eicosapentaenoic acid* (EPA) and *docosahexaenoic acid* (DHA).

Researchers measured the participants' lung function and inflammation levels before, during and after the study. While taking fish oil capsules, the asthmatics had improved lung function, lower inflammation levels and reduced bronchodilator use. There was no improvement in those who took the placebo.

Self-defense: Take a daily fish oil supplement, with a total of 1 g to 2 g of DHA and EPA. Benefits typically begin after a few months but may occur in as little as three weeks.

Caution: This dosage can have blood-thinning effects. If you take daily aspirin or a blood thinner, such as *warfarin* (Coumadin), be sure to consult your doctor before trying fish oil supplements.

•**Magnesium.** This mineral is considered a natural bronchodilator because it relaxes the muscles of the bronchial tubes that line the air passages.

Scientific evidence: In a two-month study, researchers in Brazil gave 37 asthmatic children and adolescents daily doses of either a placebo or 300 mg of magnesium. Those receiving magnesium had fewer bronchial spasms and asthma attacks, and used less asthma medication.

Self-defense: Take 250 mg to 500 mg of magnesium daily. Exceeding this dosage of magnesium can cause bloating, gas and diarrhea. Taking a calcium supplement (double the daily magnesium dose) can enhance absorption of both minerals. To ensure proper absorption of calcium, take no more than 500 mg of the mineral at a time.

•**Coenzyme Q10.** This powerful antioxidant helps cells manufacture energy and also strengthens the cells of the lungs.

Scientific evidence: Researchers in Slovakia gave 41 adult asthmatics who took steroids either a placebo or a daily dose of 120 mg of CoQ10. After 16 weeks, the asthma patients who took CoQ10 used fewer steroids.

Self-defense: Taking 100 mg to 120 mg of CoQ10 daily may be helpful—whether or not you take steroids.

Reliable brands of fish oil, magnesium and CoQ10: Allergy Research and Cardiovascular Research (both available on the Internet) or Emerson Ecologics (available at holistic doctors' offices).

Important: If you use both medications and nutritional supplements to treat your asthma, take them at least one hour apart to enhance the absorption of both.

ANTIOXIDANT-RICH DIET

It's an accepted fact among health scientists that oxidative stress—the increase in cell-damaging free radicals caused by factors as varied as fried food, air pollution and stress—plays a role in more than 50 diseases, from arthritis to cancer. Now, most scientists have concluded that oxidative stress also plays a role in asthma.

Scientific evidence: Researchers analyzed dietary data from nearly 69,000 women and found that those with the highest intake of antioxidant-rich vegetables, such as carrots and leafy greens, had the lowest incidence of asthma.

Self-defense: Each day, eat a variety of antioxidant-rich foods, including fruits…leafy, dark green vegetables, such as spinach and kale…as well as carrots, winter squash and other colorful vegetables rich in carotenoids (a family of protective antioxidants that includes beta-carotene). Aim for five to six one-half-cup servings daily of these vegetables and fruits…and juices made from them.

BREATHING EXERCISES

Breathing exercises have been shown to reduce the need for bronchodilators in people with asthma. However, few physicians are aware of the benefits, so most patients are not encouraged to try breathing exercises.

Scientific evidence: When researchers taught 57 asthmatics breathing techniques, which they practiced twice daily for 30 weeks, their use of short-acting bronchodilators declined by 82%.

Self-defense: To strengthen the lungs, prevent an asthma attack and/or help stop an attack in progress, try breathing exercises.

What to do: While sitting, place one hand on your stomach, with the palm open. Use this hand to feel your abdomen rising and falling as you breathe. Use the thumb of the other hand to feel for the pulse point of the wrist that is on your stomach. Let yourself relax.

Next, synchronize your breathing with your heart rate. Breathe in through the nose, with the pulse…breathe out through the mouth, with the pulse. Blow out through pursed lips to create a mild resistance that improves the tone and function of the diaphragm, a muscle that plays a key role in breathing. Perform for 10 to 15 minutes, twice a day—or any time you're starting to have an asthma attack.

Caution: If you are experiencing a serious asthma attack, this breathing exercise may not be effective, and you may need to use medication. But in almost all other cases, this exercise can help regulate respiration.

ACUPUNCTURE

The National Institutes of Health recognizes acupuncture as a treatment for asthma. Thousands of years of anecdotal evidence from China also confirms that acupuncture works, perhaps by balancing fundamental but unseen energy flows that affect the body.

Scientific evidence: Researchers in Beijing divided 104 asthmatics into two groups, giving one group 10 sessions of acupuncture and medications, while the other group received only medications.

Those receiving acupuncture had significantly greater improvement in their asthma symptoms and more breathing capacity. Six months later, the acupuncture group had suffered fewer asthma attacks, and had reduced their medication dosages by as much as one-third.

Self-defense: Try six to 10 initial acupuncture treatments, followed by additional treatments, if necessary. To find a qualified acupuncturist near you, consult either the American Association of Oriental Medicine at 866-455-7999, *www. aaom.org*...or the American Academy of Medical Acupuncture at 323-937-5514, *www.medical acupuncture.org.*

■ ■ ■ ■

Breathing Exercises Curb Asthma Symptoms

B reathing exercises, including shallow nasal breathing with slow exhalations, were taught by video to 57 people who used daily inhaled corticosteroids plus as-needed reliever medication (a short-acting bronchodilator) at least four times a week for mild asthma.

Result: After 28 weeks, patients had reduced the use of reliever medication by 82% and steroids by 50%.

Theory: Breathing exercises may help reduce anxiety, making asthmatics less likely to need medication.

Christine R. Jenkins, MD, PhD, clinical professor of medicine, Woolcock Institute of Medical Research, University of Sydney, Australia.

America's Top Lung Centers

John Connolly, EdD, president and CEO of Castle Connolly Medical Ltd., a consumer health research and information company in New York City, and editor and publisher of *America's Top Doctors* (Castle Connolly, *www.castleconnolly.com*). Castle Connolly's physician-led research team has extensive knowledge of the nation's leading medical centers and specialty hospitals.

M ore than 35 million Americans live with some form of chronic lung disease—asthma, bronchitis or emphysema. Each year, nearly 342,000 Americans die of lung disease, making it the third leading cause of death (following heart disease and cancer).

In the US, there are dozens of specialized lung centers. People who are treated at one of these facilities have the best possible odds of recovering from a serious lung or breathing disorder.

The following lung centers are among the finest in the US. These centers have the greatest number of pulmonary specialists listed in *America's Top Doctors* (a compilation of the top 1% of US physicians, as rated by their peers) and score high in other well-regarded, independent rankings by related professional organizations and publications. All of the following lung centers also have outstanding lung transplant facilities.

NORTHEAST

•**Brigham and Women's Hospital (Boston).** Surgeons here performed the nation's first triple-organ (two lungs and a heart) transplant in 1995. Cutting-edge care for asthma, lung cancer and chronic obstructive pulmonary disease (COPD), a group of disorders including chronic bronchitis and emphysema. 617-732-5500, *www.brighamandwomens.org.*

•**Hospital of the University of Pennsylvania (Philadelphia).** Offers an internationally recognized center for the diagnosis and treatment of rare lung diseases. 800-789-7366, *www.pennhealth.com/hup.*

•**Johns Hopkins Hospital (Baltimore).** World-renowned sleep disorders center offers comprehensive testing services for sleep-related respiratory conditions, such as narcolepsy. Also known for its aggressive approach to treating lung cancer. 410-955-5000, *www.hopkins-lungs.org.*

•**Massachusetts General Hospital (Boston).** Noted for asthma diagnosis and treatment. Patients throughout the region are referred to its Pulmonary Vascular Disease Program for pulmonary hypertension (a rare blood vessel disorder of the lungs in which the pressure in the pulmonary artery rises above normal levels). 617-726-2000, *www.massgeneral.org.*

•**NewYork–Presbyterian Hospital–Cornell/ Columbia (New York City).** Leader in diagnosing and treating asthma. Its Cardiopulmonary Sleep and Ventilatory Disorders Lab provides care for a wide range of sleep disorders related to respiratory conditions. 212-305-2500, *www.nyp.org.*

•**University of Pittsburgh Medical Center (Pittsburgh).** Noted for its state-of-the-art Center for Interstitial Lung Diseases (lung disorders caused by inflammation and scarring of the air sacs and their supporting structures). 412-802-3275, *www.upmc.com.*

SOUTHEAST

•**Duke University Medical Center (Durham, North Carolina).** Known for its interventional pulmonology program, which treats lung cancer and benign airway disorders, such as asthma. 919-416-3853, *http://pulmonary. duke.edu.*

•**Medical University of South Carolina Hospitals (Charleston, South Carolina).** Leader in diagnosing and managing acute and chronic diseases of the chest and allergic diseases. 843-792-3161, *www.musc.edu/pulmonary.*

•**Shands Healthcare at University of Florida (Gainesville).** Pulmonary specialists offer a wide range of outpatient and inpatient services, including cutting-edge cancer treatments. 800-749-7424, *www.shands.org.*

•**University of Alabama Hospital at Birmingham (Birmingham, Alabama).** Highly regarded Pediatric Pulmonary Center offers comprehensive care for children and adolescents with chronic lung disease. 205-939-9583, *http://main.uab.edu/ppc.*

•**University of North Carolina Hospitals (Chapel Hill, North Carolina).** One of the largest clinical cystic fibrosis programs in the country, with more than 500 patients in its pediatric and adult programs. 919-966-6838, *www. med.unc.edu/cystfib.*

•**Vanderbilt University Medical Center (Nashville).** Known for its specialized clinics for lung cancer, adult cystic fibrosis, allergic disorders and pulmonary hypertension. 615-322-5000, *www.mc.vanderbilt.edu.*

MIDWEST

•**Barnes-Jewish Hospital (St. Louis).** Pioneered lung volume reduction surgery, which removes lung tissue damaged by emphysema. 314-867-3627, *www.barnesjewish.org.*

•**Cleveland Clinic Foundation (Cleveland).** Noted for its Sarcoidosis Center of Excellence, and cutting-edge asthma care and research. 866-320-4573, *http://cms.clevelandclinic.org/ccfpulmonary.*

•**Mayo Clinic (Rochester, Minnesota).** A world leader in lung transplants, and COPD and lung cancer treatment. Surgeons perform more than 1,000 lung cancer surgeries annually. Access to clinical trials of experimental therapies offered for lung cancer. 507-538-3270, *www.mayoclinic. org.*

•**University of Chicago Hospitals (Chicago).** One of a handful of US centers with a dedicated interstitial lung disease program. Leader in diagnosing and treating asthma and pediatric lung disease. 888-824-0200, *www.uchospitals. edu/specialties/pulmonary.*

•**University of Michigan Health System (Ann Arbor, Michigan).** Leader in diagnosing and managing chronic lung disease, including COPD and asthma. 800-211-8181, *www.med. umich.edu.*

•**University of Minnesota Medical Center (Minneapolis).** Its Center for Lung Science and Health specializes in COPD, pulmonary fibrosis, pulmonary hypertension and cystic fibrosis. 612-624-0999, *www.med.umn.edu/pacc.*

SOUTHWEST/ROCKY MOUNTAIN

•**National Jewish Medical and Research Center (Denver).** The world's only facility dedicated exclusively to respiratory, immune and allergic disorders. 800-222-5864, *www.njc.org.*

•**University Health System–San Antonio (San Antonio, Texas).** Known for excellence in caring for patients with end-stage lung disease, such as emphysema and pulmonary fibrosis. 210-358-4000, *www.universityhealthsystem.com.*

•**University of Colorado Hospital (Denver).** Specializes in cancer prevention and early detection, smoking cessation programs, pulmonary rehabilitation and oxygen therapy. 800-621-7621, *www.uch.edu.*

WEST

•**San Francisco General Hospital (San Francisco).** Recognized for clinical care and research of infectious diseases (such as tuberculosis) and asthma. 415-206-8492, *http://pulmo nary.ucsf.edu.*

•**Stanford Hospital and Clinics (Stanford, California).** International leader in cardiopulmonary disease, where the world's first heart-lung transplant was performed. Also has new chest clinic for treatment of adults with lung diseases. 650-725-7061, *www.stanfordhospital.com.*

•**UCLA Medical Center (Los Angeles).** State-of-the-art center for asthma, chronic and acute bronchitis, interstitial lung disease, pneumonia, pulmonary vascular disease and sleep-disordered breathing. 310-825-5988, *www.lung. med.ucla.edu.*

•**UCSD Medical Center (San Diego).** Recognized worldwide as a pioneer in performing pulmonary thromboendarterectomy (PTE), a type of surgery to open an obstructed artery. Leader in treating chronic thromboembolic pulmonary hypertension (a rare outcome from blood clots in the lungs). 619-543-6222, *http:// pulmonary.ucsd.edu.*

•**UCSF Medical Center (San Francisco).** Noted center of excellence for adult cystic fibrosis and pulmonary hypertension. Also a leader in treating chest-related cancer, including lung cancer and esophageal cancer. 415-476-1000, *http://pulmonary.ucsf.edu/.*

•**University of Washington Medical Center (Seattle).** Known for diagnosing and treating rare lung diseases and genetic lung diseases, including inherited interstitial lung disease. 800-852-8546, *www.depts.washington.edu/pulmcc.*

3

Breast Cancer Treatments

Drugs That Beat Tamoxifen for Breast Cancer Survival

Postmenopausal breast cancer patients who switch from tamoxifen therapy to a new class of drugs called aromatase inhibitors may live longer. Women in the study made the switch two to three years into the typical five-year tamoxifen regimen, which is aimed at keeping recurrent breast cancer at bay.

According to the researchers, the improved performance of aromatase inhibitors means patients may also avoid the increased risk of death from other causes—such as stroke or endometrial cancer—that have been associated with tamoxifen.

"There are still a lot of questions that remain, but this study confirms that five years of tamoxifen alone is really becoming the wrong answer for most postmenopausal women," said Dr. Gary M. Freedman, a radiation oncologist at the Fox Chase Cancer Center in Philadelphia. "At this point, you have to say that aromatase inhibitors are in the mix of treatment at some point," said Freedman, who was not involved in the trial.

BACKGROUND

Tamoxifen has been in widespread use among breast cancer survivors for the last two decades. The drug is typically taken after surgery, because it targets the hormone estrogen, which can promote tumor cell growth in women with estrogen-sensitive breast cancer. A standard five-year treatment of tamoxifen has been found to reduce breast cancer death rates by as much as 31%, according to the study led by Dr. Francesco Boccardo of the National Cancer Research Institute and University of Genoa.

Aromatase inhibitors are a newer class of drugs with a different mechanism. These medicines, which include *letrozole* (Femara), *exemestane* (Aromasin), and *anastrazole* (Arimidex),

Gary M. Freedman, MD, radiation oncologist, Fox Chase Cancer Center, Philadelphia.
Lauren Cassell, MD, breast surgeon, Lenox Hill Hospital, New York City.

41

fight cancer cell growth by blocking the workings of an aromatase enzyme while also reducing estrogen.

THE STUDY

To find out if aromatase inhibitors are more effective and safer than tamoxifen, Boccardo and his colleagues conducted two trials involving a total of 828 postmenopausal Italian breast cancer patients.

Half the patients were given a five-year regimen of tamoxifen, while the other half were switched to a therapy involving one of two aromatase inhibitors around two to three years into their tamoxifen treatment.

Two aromatase inhibitors, aminoglutethimide and anastrozole, were tested. Aminoglutethimide is no longer available for the treatment of breast cancer.

RESULTS

By pooling the results of the two trials, the authors concluded that death rates due to either breast cancer or any other cause significantly improved among the patients who switched to an aromatase inhibitor.

Among full-treatment tamoxifen patients, 74 deaths were reported, of which 51 were breast cancer-related.

In comparison, 48 deaths—of which 33 were breast cancer-related—were reported among the group that switched to an aromatase inhibitor.

Boccardo and his associates also observed fewer deaths from either stroke or cardiovascular causes among the women who jumped to aromatase inhibitors.

REACTION

Freedman stressed that the study did not answer questions regarding how long aromatase inhibitors should be used for optimum effect, or whether using them before or after a tamoxifen regimen would be the best way to go.

Freedman's own research suggested that depending on disease severity, patient age and other factors, not all breast cancer survivors who've completed five years of tamoxifen would benefit from aromatase inhibitors.

"So, while in our clinical practice only premenopausal women are being recommended a full five years of tamoxifen alone, I would still say that the decision whether and when to switch to aromatase inhibitors needs to be based on the individual patient," Freedman said.

Dr. Lauren Cassell, a breast surgeon at Lenox Hill Hospital in New York City, said the Italian study reaffirms recent research.

"This finding is not surprising," she said. "There is a consensus, at least in the US, that among postmenopausal patients, aromatase inhibitors are more effective in increasing survival than tamoxifen."

Cassell pointed out that current protocols among US oncologists have already shifted toward excluding tamoxifen from newly prescribed treatment regimens in favor of aromatase inhibitors. And, most patients who are on tamoxifen treatment are now being switched over to the aromatase option, she said.

PRECAUTIONS

But, while aromatase inhibitors offer clear survival advantages, new concerns are surfacing, Cassell added.

"While aromatase inhibitors don't increase the risk for endometrial cancer or stroke associated with tamoxifen, they do increase the risk for osteoporosis and, in some cases, significant joint pain," she said. "And, they are much more pricey than tamoxifen, which is a problem for older patients on fixed incomes who don't have insurance."

info For additional information on tamoxifen and aromatase inhibitors, visit the Web site of the American Cancer Society at *www. cancer.org*. Type "medicines to reduce breast cancer risk" in the search box.

Family History Strong Predictor of Breast Cancer Risk

Journal of Medical Genetics news release.

Women who have close relatives with breast cancer but who test negative for key genetic mutations associated with the disease are still at increased risk of developing breast cancer, researchers report.

The study found that even if tests fail to detect the breast cancer-linked BRCA1 and BRCA2 gene mutations in these women, they are still about three times more likely to develop breast cancer by age 50 than women in the general population.

These women should be regularly screened for breast cancer starting at ages 35 to 40, advised researchers at St. Mary's Hospital in Manchester, England.

THE STUDY

Researchers assessed the families of 277 women with defects in the BRCA1 and BRCA2 genes. Of those 277 women, 190 had breast cancer, 48 had ovarian cancer, and 33 had both types of cancer. Six of the women were cancer-free.

Of the women's 531 female relatives tested for faults in the BRCA1 and BRCA2 genes, 49% tested negative. Of those who tested negative, 28 developed breast cancer and four developed ovarian cancer.

Faults in the BRCA1 and BRCA2 genes account for about 5% of all diagnosed breast cancer cases in developed countries. However, faults in these genes greatly increase a woman's risk of developing early breast and/or ovarian cancer compared with women in the general population.

info For more information about the genetics of breast and ovarian cancer, go to the Web site of the National Cancer Institute at *http://www.cancer.gov/cancertopics/pdq/genetics/breast-and-ovarian.*

■ ■ ■ ■

Different-Sized Breasts Linked To Cancer Risk

Researchers examined the mammograms of 252 women who later developed breast cancer and 252 women of the same age who did not develop the disease.

Result: Those who developed breast cancer had higher breast volume asymmetry (difference in volume between left and right breasts) than other women.

Theory: Estrogen, which has been linked to breast cancer, may play a significant role in breast asymmetry.

Diane Scutt, PhD, director of research, School of Health Sciences, University of Liverpool, England.

'DES Daughters' Have Double the Breast-Cancer Risk

Julie Palmer, ScD, professor of epidemiology, Boston University School of Public Health, Boston.
Jay Brooks, MD, chairman, hematology/oncology, Ochsner Health System, Baton Rouge, LA.
Cancer Epidemiology, Biomarkers and Prevention.

Women whose mothers took the synthetic estrogen *Diethylstilbestrol* (DES) while pregnant have nearly double the risk of breast cancer. This was the main finding of a study that compared women exposed to DES in utero to a group of comparably aged women who weren't exposed to the excess hormone levels.

DES was prescribed from 1938 through 1971 to prevent miscarriage and other pregnancy complications. During that time, as many as 10 million American women took DES during pregnancy, the US Centers for Disease Control and Prevention estimates.

"Women who were exposed to DES have been wondering about this for a long time," said the study's lead author, Julie Palmer, a professor of epidemiology at Boston University's School of Public Health. "We found the risk of breast cancer was about two times as high in the exposed women compared to unexposed women among those 40 years and older."

BACKGROUND

Although research published in 1953 refuted the notion that DES could prevent the loss of pregnancy or pregnancy difficulties, doctors still continued to prescribe the drug. In 1971, the US Food and Drug Administration advised doctors to stop prescribing DES because it was linked to a rare form of vaginal and cervical cancer—clear cell adenocarcinoma—in daughters of women who took DES while pregnant. These women eventually came to be known collectively as "DES daughters," according to the CDC.

Previous research had suggested that prenatal hormone levels of DES might affect the risk of breast cancer later in life. And women who took DES have higher rates of breast cancer. So, the researchers behind the new study wanted to assess what the actual risk of breast cancer was for women exposed to DES in utero.

THE STUDY

Researchers recruited 4,817 women who had been exposed to DES in utero in the 1950s and 2,073 women born in the same time period, but who had not been exposed to the drug.

The women completed questionnaires, and 102 women—76 in the DES-exposed group and 26 in the control group—reported a diagnosis of breast cancer.

After compensating for other breast-cancer risk factors, the researchers found that women who were exposed to DES in utero had a 91% higher risk for breast cancer after age 40, and a three-fold increased risk for breast cancer after age 50, when compared with women not exposed to the drug.

REDUCING BREAST CANCER RISK

Dr. Jay Brooks, chairman of hematology and oncology at the Ochsner Health System in Baton Rouge, Louisiana, said, "This is an interesting study that shows we still don't know all of the long-term effects on women who took DES and their female offspring."

Brooks said if women—all women, whether exposed to DES or not—wanted to decrease their risk of breast cancer, they should maintain a normal weight, or lose excess weight.

Palmer added that some research has shown that regular physical activity may be helpful in reducing your risk of breast cancer. Women who know they were exposed to DES in utero should carefully discuss the use of postmenopausal hormones with their doctor, she suggested. Palmer also noted that all women should have regular mammogram screenings to detect breast cancer in its earliest stages.

Depending on what additional risk factors women exposed to DES may have, Brooks said women might want to discuss the potential risks and benefits of using the medications tamoxifen or raloxifene, because these drugs block the action of estrogen, which can fuel some breast tumors.

info To learn more about the known health effects for DES daughters, visit the Web site of the Centers for Disease Control and Prevention at *http://www.cdc.gov/des/consumers/.*

■ ■ ■ ■

Chest X-rays Linked To Breast Cancer

In a study of 1,600 women who carry a mutation in the BRCA1 or BRCA2 gene (a known breast cancer risk factor), those who reported ever having a chest X-ray were 54% more likely to develop breast cancer than those who had never had one.

Theory: Genetic abnormalities can affect the body's ability to repair DNA damage caused by the ionizing radiation of chest X-rays.

David E. Goldgar, PhD, research professor, department of dermatology, University of Utah, Salt Lake City.

FDA Approves Gene-Based Breast Cancer Test

Steven Gutman, MD, director, Office of In Vitro Diagnostic Device Evaluation and Safety, Center for Devices and Radiological Health, US Food and Drug Administration.

Len Lichtenfeld, MD, deputy chief medical officer, American Cancer Society, Atlanta.

The US Food and Drug Administration (FDA) approved a new genetic test that's designed to determine the likelihood that early-stage breast cancer will recur within five to 10 years after treatment. The intended value of the test is that it could help doctors decide whether or not a woman needs chemotherapy after initial cancer treatment for early-stage disease that hasn't spread beyond the breast.

However, the test, called MammaPrint, has shortcomings, according to Dr. Steven Gutman, director of the FDA's Office of In Vitro Diagnostic Device Evaluation and Safety in the Center for Devices.

HOW THE TEST WORKS

MammaPrint is a DNA microarray-based test that measures the activity of 70 genes, providing information about the likelihood that cancer will recur. The test measures each of these genes in a sample of a woman's breast-cancer tumor and then uses a specific formula to produce a score that determines whether the patient is deemed low risk or high risk for the spread of the cancer to another site.

Women determined to be at high risk of cancer recurrence at five years have a 23% chance that the disease will reappear. Conversely, for women at low-risk, the test is 95% accurate that cancer will not return, Gutman said.

And at 10 years, women gauged at high risk for recurrence have a 29% chance their cancer will recur, while low-risk patients have a 90% chance the cancer will not return, he said.

The FDA approved of MammaPrint based on data its manufacturer—Agendia, of Amsterdam, the Netherlands—submitted from a study using tumor samples and clinical data from 302 patients at five European centers. The test has been available in Europe since 2005. Similar tests cost around $3,000.

TEST LIMITATIONS

"This information has to be used very carefully by physicians in the context of what they know about the history of the patient, the diagnostic options and the treatment options," Gutman said. "This is a complex test that requires use by people who know their business."

Dr. Len Lichtenfeld, the deputy chief medical officer at the American Cancer Society, doesn't think the test is accurate enough yet to be used in determining treatment.

"This is a first step in a long process," Lichtenfeld said. "The goal of that process is to do a test that will tell us, 'Yes, you need adjuvant therapy or, no, you don't,' and say it with 99.9% accuracy. We are not there yet."

Lichtenfeld said he isn't convinced the test has a value in deciding if a woman should have chemotherapy or not. "We don't know, at this point, whether or not this is a test that should influence the decisions that women and their doctors should be making with regard to adjuvant therapy," he said.

info For more information on breast cancer, visit the American Cancer Society's Web site at *www.cancer.org*. Click on "Choose a Cancer Topic" under "Learn About Cancer." Scroll down to "Breast Cancer."

MRI—The Test That Spots Breast Cancer Missed by Mammograms

Etta D. Pisano, MD, director, Biomedical Research Imaging Center, University of North Carolina at Chapel Hill School of Medicine.

Debbie Saslow, PhD, director, breast and gynecological cancers, American Cancer Society, Atlanta.

New England Journal of Medicine.

Women who have already been diagnosed with breast cancer should have a magnetic resonance imaging (MRI) scan of the other breast in addition to mammography. Doing so may help doctors find a small number of cancer cases missed by mammography, a new study reports.

The study found that MRI scans picked up 3% of cancers missed by mammography alone in women who had already been diagnosed with cancer in one breast.

"The results of this study will lead to changes in practice," said Dr. Etta Pisano, one of the study's authors, and director of the Biomedical Research Imaging Center at the University of North Carolina at Chapel Hill School of Medicine. "While this study does not suggest that MRI supplants mammography, I think what will end up happening is that all women with breast cancer will end up getting MRI" if they've had a normal mammography.

In fact, the American Cancer Society issued new guidelines that recommend an annual MRI screen in addition to an annual mammography for women at high risk for breast cancer.

But, because the false-positive rate of MRIs was relatively high—about 11% in the new study—the authors don't recommend MRI as a screening tool for the general population.

THE STUDY

For the new study, Pisano and her colleagues performed MRI scans on 969 women who had recently been diagnosed with breast cancer in one breast. Mammography did not detect abnormalities in the other breast of the women.

One hundred and twenty-one women had positive MRI findings, meaning they had suspected cancer in the other breast. Biopsies were done to confirm the cancer diagnosis.

Of those women, 30 (3%) were found to have cancer in the second breast—cancers that hadn't been detected with mammography.

But, the test wasn't perfect. It had a false-positive rate of 10.9%.

REACTION

"The costs of false-positives have to be weighed against the cost of missing a cancer," explained Pisano, adding that for women who've already been diagnosed with breast cancer, the additional knowledge gained from the MRI outweighs the false-positive risk.

"For these women, because they're at such high-risk, everything is worrisome. You really want to know that you're going to give them cancer therapy once, rather than twice," she said.

Robert A. Smith, director of cancer screening for the American Cancer Society (ACS), said the false-positive risk "is likely to be acceptable to women with unilateral breast cancer, since they will place a high priority on a thorough evaluation for the presence of other primary lesions."

Debbie Saslow, director of breast and gynecological cancers for the ACS, said that because of the high false-positive rate, she's "doubtful there will come a time when we recommend both mammography and MRI regardless of risk."

For the average-risk woman, she said, mammography is the screening tool of choice. And, Pisano pointed out that mammography can pick up very early cancers that an MRI scan may miss.

RECOMMENDATIONS

The ACS is recommending an MRI in addition to mammography for high-risk women, such as those with a known genetic mutation that increases the risk of breast cancer.

In the new guidelines, an annual MRI screen in addition to an annual mammography is recommended for women who...

• **Have a BRCA1 or 2 mutation,** or are untested for these mutations but have a first-degree relative with a BRCA 1 or 2 mutation

• **Have a lifetime breast cancer risk higher than 20%** (ask your doctor to assess your risk using standard risk assessment tools)

• **Have a known genetic mutation in the TP53 or PTEN genes** or have a first-degree relative with either mutation

• **Received radiation treatment to the chest between the ages of 10 and 30**

"So many women are so fearful of breast cancer, but most women aren't at high risk. Since most women aren't in this category, they need to remember that mammography is a really good test," said Saslow. "All women need to get a mammogram every year, starting at age 40."

info To learn more about breast cancer screening methods, visit *breastcancer.org* and click on "Symptoms and Diagnosis."

■ ■ ■ ■

Infrared Not a Good Alternative to Mammograms

Thermography should not be used as a substitute for mammography. In thermography, special infrared cameras are used to detect and map heat that is produced in different parts of the body. Some cancers show up as "hot spots" because new blood vessels are forming rapidly there.

However: The technique is unreliable. The rate of false-negatives (cancers that go undetected) and false-positives (nonmalignant areas that show up as hot spots and require further testing) is unacceptably high.

Mammography remains the most useful breast-cancer screening test. The American Cancer Society recommends annual mammograms for women over age 40—and earlier or more frequently for women at increased risk.

Phil Evans, MD, FACR, professor of radiology and director of the Center for Breast Care, University of Texas Southwestern Medical Center at Dallas. He is a member of the American Cancer Society's Board of Directors.

■ ■ ■ ■

Amazing Breast Cancer Breath Test

Women with breast cancer exhale higher levels of *alkanes*, a byproduct of disease-causing free radicals, than healthy women. An experimental breath test seems to be as effective as a mammogram in ruling out breast cancer but does not expose women to the radiation and discomfort associated with a mammogram.

The Breast Journal.

■ ■ ■ ■

Signs of Breast Cancer

A newly developed lump in the breast is the most common sign of breast cancer, but other red flags include…

•**Thickened, red skin** in one breast.

•**Any dimpling, puckering or retraction** (small depression) of breast skin.

•**Nipple scaling,** flaking or ulceration.

•**A newly inverted nipple.**

•**Spontaneous discharge** from one nipple.

•**A lump in the underarm.**

•**Persistent pain in one breast** (this usually indicates a benign cyst, but it should be assessed).

The Breast Journal.

What to Do If Your Mammogram Is Abnormal

Carolyn M. Clancy, MD, director, Agency for Healthcare Research and Quality, Rockville, MD.

Fran Visco, spokeswoman, National Breast Cancer Coalition, Washington, DC.

An abnormal mammogram can cause understandable worry. So what's the next best step a woman should take? New research has found that a breast biopsy is the preferred follow-up procedure, even though several other test options exist and may be offered by physicians.

A recent report by the Agency for Healthcare Research and Quality (AHRQ) compared the effectiveness of biopsy, long considered the "gold standard," with four other tests. The other four tests were magnetic resonance imaging, or MRI, ultrasonography, positron emission tomography (PET) scanning and scintimammography (a nuclear medicine test that uses a small amount of dye and a scanner to detect cancer).

The report "focuses on a very specific question," said AHRQ director Dr. Carolyn M. Clancy. "Are any of the other noninvasive tests sufficiently accurate to diagnosis cancer or to rule it out?"

BACKGROUND

A biopsy is accurate but invasive, requiring the taking of a sample of breast tissue and analyzing it for signs of cancer in a laboratory. So, researchers have been searching for noninvasive tests that would be as accurate.

NEW REPORT

The four tests assessed in the report, all suggested as substitutes for biopsies, weren't as accurate as a biopsy overall. They missed between 4% and 9% of breast malignancies in women at average risk, the report found, and probably would miss more cases than that among women at higher risk of the disease.

How accurate is accurate enough? "Some experts say a test would have to miss fewer than 2% to be considered sufficiently accurate," Clancy said.

In the AHRQ report, the researchers found that the use of MRI missed 38 cancers for every 1,000 women; ultrasound missed 50 tumors for every 1,000 women; PET scans missed 76 per 1,000 women; and scintimammography missed 93 tumors for every 1,000 women.

IMPLICATIONS

The report on the four noninvasive tests is valuable, according to Fran Visco, the first president and spokeswoman for the National Breast Cancer Coalition in Washington, DC. "My interest in the AHRQ report focuses on the fact that we move these technologies into clinical practice when we don't have the data that show they are effective. That adds to health-care costs and also doesn't serve women well."

Having access to solid data that proves a test is accurate will help women and the health-care system, she said.

Clancy added, "Findings in this study provide good information for women to have additional conversations with their doctors." If a doctor suggests one of the alternate tests after an abnormal mammogram, she said, "It would be reasonable to ask for a biopsy in lieu of these tests."

info To learn more about breast biopsies, visit the National Library of Medicine Web site at *http://www.nlm.nih.gov/medlineplus*. Click on "Medical Encyclopedia" and browse under the letter "B" for "Breast biopsy."

Hypnosis Eases Breast Cancer Biopsy Pain

Radiological Society of North America news release.

Hypnosis can help reduce a woman's pain and anxiety during breast biopsy, a new study finds. "The findings show that nonpharmacologic means can be very powerful—without side effects," said researcher Dr. Elvira V. Lang, associate professor of radiology at Harvard Medical School.

THE STUDY

The study included 236 women who were randomly assigned to one of three types of care while undergoing outpatient needle biopsy. Seventy-six of the women received standard care; 82 received structured "empathetic attention" from a person specifically assigned to be responsive to the women's needs; and 78 of the women induced self-hypnotic relaxation under instruction from a trained research assistant.

The women in the hypnosis group were instructed to roll their eyes upward, close their eyes, breathe deeply, focus on a sensation of floating and imagine a pleasant setting.

RESULTS

Before the start of their biopsies, all the women had heightened anxiety levels. During the procedure, anxiety increased significantly in the standard care group, did not change in the empathy group, and decreased significantly in the hypnosis group.

The women in the empathy and hypnosis groups reported less pain than those in the standard care group. The researchers also found that the hypnosis group had the shortest procedure times and lowest cost.

"The results extend prior assumptions about mind-body interventions, in that self-hypnotic relaxation can be learned very quickly right on the procedure table without additional cost, challenging the notion that extensive office visits or preparation are necessary," Lang said.

info To learn more about preparing for a breast biopsy, go the Web site of the American Cancer Society at *www.cancer.org*. Type "Women facing a breast biopsy" into the search line.

Red Meat May Raise Breast Cancer Risk

Eunyoung Cho, ScD, assistant professor, medicine, Harvard Medical School, Boston.

Eugenia Calle, PhD, managing director, analytic epidemiology, American Cancer Society, Atlanta.

Archives of Internal Medicine.

Steaks, hamburgers and other red meat could raise younger women's risk for an estrogen-linked form of breast cancer, researchers report. "Hormone receptor-positive" breast cancers are stimulated by higher levels of estrogen or progesterone circulating in the body. A majority of breast cancers fall into this category.

"We found that higher red meat intake might be a risk factor for hormone receptor-positive breast cancer among premenopausal women," said lead author Eunyoung Cho, an assistant professor of medicine at Harvard Medical School. "The majority of breast cancer is hormone receptor-positive, and the incidence of hormone receptor-positive tumors has been increasing in the United States," she added.

BACKGROUND

Earlier studies have looked at the association between breast cancer and red meat but only among postmenopausal women and without distinguishing between types of breast cancer. The results of these studies are largely inconclusive, Cho's team noted.

NEW STUDY

In the study, Cho's team collected data on 90,659 female nurses ages 26 to 46 taking part in the ongoing Nurses Health Study II.

The researchers excluded postmenopausal women and women who had had cancer. After 12 years, 1,021 women developed breast cancer. Of these cases, 512 were hormone receptor-positive cancers.

Cho's group found that women who had one-and-a-half servings of red meat a day had nearly double the risk for hormone receptor-positive cancer compared with women who ate less than three servings of red meat per week.

The researchers speculated that the increased risk might be linked to carcinogens found in cooked or processed red meat, hormone treatments used to spur growth in cattle and the type of iron found in red meat.

RECOMMENDATIONS

"Prevention of other chronic diseases, including colon cancer, already provides a good reason for choosing a diet low in red meat," Cho said. "So, our findings provide another reason for women to reduce their red meat intake."

One expert believes more study is needed. "This is the first study that has actually examined the association between breast cancer and the intake of red meat in premenopausal women by type of cancer," said Eugenia Calle, managing director of analytic epidemiology at the American Cancer Society. "But it's just one study."

These results need to be replicated in other studies, according to Calle.

Calle agreed that there is an association between red meat and other cancers, such as colorectal cancer. She concurs with the American Cancer Society's dietary recommendations to shun red meat.

"We recommend that people limit their consumption of processed and red meat, and eat fruits and vegetables and unrefined grains," Calle said.

info For more information on breast cancer, go to the National Breast Cancer Foundation Web site at *www.nationalbreastcancer. org*.

Low-Fat Diet Lowers Breast Cancer Recurrence Up to 42%

National Cancer Institute news release.

By reducing the amount of fat in their diet, postmenopausal women who've been treated for early-stage breast cancer may lower their risk for cancer recurrence. The study of more than 2,400 women, ages 48 to 79, found that the rate of cancer recurrence after five years was 9.8% among women who ate a low-fat diet (about 33 grams of fat per day) and 12.4% among those who ate a standard diet (about 52 grams of fat per day).

That means that, compared with those on the standard diet, the women on the low-fat diet had a 24% reduction in the relative risk of breast cancer recurrence, the study said.

The most significant risk reduction—42%—was noted in women on the low-fat diet whose tumors did not respond to the presence of the hormone estrogen. In women whose tumors did respond to estrogen, the risk reduction was 15%.

Breast cancer that doesn't respond to estrogen is called estrogen receptor-negative (ER-negative), and women with this form of cancer usually have poorer outcomes than women with ER-positive disease.

"Reductions were predicted in women with ER-positive disease because of the association between fat intake and estrogen levels, but the effect on ER-negative disease is, if verified, a surprising and potentially important observation regarding breast cancer and signals a possible new avenue of research," said John Milner, chief of the Nutritional Science Research Group at the National Cancer Institute.

info For more information on recurrent and metastatic breast cancer, go to the Breast cancer.org Web site at *http://www.breastcancer. org/rcr_intro.html.*

Pill May Help Prevent Breast Cancer

Eva Lee, PhD, professor, developmental and cell biology and biological chemistry, University of California, Irvine.
Science.

The abortion pill (RU486 or mifepristone) might ward off breast cancer in women at high risk for the disease. New research found that the chemical compound in RU486 prevented tumors from growing in mice that were genetically engineered to carry the BRCA1 breast cancer gene.

RU486 blocks the production of the hormone progesterone, and this antiprogesterone effect could have prevented the growth of tumors in these mice, the authors speculated. RU486 aborts a pregnancy via the same mechanism.

Still, experts are far from recommending RU486 as breast cancer therapy in people.

THE STUDY

Researchers studied mice that carried the mutated form of BRCA1, which caused them to be highly susceptible to breast cancer.

The mice's mammary cells accumulated high levels of progesterone receptors and then divided and proliferated at an abnormally rapid rate.

However, mice treated with RU486 did not develop breast tumors by the time they reached one year of age. On the other hand, untreated mice developed tumors by eight months.

Progesterone may encourage the proliferation of mammary cells that carry a breast cancer gene, the researchers said.

IMPLICATIONS

Although the study was done in mice, the same mechanism occurs in human cells, said study author Eva Lee, a professor of developmental and cell biology and biological chemistry at the University of California, Irvine.

She speculated that clinicians might one day be able to use progesterone-blocking compounds to prevent breast cancer in women with a genetic predisposition.

But RU486 may not be the best candidate, however.

"It is the most widely available antiprogesterone drug," Lee said. "We are currently testing a more specific antiprogesterone drug to see whether it has the same effect and if that's proven, we'll go to a small clinical trial to see if that antiprogesterone drug is effective in a high-risk population."

info For more information about breast cancer, go to the Web site of the National Cancer Institute at *www.cancer.gov/cancertopics/ types/breast.*

FDA OKs New Drug to Slow Breast Cancer

US Food and Drug Administration news release.
Len Lichtenfeld, MD, deputy chief medical officer of the American Cancer Society, Atlanta.
American Society of Clinical Oncology news conference.

US regulators approved a new drug that in clinical trials delayed breast cancer progression in women no longer responding to *trastuzumab* (Herceptin), a drug effective against tumors with too much of a protein called HER-2. When given in combination with chemotherapy, the new drug, *lapatinib* (Tykerb), did a better job of curtailing cancer growth than did the chemotherapy alone.

"Today's approval is a step forward in making new treatments available for patients who have progression of their breast cancer after treatment with some of the most effective breast cancer therapies available," said Dr. Steven Galson, director of the Center for Drug Evaluation and Research at the US Food and Drug Administration (FDA). "New targeted therapies such as Tykerb are helping expand options for patients."

About 8,000 to 10,000 American women die from metastatic HER 2-positive breast cancer each year, the FDA said.

HOW IT WORKS

Tykerb, among a class of drugs called kinase inhibitors, deprives tumor cells of signals they need to grow. But it differs from other cancer drugs in that it actually enters cells and blocks the function of the HER-2 protein, the agency said.

Tykerb, which comes in pill form, is made by GlaxoSmithKline, which funded the clinical trial.

THE STUDY

The drug was tested in a trial involving 400 women with advanced or metastatic breast cancer that was HER-2 positive. Common side effects included diarrhea, nausea, vomiting and a rash. A small percentage of participants also had a decrease in heart function that may have been characterized by shortness of breath. This condition generally was reversible, the FDA said.

Some 20% to 25% of breast cancers have abnormally high levels of the HER-2/neu receptor and, as a result, are generally more aggressive. Herceptin blocks activity of the receptor by binding to the part of the receptor outside the cell. Tykerb, by contrast, binds to a part of the receptor inside the cell.

The clinical trial included a plan for an independent monitoring committee to analyze data at the halfway point to see if the benefits were larger than anticipated, in which case the committee would recommend the study be closed.

The monitoring committee made a unanimous recommendation to terminate the trial because the results were so encouraging.

Women in the combined therapy group had almost double the time of disease progression as did women receiving chemotherapy alone: 36.9 weeks versus 19.7 weeks.

Responding to the FDA's approval of Tykerb, Dr. Len Lichtenfeld, deputy chief medical officer of the American Cancer Society, said, "The approval of Tykerb is a significant step forward because it once again demonstrates the promise of targeted therapies, where we take our understanding of how cancer cells work and apply that knowledge to new drug development. We

now have a new drug that offers promise and hope to women who have a more aggressive form of breast cancer, where until very recently we had little to offer."

info For more information, visit the Web site of the National Cancer Institute at *http:// www.cancer.gov/clinicaltrials* and click on "Clinical Trial results."

■ ■ ■ ■

Better Breast Cancer Recovery

Women with breast cancer who walked for at least one hour a week were 20% less likely to die from breast cancer compared with those who didn't exercise at all.

Theory: Exercise lowers hormone levels, which suppresses cancer growth recurrence.

For maximum benefit: Women with breast cancer should walk (or perform equivalent exercise, such as bicycling) a total of three to five hours per week.

Michelle D. Holmes, MD, assistant professor of medicine, Harvard Medical School, Boston.

Men with Breast Cancer at High Risk Of Other Cancers

Hoda Anton-Culver, PhD, director, epidemiology, University of California, Irvine.

Breast Cancer Research.

Men who have breast cancer have a significantly increased risk for a second cancer, malignant melanoma and stomach cancer, according to the largest study ever done on the subject. "We looked at the risk not only of a second breast cancer but also of other cancers. We found the risk of other cancers increased as well," said lead researcher Hoda Anton-Culver, director of epidemiology at the University of California at Irvine.

BACKGROUND

Breast cancer remains rare among men. About 1,400 new cases are reported in the US each year, according to the American Cancer Society.

Because of the relatively small incidence of male breast cancer, "not one study until now has looked at large numbers," Anton-Culver said. However, "our study looks at a very large number of men," she said, "so there can be validity to large numbers of a rare cancer like this one."

The researchers analyzed data on 1,926 men with breast cancer. Of these, 221, or 11.5%, developed a second cancer at least two months after their breast cancer diagnosis.

One significant second cancer was malignant melanoma, with an incidence that was 50% higher than normal, as well as an elevated risk of stomach cancer, according to Anton-Culver.

POSSIBLE EXPLANATIONS

There are several possible explanations for the increased risk, she said. It might be due to the side effects of treatment of the primary breast cancer, for example. But the most probable cause is genetics, she said, with the men being at "higher risk of developing cancer in general."

And studies by the group have shown a high incidence of a breast cancer-related gene, BRCA2, in the men, Anton-Culver said.

"We definitely do see an association between breast cancer in men and an increased risk of being a carrier of a cancer-related gene," Anton-Culver said. That relationship indicates that a screening program looking at close relatives of men with breast cancer could help with the early detection of malignancies, she said.

info For more information on male breast cancer, go to the Web site of the National Library of Medicine at *http://www.nlm.nih.gov/medlineplus/malebreastcancer.html*.

■ ■ ■ ■

Risk Factors for Men

Although breast cancer is approximately 100 times more common in women than in men, it will be diagnosed in an estimated 2,030 American men this year. Among men, those between the ages of 60 to 70 are at greatest risk.

Breast cancer risk factors for men include a family history of breast cancer (in women or men), obesity, physical inactivity, radiation exposure, heavy alcohol consumption and estrogen treatment. Men who notice a lump or swelling…skin dimpling…a nipple that turns inward…redness or scaling of the nipple or breast skin…or nipple discharge should see a doctor as soon as possible.

American Cancer Society.

Compound Boosts Tamoxifen's Cancer-Fighting Power

V. Craig Jordan, PhD, ScD, vice president and scientific director, medical science division, Fox Chase Cancer Center, Philadelphia.

William L. Farrar, PhD, head, Cancer Stem Cell Section, Laboratory of Cancer Prevention, US National Cancer Institute-Frederick, Frederick, MD.

Cancer Cell.

Scientists at the National Cancer Institute report that adding a second drug molecule to tamoxifen, the breast cancer drug used successfully for more than 20 years, helps it retain its full strength.

Over time, tamoxifen can lose its effectiveness. But the new molecule, called disulfide benzamide or DIBA, could provide a way to overcome that acquired resistance and restore tamoxifen's effectiveness.

DIBA "is not a new molecule," noted William Farrar, head of the Cancer Stem Cell Section of the National Cancer Institute's Center for Cancer Research at Frederick, Maryland, and the study's lead author. "It's been around a while."

Farrar's team gave DIBA to mice engineered to develop tamoxifen-resistant tumors and then to human breast cancer cells in the laboratory. Tumor growth slowed in both cases.

Tamoxifen is the standard of care for women who have what's known as "estrogen receptor-positive breast cancer." When estrogen binds to the estrogen receptor, a series of events that promote rapid cell division ensues. If that cell happens to be a breast cancer cell, the cascade of events can lead to tumor growth.

Tamoxifen acts to block the effects of estrogen on breast tissue. It is routinely used in advanced breast cancer or as additional therapy after primary treatment for early-stage breast cancer.

In Farrar's study, when DIBA was added to the mix, tamoxifen easily inhibited the growth of breast cancer cells.

DIBA "switches off everything, all the molecular machinery of estrogen receptors, which results in breast cancer cell death," Farrar said. And, in the human breast cancer cell lines, "we got a 90 percent reduction in tumors," he added. In the mice studies, DIBA reduced tumor volume almost 50 percent.

DIBA is what is known as a "lead" compound, Farrar said, which means it merely opens the door to suitable drugs. DIBA itself "is probably not appropriate for humans, because of solubility problems." Farrar's team will try to develop or find another compound more suitable for human use, fashioning it after the properties of DIBA.

As research progresses from the laboratory to human clinical trials, "our goal is to develop a molecule that can be orally administered," Farrar said.

V. Craig Jordan, vice president and scientific director of the medical science division of the Fox Chase Cancer Center in Philadelphia, views the new research as promising. Jordan, known as the "father of tamoxifen," notes that tamoxifen is life-saving but also beset with resistance problems.

For example, Jordan said, "if 100 women had advanced breast cancer, 20 would have estrogen receptor-negative [cancer], and tamoxifen would not be indicated. Eighty would be estrogen receptor or ER positive, and 40 would get an initial response from tamoxifen while 40 would not. Of the 40 [who got a response], ultimately all would get acquired resistance. It would take two to five years for that to happen."

According to Jordan, members of the NCI team "have created an opportunity to move from the laboratory to the clinic." Eventually, he said, a DIBA-like compound might boost responses in those who acquired tamoxifen resistance and

perhaps in those who initially did not respond to tamoxifen.

The current research, however, focused only on acquired resistance, not initial or intrinsic resistance, he added.

Next, the compound or a similar compound must be tested in humans, Jordan said.

info There's more information on tamoxifen at the National Cancer Institute Web site, *www.cancer.gov/cancertopics/factsheet/therapy/tamoxifen.*

35% of Breast Cancer Patients Stop Taking Tamoxifen Too Early

Thomas I. Barron, MSc, department of pharmacology and therapeutics, Trinity College Dublin and St. James's Hospital, Dublin, Ireland.

Robert Smith, PhD, director, cancer screening, American Cancer Society, Atlanta.

Nearly one-quarter of breast cancer patients stop taking the drug tamoxifen within the first year of a standard five-year regimen, a new study reveals. Doctors routinely prescribe tamoxifen—which inhibits estrogen's stimulatory effect on cancer cells—to patients after breast cancer treatment, to help prevent a recurrence. But the new study found a steep drop-off in drug adherence—about twice the rate observed in previous studies. Treatment nonadherence rose over time and shifted with patient age, the researchers added.

In fact, the study found that more than one-third of patients ceased taking their medication within three-and-a-half years of treatment. Younger women between ages 35 and 44, and those over the age of 75, were the most likely to discontinue tamoxifen.

"We now know that there are a considerable number of women who stop taking their tamoxifen early," said study author Thomas I. Barron, from the department of pharmacology and therapeutics at Trinity College Dublin and St. James's Hospital in Ireland. That's troubling, he said, because "women discontinuing their tamoxifen early may not receive the full benefits of their treatment."

BACKGROUND

Barron's group believes that the "surprisingly high" lack of adherence stems from the relatively long time periods that women are placed on the drug and its often troublesome side effects.

Tamoxifen, a "selective estrogen receptor modulator," is typically prescribed for a five-year period following a diagnosis of breast cancer, although in some cases a longer regimen is recommended. Taking the medication for less than five years can undercut the drug's effectiveness and is associated with more frequent cancer recurrence and, ultimately, a higher risk of death, experts say.

About 75% of women diagnosed with breast cancer are prescribed a hormonal agent such as tamoxifen as part of their overall treatment, according to Barron and his colleagues. Research suggests that tamoxifen prevents more than 40,000 breast cancer recurrences worldwide each year.

However, side effects that mimic menopausal symptoms are prevalent among some, but not all, women who take the drug. These include hot flashes, vaginal discharge, irregular menstruation, headaches, fatigue, nausea and vaginal itching.

THE STUDY

To gauge patient adherence with prescribed tamoxifen, Barron and his team reviewed pharmacy database records to examine the prescription-filling habits of more than 2,800 breast cancer patients over the age of 35 on a tamoxifen regimen.

According to researchers, all patients received free health services and free medicine, so cost was not an obstacle to continued treatment. None of the patients took any other hormone therapy with tamoxifen.

FINDINGS

More than 11% of the women stopped taking the medication within 30 days of treatment, a figure that rose to almost 15% by 90 days.

The one-year dropout rate was 22% and by the second year more than 28% of the women were off the drug. By three-and-a-half years that number had risen to just over 35%.

In total, a little more than 31% of the patients continued with tamoxifen as prescribed throughout the study period.

EXPLANATION

Though no single reason was offered for the high dropout rates, the authors believe that, among the elderly, a drop in social support and an increase in functional impairment might play a role. Younger patients may simply be less willing to put up with side effects and be less accepting of their breast cancer diagnosis overall, relative to older women, the researchers said.

Barron pointed out that, due to patient demand and preference, the number of new oral anticancer medicines is increasing, and adherence problems regarding tamoxifen might apply to a much broader range of cancer treatments.

"The effectiveness of these new and powerful treatments over the more traditional intravenous chemotherapies depends very much on patients' ability to adhere to treatments," he cautioned.

ADVICE

Barron said patients contemplating the cessation of their tamoxifen regimen due to harsh side effects should talk to their doctors first.

"It may be possible to alleviate any troublesome side effects they are experiencing or, in some cases, alternative hormonal treatment may be available," he said.

Robert Smith, director of cancer screening for the American Cancer Society in Atlanta, seconded the need for continuous physician oversight.

"My impression is that most women are not particularly happy with the side effects, although they experience them at different levels," said Smith. "And five years is a long time to take a drug. So for doctors maintaining the protocol—making sure the women complete it—becomes as much a standard of care as prescribing the treatment in the first place."

 For additional information on tamoxifen, visit *www.drugs.com/pdr/tamoxifen-citrate. html.*

Breast Cancer Responds to Shorter-Course Radiation

Fox Chase Cancer Center news release.

Ashorter course of external beam radiation therapy for early-stage breast cancer is both safe and effective, new research shows.

BACKGROUND

Many women with early breast cancer have breast-sparing surgery (lumpectomy) followed by treatment with external beam radiation five days a week for six to seven weeks.

NEW STUDY

This study of 75 patients concluded that intensity modulated radiation treatment (IMRT) can be safely done in four weeks by increasing the daily dose of radiation.

"We know the standard regimen of daily radiation five days a week for six to seven weeks is a tremendous time commitment for women who are often still working or providing family care or both," said study lead author Dr. Gary Freedman, a radiation oncologist at Fox Chase Cancer Center in Philadelphia.

"Our goal in this research was to reduce the burden of treatment time while maintaining a high level of quality of life," Freedman said.

He and his colleagues measured toxicity, pain and cosmetic outcomes for the women who received the shorter course of IMRT and compared those results to data on women who had the usual course of therapy.

RESULTS

The researchers found little or no difference between the two groups.

"These results demonstrate that the increased daily radiation given to the breast does not result in significant increased side effects, but it allows us to dramatically reduce the time needed for treatment," Freedman explained.

"Longer follow-up is needed to compare the outcomes at five years after treatment," he added.

info For more information on radiation treatment for breast cancer, go to *www.breast cancer.org*. Click on "Radiation Therapy" under the "Treatment" section.

■ ■ ■ ■

Hot Cancer Treatment

Heating tumors after radiation is more effective than radiation alone. A study of patients with breast, melanoma or other cancers found that radiation plus heat destroyed tumors in 66% of patients, compared with 42% of those getting only radiation.

Science News.

Delaying Chemo After Breast Cancer Surgery Can Be Safe

Journal of Clinical Oncology news release.

Women with early-stage breast cancer may safely wait up to 12 weeks after cancer surgery before they begin chemotherapy, a new study shows. However, waiting any longer than that increases the risk of cancer recurrence and reduces overall survival by 60%, a Canadian team concluded.

THE STUDY

Researchers analyzed the records of nearly 2,600 breast cancer patients.

The women received chemotherapy after surgery for stage I and II breast cancer. Among women who started chemotherapy within four weeks of surgery, 84% were alive five years after their breast cancer diagnosis. Survival rates were similar for women who began chemotherapy four to eight weeks (85%) and eight to 12 weeks (89%) after surgery.

But five-year survival dropped to 78% among women who didn't start chemotherapy until more than 12 weeks after breast cancer surgery. These women also had a higher rate of cancer recurrence (31%) than women who started chemotherapy within 12 weeks (18% to 26%).

ADVICE

"Our findings can reassure women with early-stage breast cancer that it is okay to take some time before they start chemotherapy to gather information and be actively involved in treatment decision-making. These steps have been shown to reduce anxiety and depression associated with breast cancer," said study lead author Dr. Caroline Lohrisch, a medical oncologist with the British Columbia Cancer Agency.

"However, to achieve the full benefit of chemotherapy, patients should not delay further, and should ensure that they start treatment within three months of surgery," she added.

 For more information on chemotherapy, go to *www.medicinenet.com/chemotherapy/*.

What Most Women Still Don't Know About Breast Cancer

Carolyn M. Kaelin, MD, MPH, founding director of the Comprehensive Breast Health Center at Brigham and Women's Hospital, surgical oncologist at Dana Farber Cancer Institute and an assistant professor of surgery at Harvard Medical School, all in Boston. Dr. Kaelin is author of *Living Through Breast Cancer* and coauthor of *The Breast Cancer Survivor's Fitness Plan*. McGraw-Hill.

Most women know to tell their doctors about any new breast lumps. But a lump is not the only potential warning sign of breast cancer. As a breast cancer surgeon who also has survived this disease, I know many subtle signs of breast cancer that initially may go unnoticed.

In my own case, the first clue was not a lump —but rather a tiny area of retracted skin on my breast. The mammogram I received the next day appeared normal, but I knew to follow up with an ultrasound (an imaging test using high-frequency sound waves). This test revealed a tumor, which a biopsy later confirmed was malignant.

Important facts that could save your life—or that of a loved one...

•**A swollen, red, warm and/or tender breast can indicate breast cancer.** Such symptoms can mean an infection, but they also can be caused by inflammatory breast cancer, a rare condition in which cancer cells clog the lymphatic channels in the breast skin, preventing the lymph fluid from draining.

Self-defense: If you're diagnosed with a breast infection that doesn't clear within one week of antibiotic treatment, your doctor should order a mammogram and arrange for a skin biopsy to check for inflammatory breast cancer.

Mammograms miss about 10% to 20% of breast cancers. Even so, studies suggest that among women who undergo annual screenings, mammograms may reduce the breast cancer death rate by as much as 65%. And the technology continues to improve. According to a study published recently in *The New England Journal of Medicine*, newer digital mammography (which provides computer-generated images that can be enlarged and/or enhanced) is up to 28% more accurate than film mammography in detecting cancers in women who are under age 50, premenopausal or who have dense breast tissue (breasts that have a much greater proportion of dense tissue than fat). Digital mammography is not yet widely available in the US.

Self-defense: If you have a lump or another suspicious symptom and have already had a normal mammogram, request an ultrasound. This test can distinguish between fluid-filled and solid masses. It's a rare breast cancer that eludes both a mammogram and ultrasound.

•**Some breast cancer risk factors are not well-known.** More than 75% of breast cancers occur in women over age 50. You're at higher risk if you've been taking combination estrogen/progesterone hormone replacement therapy for at least five years…if you began menstruating before age 12 or stopped after age 55…if you've never had children or had your first child after age 30…and/or if you consume more than one to two alcoholic drinks daily. Dense breast tissue on a mammogram has recently been identified as an independent risk factor.

You also are at higher risk for breast cancer if one or more of the following is true: A first-degree relative (mother, sister or daughter) has had breast cancer…a family member was diagnosed with breast cancer when younger than age 40 or before menopause…a family member had cancer in both breasts…or you have a family history of ovarian cancer. This constellation of factors could suggest the presence of a mutated gene, such as the BRCA1 or BRCA2, which may be inherited.

STAY-WELL STRATEGIES

There's no way to predict or prevent every breast cancer, but you can lower your chances of developing or dying from the disease.

Here's how…

•**Maintain a healthy weight.** Gaining weight and being overweight raise the likelihood of developing a breast malignancy—and worsen your prognosis if you already have this type of cancer.

Reason: Body fat produces estrogen, which is one of the factors that increase breast cancer risk.

•**Stay active.** Exercise helps prevent breast cancer—probably by decreasing circulating estrogen. Newer research suggests that it also may improve long-term survival odds for those previously treated for the disease. In a recently published *Journal of the American Medical Association* study, breast cancer patients who walked or engaged in another moderate exercise three to five hours weekly were 50% less likely to have a recurrence or to die prematurely than women who exercised less than one hour weekly.

Best choice: Aerobic exercises, such as walking, jogging or cycling.

Weight-bearing exercises, such as walking or weight-lifting, also help to minimize bone loss—a significant advantage, since chemotherapy can lead to osteoporosis. (Chemotherapy can damage the ovaries, reducing estrogen levels and inducing early menopause in premenopausal women, which greatly accelerates bone loss.)

Self-defense: In addition to performing regular weight-bearing exercise, women with breast cancer should take a daily calcium supplement (1,000 mg for those ages 31 to 50…and 1,200 mg for those ages 51 or older) plus at least 200 international units (IU) of vitamin D. If you've had chemotherapy, experienced premature menopause or take an aromatase inhibitor

(a drug used to treat postmenopausal breast cancer patients), ask your doctor what levels of calcium and vitamin D intake are right for you.

Tamoxifen (Nolvadex), the only FDA-approved breast cancer preventive drug, also has been shown to conserve bone while reducing malignancies in high-risk women by as much as 50%.

Downside: Tamoxifen increases risk for blood clots, stroke and uterine cancer.

Some recent studies have shown the osteoporosis drug *raloxifene* (Evista) to be as effective as tamoxifen for preventing breast cancer and preserving bone in postmenopausal women—with lower risk for uterine cancer. But Evista has not yet been approved by the FDA as a breast cancer preventive or for premenopausal women, so it is prescribed "off-label."

Best: Ask your doctor if either drug may be appropriate for you.

LATEST ADVANCES

•**Aromatase inhibitors (AIs)** may offer even more powerful protection against breast cancer recurrence and death for postmenopausal women than tamoxifen. Whereas tamoxifen works by blocking estrogen from binding with cancer cells, AIs work by inhibiting estrogen production in fat tissues—our primary source of the hormone after menopause.

In a recent British study, breast cancer patients who switched from tamoxifen to an AI called *exemestane* (Aromasin) were 17% less likely to see their breast cancer spread to other organs, had a 15% lower chance of dying within about five years than women who stayed on tamoxifen, and had a 44% lower risk of developing cancer in the opposite breast. AIs do not appear to raise risk for endometrial cancer as tamoxifen does, but AIs do speed bone loss and are not effective for premenopausal women.

•**Newly developed tests** are enabling doctors to look at the genetic makeup of tumors and predict with increasing accuracy which are likely to recur or metastasize.

In the past, breast cancer patients had been routinely prescribed chemotherapy, usually following surgery, since doctors had no way of knowing which cancers would return and become fatal. New tests, which include "tumor profiling" (a more detailed analysis of the tumor than biopsy alone), take some of the guesswork out of deciding who will benefit most from chemotherapy and who is most likely to do just fine without it.

Breast Cancer Vaccine Shows Promise

Mayo Clinic news release.

Scientists have developed a breast cancer vaccine that stimulates a powerful immune system response to tumor cells. In mice, the "synthetic peptide" vaccine stimulated an anti-tumor T-cell response that identified and prevented the spread of breast cancer cells. T-cells are white blood cells that play an important role in immune response.

THE STUDY

A team at the Mayo Clinic in Rochester, Minnesota, tested the vaccine on female mice that had the cancer-producing oncogene HER-2/neu. The mice received the vaccine at the early stage of tumor development. The vaccine either slowed or stopped the progression of breast cancer in all the mice.

HOW THE VACCINE WORKS

Because synthetic peptides alone do not usually trigger a strong immune response, the vaccine was given in combination with a "Toll-like receptor" stimulant, which mimics the way invading bacteria would spur the immune system into action.

"We found that we could train the immune system to recognize these synthetic peptides as dangerous foreign agents of the HER-2/neu gene by mimicking what the bacteria would do in your body. The body responded by killing everything that expressed HER-2/neu in high amounts," said study author Dr. Pilar Nava-Parada.

Using this approach, it would likely take only one immunization to build an immune system response powerful enough to destroy a tumor.

To date, attempts at creating effective cancer vaccines have produced mixed results. This and other new studies suggest that scientists are moving closer to creating viable cancer vaccines, the Mayo researchers said.

info For more information about cancer vaccines, go to the Web site of the National Cancer Institute at *http://www.cancer.gov/news center/pressreleases/cancervaccines.*

Decline in HRT Use Linked to Drop in Breast Cancer

Donald Berry, PhD, chairman, department of biostatistics, University of Texas M.D. Anderson Cancer Center, Houston.
Julia Smith, MD, PhD, director, New York University Cancer Institute Breast Cancer Screening and Prevention Program, and director, Lynne Cohen Breast Cancer Preventive Care Program, New York University Cancer Institute and Bellevue Hospital, New York City.
New England Journal of Medicine.
The Lancet.

When millions of US women threw out their prescriptions for hormone replacement therapy (HRT) in 2002, the rates of breast cancer started dropping almost immediately, according to US researchers. Their findings coincided with a report from the UK that showed women who took HRT after menopause were 20% more likely to develop ovarian cancer or die from it than postmenopausal women who never took HRT.

THE US AND UK STUDIES

The breast cancer report looked at the incidence of breast cancer both before and after the news broke from the long-term Women's Health Initiative (WHI) study that HRT might be more damaging than helpful to a woman's health. Between 2001 and 2004, it shows, the overall incidence of breast cancer decreased by 8.6% in postmenopausal women.

The UK study determined that 1,000 additional women died from ovarian cancer between 1991 and 2005 because they were using HRT, and that 1,300 extra cases of ovarian cancer were diagnosed in the same period.

The researchers, from the Cancer Research UK Epidemiology Unit in Oxford, also found that after women stopped taking HRT, their risk of ovarian cancer returned to the same level as those who never used HRT.

For the US study, experts suspect that HRT may have been fueling some breast cancers because that decline began soon after many women stopped using HRT.

"From 1975 to 2000, breast cancer incidence increased rather dramatically. While part of that increase was clearly due to the introduction of screening mammography (due to increased detection), once you take out that effect, there is still a rather astounding increase of 30%," said Dr. Donald Berry, chairman of the department of biostatistics at the University of Texas M.D. Anderson Cancer Center in Houston.

"While there have been a number of theories put forward to explain the increase, it now looks like some of that increase is due to the use of HRT," Berry said. "When women stopped using HRT, it looked kind of like a market correction and the numbers went back down."

BACKGROUND

Initially, it appeared as if combination estrogen-progestin hormone replacement therapy was the answer to many ills. Researchers hoped that HRT would lower the risk of such serious illnesses as heart disease and dementia.

However, the WHI study, which included more than 16,000 postmenopausal women, was halted early in May 2002 because HRT was increasing the risk of coronary disease, stroke and blood clots.

After the WHI trial was halted, many women stopped taking hormones. In fact, the use of HRT had dropped by 38% in the US by the end of 2002. In 2001, 61 million prescriptions were written for hormone replacement therapy. In 2002, there were about 47 million prescriptions. By 2003, that number had fallen to 27 million, and by 2004 just 21 million, the study authors noted.

BREAST CANCER RATES DROPPING

The rate of breast cancer started dropping soon after the WHI results in 2002, according to the new study.

Between 2001—the last full year of combination HRT use—and 2004, rates of breast cancer in the US dropped by 8.6% in postmenopausal women. The rates of estrogen receptor-positive breast cancer—those cancers fueled by the

hormone estrogen—dropped by 14.7% in women between the ages of 50 and 69. Yet, rates of estrogen receptor-negative cancers dropped only 1.7% in the same time period, which further suggests that stopping HRT played a role in the decline.

"HRT is probably not something that causes cancer; it probably just fuels existing cancers," explained Berry. "If you feed it, it grows, and if you stop feeding it, it stops growing."

Berry said the Emory researchers looked at other potential causes for the decline in breast cancer rates, including whether fewer women were getting screening mammograms to detect tumors. The researchers also checked for environmental factors and the use of breast cancer drugs such as tamoxifen and raloxifene. But none of these factors had changed significantly enough to cause such a drop in breast cancer rates, the study authors said.

The breast cancer rates leveled off by 2004, to rates not seen since 1987, the study authors said.

REACTION

"Overall, this is very encouraging news," said Dr. Julia Smith, director of the New York University Cancer Institute Breast Cancer Screening and Prevention Program in New York City.

However, Smith said she'd like to know if this drop would affect survival rates in the future. "Have these cancers been eliminated, or are they just below our level of detection now, but will rise up again?" she asked.

IS HRT EVER SAFE?

Both Berry and Smith pointed out that if a woman is suffering from menopausal symptoms, such as hot flashes, short-term use of hormone replacement therapy is likely safe.

"You can give low-dose HRT for short periods of time for women who really have a quality-of-life issue," Smith said. She added that individual risk needs to be assessed on a case-by-case basis, but even some women at high risk of breast cancer may be able to use HRT for short-term relief.

"It doesn't make sense to do something in the name of prevention and protection—(withholding HRT)—that ends up hurting the person," Smith said.

Berry said, "If you're taking HRT for long-term health effects, it's not worth it. But, if you're taking

HRT for menopausal symptoms and it works for you, it's probably a reasonable thing to continue. I'd stop it occasionally to see if the hot flashes are still there, but short-term use for a year or two probably won't affect your risk in the long run."

MORE INFORMATION

info To learn more about preventing breast cancer, visit the American Cancer Society's Web site at *www.cancer.org*. Type "Can Cancer Be Prevented?" in the search box.

draw cells together enhances the transformation of normal cells to cancerous cells, thus stimulating tumor growth.

Ando and his colleagues say that this increased cell growth can be halted when an E-cadherin antibody or a calcium-chelating agent is used to block E-cadherin function in the presence of estradiol.

It's the first step in what may lead to new drugs.

Shocking Way Fat Hormone Spreads Breast Cancer

Sebastiano Ando, professor, department of cell biology, University of Calabria, Italy.
Federation of American Societies for Experimental Biology.

New clues have surfaced on how leptin, a hormone found in fat cells, may play a major role in the development and progression of breast cancer.

Italian researchers have identified a new mechanism that helps explain how obesity boosts risk of breast cancer, a discovery that may lead to new drugs to specifically combat the problem.

Research team leader Dr. Sebastiano Ando notes that obesity increases the risk of breast cancer in postmenopausal women, shortens the time between cancer recurrence, and lowers overall survival rates. His team finds that leptin increases the amount of estradiol (a type of estrogen) in breast tissue.

HORMONE FEEDS TUMORS

Ando's research team finds that combined exposure to leptin and estradiol increases the size of breast cancer tumors in both mice and in tissue cultures. This growth in tumor size was accompanied by an increase in E-cadherin, an intracellular adhesion molecule generally regarded as a tumor suppressor.

But the new twist is that E-cadherin may act as a tumor *enhancer* when it's exposed to leptin and estradiol. In that case, E-cadherin's ability to

Estrogen Blocks Immune System from Attacking Breast Cancer

David J. Shapiro, professor of biochemistry, University of Illinois at Urbana-Champaign.
Oncogene.

There's more evidence pointing to a connection between estrogen and breast cancer. New research indicates that the female hormone appears to shield breast cancer cells from attack by the body's immune cells.

It was already known that estrogen enhances the growth and migration of breast cancer cells. But this study, by researchers at the University of Illinois at Urbana-Champaign, finds that estrogen also stimulates a certain chemical—called protease inhibitor 9 (PI-9)—that hinders the ability of immune cells to kill tumor cells.

This cause-and-effect mechanism may lead to new breast cancer therapies.

"The amounts of estrogen required to do this are quite small," notes researcher David J. Shapiro, professor of biochemistry at the University of Illinois at Urbana-Champaign.

PI-9 has already been implicated in other kinds of cancers. For example, high levels of PI-9 in some lymphomas are associated with poor patient prognoses.

But this is the first time that estrogen's role in shielding breast cancer cells from immune cells has been identified.

4

Cancer Breakthroughs

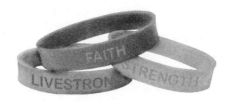

Daily Aspirin Reduces Cancer Risk Up to 15%

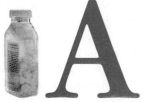 A daily aspirin may lower the odds of developing colon, prostate and breast cancer for people at high risk for those malignancies, researchers at the American Cancer Society (ACS) report.

"Men and women who used adult-strength aspirin daily for five or more years had about a 15% lower overall rate of developing cancer, particularly colon, prostate and possibly breast cancer," said study lead author Dr. Eric Jacobs, an epidemiologist at the ACS.

However, his team said there's not enough evidence that aspirin's value as a cancer preventive outweighs its potential toxic side effects, which include a higher risk for bleeding.

THE STUDY

In the study, researchers looked for a link between long-term aspirin use—dosed at 325 milligrams or more a day—and cancer in nearly 70,000 men and more than 76,000 women.

During 12 years of follow-up, more than 18,000 men and women were diagnosed with cancer.

The researchers found that taking daily aspirin for at least five years was linked with about a 15% relative reduction in overall cancer risk. This decrease did not reach statistical significance in women, however.

In addition, aspirin was associated with a 20% reduction in the risk for prostate cancer in men and a 30% reduction in the risk for colorectal cancer in both men and women, compared with people who didn't take the medicine, Jacobs's team found.

Aspirin had no effect on risk for lung cancer, bladder cancer, melanoma, leukemia, non-Hodgkin's lymphoma, pancreatic cancer, and kidney cancer, the researchers noted. Also, aspirin

Eric Jacobs, PhD, epidemiologist, American Cancer Society, Atlanta.

Maria Elena Martinez, PhD, Arizona Cancer Center, Tucson.

Journal of the National Cancer Institute.

use for *less* than five years did not lower the risk for cancer.

MORE RESEARCH NEEDED

If more evidence comes to light suggesting that aspirin curbs cancer risk, American Cancer Society recommendations might someday change, Jacobs said. "Future recommendations could take cancer prevention into account when deciding on the best dose for people who already need to take aspirin for cardiovascular protection," he said. "We're not there yet."

EXPERT REACTION

One expert agreed that aspirin should not be taken to prevent cancer, at least for now.

"The jury is still out about making recommendations about aspirin for the prevention of cancers. Even those cancers where we do see significant protection," said Dr. Maria Elena Martinez, from the Arizona Cancer Center, Tucson.

It is difficult to make recommendations when there are significant toxicities associated with aspirin, Martinez said. "People should not take aspirin for the protection against colon cancer or any cancers at this point," she said.

Martinez said that unlike cardiovascular protection—where low-dose aspirin appears to be effective—cancer protection is only seen when high doses are taken. "It's with the higher doses where we see the toxicity and side effects," she said.

"If there were evidence that aspirin protected against a multitude of cancers, then we might get to the point where we say it's time to start considering it," Martinez said. "But you have to keep in mind that it comes with side effects. At this point, we are not ready to say, 'Take aspirin,' as we do with cardiovascular disease," she added.

info For more information on the benefits of daily aspirin use, visit *www.medscape. com* and search "daily aspirin use."

Protect Yourself from The Fastest-Growing Cancer Threat

Herman Kattlove, MD, a medical oncologist and medical editor with the American Cancer Society. He is based in Los Angeles.

Cancer rates are declining in the US, but the incidence of adenocarcinoma, the most common type of esophageal cancer, has increased more rapidly since the 1970s than any other cancer.

Until recently, cancer of the esophagus—the foot-long muscular tube that carries food from the mouth to the stomach—has been considered deadly, though relatively rare. Now both of these beliefs are being challenged.

At one time, people diagnosed with esophageal cancer who underwent surgery had a low chance of surviving for five years. That survival rate is now as high as 50%, most likely due to earlier screening and diagnosis.

Fortunately, healthy lifestyle changes can reduce your risk of developing esophageal cancer.

WHO IS AT RISK?

As with many cancers, the risk for esophageal cancer increases with age—nearly 80% of new cases are diagnosed in people ages 55 to 85.

There are two main types of esophageal cancer—squamous cell carcinoma, which develops in the cells that line the entire esophagus, and adenocarcinoma, which occurs in the part of the esophagus closest to the stomach.

More than half of all squamous cell carcinomas are linked to smoking. Risk of adenocarcinoma is doubled in people who smoke a pack of cigarettes or more per day. Carcinogens in tobacco are believed to enter the bloodstream and contribute to the development of esophageal cancer. Excessive alcohol consumption—more than two drinks daily—also increases the risk for the squamous cell type of cancer, although it is not known why.

Tobacco and alcohol are a potentially deadly combination. A person who drinks excessively and smokes one to two packs of cigarettes a day has a 44 times higher risk of getting esophageal cancer than someone who does neither.

A diet low in fruits and vegetables accounts for approximately 15% of esophageal cancer risk. To help avoid the disease, eat at least five daily servings. Some scientific evidence suggests that berries, particularly black raspberries, which are rich in cancer-fighting antioxidants, protect against esophageal cancer.

Body weight also is a factor. Obese men are twice as likely to die from adenocarcinoma of the esophagus as men of normal weight.

THE HEARTBURN CONNECTION

Frequent heartburn, known as *gastroesophageal reflux disease* (GERD), is caused by stomach acid backing up into the esophagus. Up to 14% of Americans experience heartburn at least weekly, while 44% suffer from it monthly. GERD is linked to nearly one-third of esophageal cancer cases.

An additional factor for esophageal adenocarcinoma is a condition called Barrett's esophagus, in which cells of the esophagus begin to resemble those that line the stomach. People with Barrett's esophagus are about 50 times more likely to develop esophageal cancer than those without the condition.

People who suffer from chronic heartburn (three or more times per week for more than three months) should be screened for Barrett's esophagus. If they are found to have the condition, screenings every year may be recommended to detect esophageal cancer.

Screening involves the use of endoscopy, an invasive procedure that requires sedation. During the test, the doctor passes a thin, flexible tube (endoscope) through the mouth to view the entire length of the esophagus.

Prompt and effective treatment of GERD might reduce the risk for esophageal cancer, although this has never been proven. A number of effective prescription and over-the-counter GERD remedies, which block the production of stomach acid, are available. These include H2 blockers, such as *ranitidine* (Zantac) and *famotidine* (Pepcid), and proton pump inhibitors, such as *omeprazole* (Prilosec).

SYMPTOMS AND DIAGNOSIS

Difficulty swallowing is the most common symptom of esophageal cancer. If you notice that swallowing has become even slightly harder—you must swallow more firmly or food doesn't go down properly—see your doctor immediately. It could save your life.

Weight loss commonly occurs because of difficulty swallowing and loss of appetite. Frequent bouts of hiccups, another sign of esophageal cancer, may result when cancer irritates the nerves leading to the diaphragm. More advanced cancer may compress the nerves that control the vocal cords, which can lead to hoarseness.

If your doctor suspects cancer, endoscopy will be performed and a biopsy taken. Additional tests may be necessary—endoscopic ultrasound, a procedure that involves the use of high-frequency sound waves, to pinpoint the tumor thickness...and a computed tomography (CT) scan and a positron emission tomography (PET) scan to determine whether the tumor has spread to nearby lymph nodes.

TREATMENT

Surgery is the main treatment for esophageal cancer. Most often, the surgeon will perform esophagectomy, in which the cancerous part of the esophagus and nearby lymph nodes are removed, or esophagogastrectomy, in which the lower part of the esophagus and upper part of the stomach are removed. With both procedures, the remaining part of the esophagus is reconnected to the stomach, often with a segment of the large intestine.

These procedures are extremely complex and demand a high degree of surgical expertise, as well as a skilled team of nurses and other personnel to provide after-care. Choose a major cancer center that performs more than 10 esophageal cancer surgeries a year.

Chemotherapy and radiation before surgery have been shown to improve the outcome, possibly because they destroy microscopic tumor tissue before it can spread.

In one study of 802 patients, 42% of those who had two rounds of chemotherapy before surgery were still alive two years later, compared with 34% of those who had surgery alone.

New finding: A long-term clinical trial showed that esophageal cancer patients who received so-called "triple therapy"—treatment with two cancer drugs (5-fluorouracil and cisplatin) and daily radiation for five weeks before surgery—had a

39% chance of surviving for five years, compared with 16% of patients who received only surgery.

The Ideal Cancer Protection Plan

D. Barry Boyd, MD, director of the Integrative Medicine Program at Greenwich Hospital-Yale New Haven Health System, and the Boyd Center for Integrative Health, both in Greenwich, CT. He is the author of *The Cancer Recovery Plan: Maximize Your Cancer Treatment with This Proven Nutrition, Exercise and Stress-Reduction Program*. Avery.

The best surgery, chemotherapy and radiation therapy are not always enough to prevent a cancer recurrence. In an estimated four out of every 10 cancer cases, the malignancy comes back despite state-of-the-art medicine.

To maximize the effectiveness of standard cancer treatment, you need an integrative program that includes a healthful diet, emotional support and regular exercise. This type of approach may give the 9.8 million Americans who are cancer survivors the best possible chance of avoiding a recurrence—and help protect people who have never had cancer and want to do all they can to prevent it.

THE MYSTERY OF METABOLISM

Conventional oncologists usually advise patients to avoid weight loss, a significant side effect of chemotherapy and radiation. But for most people with cancer, avoiding weight gain is just as important. Research shows that excess weight increases the risk for the development and recurrence of many cancers as well as associated mortality.

What's the link between weight and cancer? Insulin resistance is one theory that is being extensively studied. Insulin, a hormone produced by the pancreas, is vital for glucose (blood sugar) metabolism—it brings this simple sugar into the cells to be broken down for energy. Trouble develops when the cells become less sensitive to insulin, usually as a result of a

person being overweight and/or underactive. The pancreas responds by producing more insulin, and higher levels of the hormone remain in the bloodstream.

Excessive insulin levels have been linked to persistent, low-grade inflammation, which releases chemicals that stimulate the growth of cells. Many experts believe that inflammation also stimulates the growth of cancer cells. Cancer and some cancer treatments, such as hormone therapy, may increase insulin resistance as a result of decreased metabolism, reduced activity levels and changes in nutritional intake.

People diagnosed with cancer, especially if they are overweight, should be tested for insulin resistance by checking levels of fasting blood sugar, insulin and lipids, and seek treatment with medication if necessary.

A CANCER-FIGHTING DIET

Weight control is one of the most important ways to help your body fight cancer and promote recovery. Unfortunately, many cancer patients seek fattening comfort food, or their doctors tell them to eat whatever they want.

The ideal cancer-fighting diet consists of 45% complex carbohydrates, 25% protein and no more than 30% fat. Strong evidence has shown that this kind of balanced diet is associated with lower rates of cancer and cancer recurrence.

The Mediterranean diet—including ample amounts of fruits and vegetables, whole-grain cereals and olive oil—is a wise choice. Small meals eaten four to six times a day also are recommended. That's because people who consume their food over the course of the day—rather than in one to three big meals—tend to take in fewer calories and stay healthier.

The same guidelines are important if your appetite is diminished by nausea caused by chemotherapy or the cancer itself. In these cases, a balanced diet is important because it helps prevent nutritional deficiencies that can result from appetite loss.

To create a cancer-fighting diet...

•**Choose the right carbs.** The amount of carbohydrates you consume isn't as critical as the kind. Sharply limit pastries, candies, beverages containing high-fructose corn syrup, such as soft drinks and some fruit-juice drinks, and refined grain products, such as white rice and bread made from white flour. The carbohydrates in these foods are broken down immediately and deposited into the bloodstream, triggering an insulin surge. With repeated exposure to insulin peaks, cells become less sensitive to the hormone.

Complex carbohydrates, such as fruits and vegetables, beans, brown rice, whole-grain cereals and whole-grain baked goods, are digested and absorbed gradually. Insulin is produced at a steady, moderate rate, fueling the body's cells with maximum efficiency. What's more, the fiber in complex carbs fills you up, so you can satisfy your hunger with fewer calories.

Eat a variety of vegetables and fruits. Specific "superfoods," such as beans and blueberries, have received a great deal of attention for their healing properties, but it's crucial to get a broad selection of healthful foods.

Fruits and vegetables should be a mainstay of your diet—the American Cancer Society recommends at least five daily servings. Nine daily servings are even better. One-half cup is the standard serving size. In addition to fiber and complex carbohydrates, fruits and vegetables contain chemicals known as phytonutrients that protect against carcinogens and enhance the body's own healing powers.

Broccoli, cauliflower and cabbage have different phytonutrients than garlic and onion. Berries, citrus fruits and leafy, green vegetables each have their own nutrients. Eating a variety of fruits and vegetables ensures that you get them all.

•**Avoid dangerous fats.** Saturated fats, found mostly in meats and high-fat dairy products, promote insulin resistance, so limit your meat intake to two servings (three ounces per serving) of lean red meat per week and consume only low-fat or nonfat dairy products (one to three servings daily). Good protein sources include poultry, fish, nuts and legumes.

Trans fat, found in many baked goods and processed foods, also causes inflammation.

Beware: Even in food products that claim "0" trans fat on the food labels, small amounts may be present and listed as "partially hydrogenated oil."

On the other hand, omega-3 fatty acids, found in cold-water fish, such as salmon, sardines and herring, have been shown to reduce inflammation and provide a range of other anticancer benefits. Other sources of omega-3s include walnuts and flaxseed.

Important: Food is the best way to get vitamins, minerals and other nutrients. High-dose supplements should be taken only under the supervision of a health-care professional who is knowledgeable about nutrition and cancer care.

BE SURE TO FIND EMOTIONAL SUPPORT

Serious illness, such as cancer, can trigger the release of stress hormones that increase your risk of developing excessive insulin levels.

My advice…

•**Get emotional support.** In a Yale study that followed more than 300 women with breast cancer for 10 years, those who felt free to talk about their illness with others were significantly more likely to survive. Don't be reluctant to ask friends and family for help in performing difficult chores and for company during doctor visits.

•**Choose a doctor who gives you hope.** Hopelessness and helplessness are the worst stressors for people with cancer. Make sure your care is directed by a medical professional who focuses on the most positive possible outcome, even if the disease is severe.

EXERCISE IS ESSENTIAL

Exercise reduces insulin resistance by building up lean, metabolically active tissue—which is better than fat tissue for cancer prevention.

In a recent study of 2,987 breast cancer patients, women who walked three to four hours a week had a 50% lower risk of dying from breast cancer than women who did little or no exercise. Researchers believe that physical activity also helps fight other types of malignancies.

For cancer prevention, strive for 30 minutes of brisk walking per day—or its equivalent in comparably strenuous activities, such as swimming or cycling.

Breakthroughs for Brain Tumor Patients

Michael Vogelbaum, MD, PhD, associate director of neurosurgical oncology and vice chairman of the Brain Tumor Institute at the Cleveland Clinic in Ohio. Dr. Vogelbaum is also director of the institute's Center for Translational Therapeutics, which conducts laboratory and clinical studies to evaluate the ability of new drugs to reach their targets in brain tumors, as well as to identify genetic factors that may predict patients' responses to treatments.

Primary brain tumors—those that originate in the brain rather than metastasizing from other parts of the body—are among the most virulent of cancers. The most common type, glioma, tends to strike otherwise healthy adults with seeming randomness and is often fatal.* An estimated 17,000 to 20,000 Americans will be diagnosed with a primary brain tumor this year.

Good news: Recent research is giving these patients reason for hope. If you or a loved one has been diagnosed with a brain tumor, here's what you need to know...

TREATMENT ADVANCES

The most aggressive of all gliomas, Glioblastoma multiforme (GBM), is also the most common, with about 10,000 to 12,000 diagnosed in the US annually, most after age 50. The median survival time for someone with GBM is about one year.

These tumors rapidly spread and infiltrate normal parts of the brain, so it's impossible to excise them completely. The traditional approach to treating GBMs has been to surgically remove as much of the tumor as possible and then administer radiation therapy. When the tumor regenerates, as GBMs often do, doctors have prescribed chemotherapy to slow the growth.

Breakthrough: In a recent trial by Canadian and European researchers, GBM patients who were given radiation therapy and the chemotherapy drug *temozolomide* (Temodar) following surgery did significantly better than those who received radiation alone. A full 26.5% of the patients who received combination therapy were living two years after their diagnoses, versus only

*Meningioma, a type of brain tumor that is usually benign, is about twice as common as glioma.

10.4% of the control group. These results were so positive that this approach is now the standard of care for all GBM patients in North America and Europe. More studies are needed to determine its long-term efficacy and safety.

On the horizon: It may soon be possible to identify which GBM tumors will respond optimally to the new protocol. In reviewing their trial data, Canadian and European researchers noticed that patients whose tumors had an inactivated gene, known as 06-methyl-guanine-DNA methyltransferase (MGMT), did markedly better on the combination therapy than those whose tumors had an active MGMT gene. The median survival among patients with inactive MGMT was nearly 22 months, and an astounding 46% of them were alive at two years. Those who had an active MGMT gene survived for a median of nearly 13 months. The gene enables cancer cells to repair themselves after being damaged by certain chemotherapy drugs, rendering the chemotherapy ineffective. We're exploring ways to safely "turn off" the gene in patients for whom it remains active.

OTHER RESEARCH ADVANCES

All cancers are in part genetic, since genes play a role in the development and progression of the disease. Genetic variations also appear to affect whether and to what extent another type of tumor, called an oligodendroglioma, will respond to chemotherapy. This slow-growing tumor is rare and typically occurs in middle-aged adults.

We've long known that an estimated two-thirds of these tumors are sensitive to chemotherapy drugs, while the remaining one-third are largely impervious. Researchers at Massachusetts General Hospital, in collaboration with Canadian colleagues, discovered in 1998 that responsive oligodendrogliomas had one thing in common—loss of parts of chromosomes (cell structures that carry genetic information), specifically chromosomes 1p and 19q. For reasons that are not yet clear, parts of these chromosomes "disappear" in some of these tumors. About 50% of patients with oligodendrogliomas lack these chromosomes. Virtually all oligodendrogliomas lacking both of these chromosomes will have a prolonged response to treatment, while those that retain them, particularly the

1p chromosome, are unlikely to have durable responses to treatment.

While patients with oligodendrogliomas are now routinely screened for loss of 1p and 19q chromosomes, doctors have yet to reach a consensus on how best to treat tumors lacking them. Some still recommend aggressive surgery to remove the bulk of the tumor, followed by radiation and chemotherapy. Others suggest starting with chemotherapy, hoping that patients may be able to avoid surgery and radiation. Both approaches are meeting with success. The median survival rate for these patients now exceeds seven years. Clinical trials are under way to study these treatment approaches.

CLINICAL TRIALS MATTER

All new therapies—surgical, radiological, pharmacological—must prove safe and effective in clinical trials before being prescribed to the general patient population.

One big challenge we face in advancing brain cancer therapies is making patients aware of the clinical trials that may benefit them personally …or lead to lifesaving treatments for future generations. For patients whose brain tumors do not respond to traditional treatment, an investigational therapy may be their best hope.

info To learn more about clinical cancer trials, or to find a trial that may be right for you or a loved one, consult the National Cancer Institute, 800-422-6237, *www.cancer.gov*, or the American Cancer Society, 800-227-2345, *www.cancer.org*.

■ ■ ■ ■

Brain Tumor Symptoms

Symptoms usually emerge over the course of a few days or weeks, and may include…

- **Seizures in patients without a history of seizures**
  - **Headaches**
  - **Personality changes**
  - **Weakness on one side of the body**
  - **Changes in speech**
  - **Changes in vision**

Some of these symptoms are associated with other serious conditions, including stroke, so it's important to report them immediately to your doctor. If he/she suspects a brain tumor, he will perform a neurological exam and may order a computed tomography (CT) or magnetic resonance imaging (MRI) scan, followed by a biopsy to confirm the diagnosis.

Best Foods for Fighting Cancer

Karen Collins, RD, a registered dietitian and nutrition adviser to the American Institute for Cancer Research (AICR) in Washington, DC. She is the author of *Planning Meals That Lower Cancer Risk,* AICR, available at many college libraries, and "Nutrition Notes" and "Nutrition-Wise," weekly columns syndicated to more than 700 newspapers nationwide. She maintains a private practice in Jamestown, NY.

Only about 10% of all cancers are caused by genetics. The remaining 90% of malignancies are related to diet, weight and exercise…smoking…and/or environmental factors.

Even though most people realize that diet can affect cancer risk, few regularly consume a variety of the foods that contain large amounts of phytochemicals, substances that actually can inhibit the cellular damage that leads to cancer.

Eating a combination of cancer-fighting foods is the best approach because no single food supplies all the available protective substances —vitamins, minerals, phytochemicals and fiber.

BLACK BEANS

Beans (legumes) have high levels of a cancer-fighting compound called phytic acid. They're also rich in fiber and saponins, chemical compounds that reduce the ability of cancer cells to proliferate.

The landmark Nurses' Health study found that women who ate four or more servings of legumes weekly were 33% less likely to develop colon polyps than those who consumed one or fewer weekly servings. In people already diagnosed with colon polyps, those who ate more beans reduced their risk for a recurrence by 45%, compared with those who ate fewer beans.

Bonus: Beans are very high in protein. They're a good substitute for people who want to reduce their consumption of red meat—a major source of saturated fat, which can increase cancer risk.

Other cancer-fighting legumes: Small red beans, red kidney beans, pinto beans and garbanzo beans.

Helpful: If you don't want to spend time cooking dried beans, you can get many of the same benefits by eating canned. To reduce the sodium in canned beans, empty them into a colander and rinse thoroughly with cold water.

Recommended: Eat one-half cup of beans at least four times weekly.

BLUEBERRIES

Berries are rich sources of vitamin C and other antioxidants. People who regularly eat berries have a lower risk for malignancies of the colon, bladder, esophagus and prostate. Berries also may lower the risk for lymphoma and premenopausal breast cancer.

Blueberries are an excellent choice for cancer prevention because they are among the richest sources of antioxidants, chemical compounds that protect cells from free radicals that can damage cell DNA—the first step in cancer.

Development: Much of this nutritional power comes from their high levels of anthocyanidins, a type of antioxidant that reduces the ability of carcinogens to damage DNA.

Bonus: Because berries are both filling and low in calories, they can be substituted for other sweet snacks to promote weight loss—which further reduces the risk for many cancers.

Other cancer-fighting berries: Blackberries, strawberries, raspberries and cranberries.

Helpful: Keep frozen berries in the freezer. They can be kept almost indefinitely without spoiling and provide virtually the same nutritional benefits as fresh berries.

Recommended: Aim for at least one half-cup serving of berries per week.

BROCCOLI

Broccoli is a cruciferous vegetable that is rich in isothiocyanates, a family of phytochemicals linked to a reduced risk for colon, prostate, lung and premenopausal breast cancer. One of these phytochemicals, sulforaphane, reduces the ability of carcinogens to cause cell damage—and

may increase the tendency of cancer cells to self-destruct, a process called apoptosis.

A study published in the *Journal of the National Cancer Institute* reports that men who consumed three or more weekly servings of broccoli (raw or cooked) were 41% less likely to get prostate cancer than those who consumed less than one weekly serving.

Other cancer-fighting cruciferous vegetables: Cauliflower, brussels sprouts, cabbage and kale.

Helpful: If you don't like the strong taste (and smell) of cooked broccoli and other cruciferous vegetables, eat them raw or lightly sauté them in olive oil or canola oil for three to four minutes.

You also can microwave or steam them. (Long cooking, such as boiling for 15 minutes or more, causes the release of strong-smelling/ tasting sulfur compounds.)

Recommended: Aim for three to five half-cup servings per week of cruciferous vegetables.

GARLIC

Garlic is an allium, which is a family of plants that contain allyl sulfides, phytochemicals not found in any other foods.

The Iowa Women's Health Study found that people with the highest intake of garlic (at least one serving weekly) had a 32% lower risk of developing colon cancer than those who never ate garlic. Garlic has also been linked to a lower risk for prostate, lung, breast and skin cancers.

Bonus: Garlic can be used as a flavor enhancer to make healthful foods—vegetables, beans, whole grains, etc.—more enjoyable… and it reduces the need for unhealthful flavorings, such as salt and butter.

Other cancer-fighting alliums: Onions (all types), leeks and chives.

Helpful: To reduce the strong taste, use cooked garlic (by sautéing or roasting it, for example) rather than raw. The flavors mellow with long cooking. Wait 10 to 15 minutes after chopping garlic before cooking, to allow the active form of the protective phytochemicals to form. The cancer-fighting properties of jarred garlic are unknown.

Recommended: Aim to eat one to three cloves of garlic per week.

WALNUTS

Walnuts provide fiber and are rich in omega-3 fatty acids, the same healthful, anti-inflammatory fats that are found in fish. Reducing inflammation in the body helps prevent cell damage that can lead to cancer.

Other cancer-fighting nuts: Almonds and hazelnuts.

Helpful: Buy packaged or bulk shelled, unsalted nuts (raw or roasted). Substituting nuts for other snacks improves the body's ratio of omega-3 to omega-6 fatty acids—important for lowering inflammation and cancer risk.

Recommended: Eat three to five one-third-cup servings weekly.

WHOLE-GRAIN BREAD

Whole-grain bread is high in fiber. As fiber and certain starches resistant to digestion are fermented in the colon, substances are produced that block the cancer-promoting effects of bile acids. In addition, whole grains are higher in antioxidant vitamins (including vitamin E) and phytochemicals, called phenols, than are refined grains.

When scientists analyzed and combined the results from 40 different studies, they found that people who ate the most whole-grain bread and/or other whole grains had a 34% lower risk for cancer overall than those who consumed less.

Other cancer-fighting whole grains: Whole-wheat pasta, whole-grain breakfast cereal, brown rice, bulgur, kasha and quinoa.

Helpful: When shopping for whole-grain bread or cereal, don't be misled by terms like multigrain, which merely means that more than one type of grain is included…and don't judge by brown color, which can result from added caramel coloring. Check the ingredients list to make sure a whole grain is listed first, such as whole wheat or whole rye. "Flour" or "wheat flour" means that the product contains refined flour made from wheat—not whole-grain flour.

Recommended: Aim for three daily servings —one-half cup of whole grains or a slice of whole-grain bread counts as one serving.

New Therapies to Fight Blood Cancer

Brian G.M. Durie, MD, a hematologist/oncologist who specializes in multiple myeloma and related disorders at Cedars-Sinai Outpatient Cancer Center at the Samuel Oschin Comprehensive Cancer Institute and national program director and senior adviser at Aptium Oncology, both in Los Angeles. He is also medical director and chairman of the board of the International Myeloma Foundation, www.myeloma.org.

One in four patients who has the blood cancer known as multiple myeloma has no major symptoms at the time of diagnosis. The disease, which usually develops after age 60, occurs when a type of white blood cell (a plasma cell) found in the bone marrow becomes abnormal, producing cells that multiply uncontrollably (myeloma cells). The result is bone erosion, anemia and other complications.

Latest development: With recently discovered drug therapies, more than 90% of patients suffering from this incurable yet treatable cancer can achieve at least a 50% reduction in the size and number of tumors—or even a complete remission, sometimes lasting for up to 10 years.

ARE YOU AT RISK?

The exact cause of multiple myeloma is unknown, but there is a small increased risk within families, and an approximately 5% occurrence rate within extended families. A combination of environmental factors, including exposure to agricultural chemicals (such as dioxins) and benzene-related chemicals (such as solvents), is believed to contribute most.

A primary symptom of multiple myeloma is a deep and persistent pain in the spine, ribs and/or hips. Although the pain initially can be intermittent, a progressive, persistent pain ultimately develops.

Important: Anyone who suffers from back or bone pain that isn't related to an injury and that lasts longer than four to six weeks needs a checkup, possibly including X-rays and/or other scans, such as computed tomography (CT). It's best to start by seeing an internist, who may refer you to an orthopedist or rheumatologist. *In addition to bone pain, symptoms include…*

•**Fatigue.** The multiplication of myeloma cells can reduce red blood cell production in bone marrow, causing anemia and weakness.

•**Fractures.** Multiple myeloma causes loss of bone density, which increases the risk for bone fractures—even from minor accidents, such as bumping into furniture.

•**Frequent infections.** Kidney and/or bladder infections often occur in multiple myeloma patients. That's because the proliferation of abnormal cells can inhibit the production of immune cells that are needed to fight infection.

DIAGNOSING MULTIPLE MYELOMA

Simple blood and urine tests that are performed during a routine physical exam can reveal signs of multiple myeloma. However, more detailed follow-up testing is required if the disease is suspected.

What the doctor looks for…

•**Elevated M proteins.** Abnormal plasma cells secrete large amounts of monoclonal *immunoglobulin* (M protein). If these proteins are present in blood (or in urine), other blood tests may be necessary.

Important: Many patients have *smoldering myeloma*—slight abnormalities that progress slowly over a period of years. They are at higher risk of progressing to multiple myeloma and need frequent monitoring, including blood tests every one to two months.

•**Anemia.** This is the most common indicator of myeloma cell buildup in bone marrow.

Other warning signs: Low white blood cell or platelet counts or elevated serum levels of *beta-2-micro-globulin* (another protein produced by myeloma cells).

If blood and urine tests point to multiple myeloma, X-rays, a CT scan or a magnetic resonance imaging (MRI) scan will be needed to check for a loss of bone density. A bone marrow biopsy can be performed to confirm the presence of myeloma cells.

BEST TREATMENT OPTIONS

When a diagnosis of multiple myeloma is established, drug treatment is required, even if the patient has no symptoms. Treatment can delay the onset of symptoms…or relieve discomfort and minimize complications once symptoms start. Treatment includes oral or intravenous drugs that eliminate myeloma cells. Other measures include radiation treatments and bone therapy with bisphosphonate drugs, such as *pamidronate* (Aredia), to improve bone healing and strength. *Main drug therapies…*

•**Thalidomide/dexamethasone.** Thalidomide, used to treat morning sickness in the 1950s, was withdrawn from the market when it was found to cause severe birth defects. It's recently been found to be extremely effective for multiple myeloma—and very safe as long as it's not taken by pregnant women.

When combined with the steroid dexamethasone, thalidomide inhibits the growth and spread of myeloma cells—and doesn't cause the side effects of chemotherapy. About 70% of patients who take this drug combination improve significantly, and about 35% have excellent results or even a remission.

•**Velcade/Revlimid.** Both are new drugs developed for multiple myeloma—particularly for resistant forms that don't respond to other treatments. Like thalidomide, they're combined with dexamethasone, but they have a higher success rate…and are better tolerated than older chemotherapy drugs.

•**High-dose chemotherapy/stem-cell transplant.** Until new drugs were discovered in the late 1990s, this was considered one of the best treatments—and it still is the standard of care following initial therapy with other drugs.

How it works: Patients take drugs for three to six months to achieve a partial remission. Injections are given to stimulate the release of immature blood cells (stem cells) from the bone marrow into the blood, and the stem cells are then "harvested." Next, patients take very high doses of a chemotherapy drug to wipe out the myeloma cells remaining in the bone marrow. The original stem cells are then reintroduced intravenously to replace the damaged bone marrow.

About half of patients who receive high-dose chemotherapy and stem-cell transplant can achieve a remission, and most have a significant reduction in symptoms.

■ ■ ■ ■

A Persistent Itch May Be A Sign of Skin Cancer

Any skin irritation that persists for weeks may be early-stage skin cancer, especially if it increases in size, changes color or bleeds. See a dermatologist—he/she usually can tell quickly whether an irritation is benign or cancerous.

Perry Robins, MD, dermatologist and professor of dermatology at New York University Medical Center, New York City, and president of The Skin Cancer Foundation.

Natural Ways to Fight Side Effects of Cancer Treatment

Dr. Mark Stengler is a licensed naturopathic medical doctor and a leading authority on the practice of alternative and integrated medicine. An associate clinical professor at the National College of Naturopathic Medicine in Portland, OR, Dr. Stengler has served on a medical advisory committee for the Yale University Complementary Medicine Outcomes Research Project and is the author or coauthor of 16 books, including two best sellers—*The Natural Physician's Healing Therapies* and *Prescription for Natural Cures*. Dr. Stengler is the founder and director of the La Jolla Whole Health Clinic in La Jolla, CA. *www.DrStengler.com.*

The American Cancer Society estimates that over 1.4 million Americans will be diagnosed with some form of cancer in 2007. The vast majority will choose to be treated with conventional therapies, such as chemotherapy, radiation, surgery or a combination. I often advise patients who are undergoing these treatments and want to reduce their risk of side effects and optimize their outcome. It is gratifying to help these people who are in physical and emotional turmoil. An example is Yolanda, a 62-year-old woman who was diagnosed with a form of lymphoma (cancer of the lymphatic system). A program of nutrition and dietary supplements gave her more energy, promoted bowel regularity and boosted her immunity. Her oncologist was quite surprised with how well she tolerated her chemo treatments and remarked on her quick recovery.

UNDERSTANDING CHEMOTHERAPY AND RADIATION

Chemotherapy involves the use of one or more drugs to destroy cancer cells. The treatments are given intravenously (IV) through a vein, orally or by injection into a muscle. These medications not only attack cancer cells but also harm healthy cells. This causes a variety of side effects, depending on the chemotherapeutic agents being used and the individual's response.

Examples of short-term side effects include loss of appetite, memory impairment, constipation, diarrhea, hair loss, nausea, mouth sores, easy bruising, fluid retention and pain in muscles, bones, nerves and joints. It also can result in bone marrow suppression, which can lower white and red blood cell counts, causing fatigue and increasing a patient's susceptibility to infection. Long-term side effects can include infertility, chronic fatigue and continued bone marrow suppression. In addition, chemotherapy can result in secondary cancers—for example, a breast cancer patient might develop acute leukemia.

Radiation therapy also kills cancer cells and shrinks tumors. It is mainly used to attack localized cancers as opposed to cancer that has spread. Radiation treatments can be administered externally by a machine, internally through radioactive material placed in the body near cancer cells or via radioactive substances that are injected and circulate throughout the body. Side effects can be similar to those caused by chemotherapy, but symptoms such as redness, swelling and a burning sensation often are specific to the region being treated. Burned or reddened skin also can develop at the treated area.

SUPPLEMENTS THAT HELP

The following supplements are recommended for people undergoing chemotherapy or radiation therapy. You can take all of them at once —with the exception of the mushrooms listed, which are typically taken one at a time, as directed. Always consult with your oncologist before taking any supplement. Supplements work best in conjunction with a healthful diet and lifestyle.

71

DETOXIFICATION THERAPIES

Toxic by-products are formed by cancer treatments. You can help eliminate these toxins from your body by supporting liver and kidney detoxification.

•**Milk thistle** is an excellent herb that supports liver detoxification and protects against liver and kidney cell damage. Studies show that it actually helps liver cells regenerate. I recommend a 175-mg to 250-mg capsule of standardized extract (70% to 85% silymarin) taken three times daily. It can also be taken in liquid form. An excellent product is Thisilyn by Nature's Way, available in capsule form at most health-food stores, or you can contact the manufacturer to find a retailer (800-962-8873, *www.naturesway. com*).

•**Chlorella, spirulina, wheatgrass** and other "super greens" are nature's great detoxifiers. You can take chlorella by itself—it contains chlorophyll and a host of other detoxifying nutrients. A good choice, SunChlorella A, is available at health-food stores or from Sun Chlorella USA (800-829-2828, *www.sunchlorellausa.com*). Follow label instructions. KyoGreen Energy by Kyolic is a good formula that contains a mixture of greens. It is available in tablet or powder form. To locate a store or mail-order company, contact Wakunaga (800-421-2998, *www.kyolic. com*).

BOOSTING IMMUNITY

Because cancer treatments, especially chemotherapy, have a suppressive effect on the immune system—which makes you more vulnerable to infection—immunity boosting is critical. The following natural therapies can be used to support normal immune function without interfering with treatment.

•**Coriolus versicolor mushroom extract** is routinely used in Japan and China to support the immune function of people with cancer. It also is helpful in reducing the side effects of chemotherapy and radiation.

A study published in *The Lancet* examined the effects of coriolus on patients undergoing chemotherapy after surgical removal of stomach cancer. The 262 patients were randomly assigned chemotherapy alone or with coriolus extract. The survival rate of the group using the combination was 73% after five years, while the chemotherapy-only group had a survival rate of 60%. Researchers concluded that coriolus had "a restorative effect in patients who had been immunosuppressed by both recent surgery and subsequent chemotherapy." The recommended dose is 2,000 mg to 3,000 mg daily. The Mushroom Science brand of coriolus duplicates the formula that was used in the study and is available at health-food stores or by contacting Mushroom Science (888-283-6583, *www.mush roomscience.com*).

•**Maitake mushroom extract** is one of the most-studied mushroom extracts. Since the 1980s, Hiroaki Nanba, MD, a professor of microbiology at Kobe Pharmaceutical University, Kobe, Japan, has been researching maitake extract. It has been shown to enhance the activity of the body's natural killer cells against cancer cells. In addition, maitake extract has been shown to reduce the side effects of chemotherapy. A survey of 671 patients showed that the use of maitake during chemo reduced adverse effects such as hair loss, pain and nausea. Maitake Gold 404 is the form recommended by Dr. Nanba. Typical dosage is 1 mg per two pounds of body weight daily. It is available in capsule or liquid form at health-food stores. For a store locator, consult Natural Factors (800-322-8704, *www.natural factors.com*). Or you can buy Cellular Essentials NK-5 from Swanson Health Products (800-824-4491, *www.swansonvitamins.com*)—it contains Maitake Gold 404.

Note: Choose either coriolus or maitake based on the type of cancer being treated. Coriolus is a good general choice, especially for people with cancers of the throat, lungs and digestive tract. Maitake is better studied for cancers of the breast, prostate and liver.

•**Curcumin** is the yellow pigment found in turmeric, a prime ingredient in curry. It has been shown to have anticancer properties and to enhance the effectiveness of some chemotherapy drugs, such as *cisplatin* (Platinol). It has no known side effects. The recommended supplement dose is 400 mg twice daily. Many brands are available at health-food stores.

•**Whey protein,** derived from cow's milk, supplies all the essential amino acids the body needs for repair, including the amino acid *glutamine*, which prevents mouth sores and strengthens immunity. Take 20 g of whey protein powder twice daily, in water or a shake.

DIGESTIVE HELP

Digestive function often is compromised by cancer treatments, particularly chemotherapy and radiation for cancers in the abdominal area. These treatments destroy "friendly" bacteria, which are important for digestion, detoxification and immune function.

•**Probiotics** contain beneficial bacteria, such as *Lactobacillus acidophilus* and *Lactobacillus bifidus*. Take a daily dose of 10 billion or more active organisms. Good products include DDS Plus by UAS Laboratories (800-422-3371, *www. uaslabs.com*) and Bio-K Plus by Bio-K Plus International (for a store locator, go to *www.biok plus.com* or call 800-593-BIOK).

•**Ginger** helps relieve indigestion, nausea, bloating and diarrhea. Sip ginger tea throughout the day, or take two 300-mg capsules twice daily.

•**Homeopathic Nux vomica,** derived from the poison nut tree, combats nausea and constipation. Take two pellets of a 30C potency twice daily until symptoms subside, usually within two to three days.

Childhood Cancer Survivors Face Higher Sarcoma Risk

Tara O. Henderson, MD, department of pediatrics, section of Hematology-Oncology, University of Chicago Pritzker School of Medicine, Chicago.

Kevin Oeffinger, MD, director, Program for Adult Survivors of Pediatric Cancer, Memorial Sloan-Kettering Cancer Center, New York City.

Journal of the National Cancer Institute.

S urvivors of pediatric cancer face nine times the normal risk for developing sarcoma—a cancer of the connective or supportive tissue—at least five years after treatment for the initial cancer, a new study reveals.

The risk for developing sarcoma is particularly elevated among patients with a family history of cancer or whose primary childhood bout was a form of sarcoma, a bone tumor or Hodgkin's lymphoma, the researchers found. The use of radiation and certain kinds of chemotherapy drugs was also associated with higher sarcoma risk.

"This study is a red flag," said lead author Dr. Tara O. Henderson, of the department of pediatrics within the hematology-oncology section at the University of Chicago's Pritzker School of Medicine. "And it shows that, if a patient with a history of childhood cancer later presents with a lump and a bump anywhere on their body, you need to be more suspicious of sarcoma than you would be for someone in the general population."

According to the American Cancer Society, more than three-quarters of all pediatric cancer patients now survive five years or more.

The authors note that previous research has shown that among such survivors, a secondary cancer of some kind is the leading cause of death. Sarcoma is known as a particularly stealthy though rare threat, whose nonspecific symptoms make it difficult to diagnose.

THE STUDY

Henderson and her team analyzed data on more than 14,000 American and Canadian patients participating in the Childhood Cancer Survivor Study—the largest ongoing analysis of pediatric cancer patients conducted to date.

All the patients in the study were under the age of 21 when they were diagnosed with cancer between 1970 and 1986. All lived at least five years past their initial diagnosis of leukemia, Hodgkin's lymphoma, non-Hodgkin's lymphoma, neuroblastoma, sarcoma, kidney or bone cancer, or cancer of the central nervous system.

RESULTS

Henderson and her colleagues found that 751 secondary cancers developed among the study participants, of which 108 were sarcomas affecting 104 patients. Such sarcomas were diagnosed an average of 11 years after the pediatric cancer diagnosis.

Secondary sarcomas, new cancers that start after primary cancer has been treated, were determined to be the ultimate cause of death for more than one-third of the 104 secondary sarcoma patients.

The sarcoma patients were also found to be more likely to have received radiation for their pediatric cancer; have received higher doses of two chemotherapy drugs (anthracyclines or alkylating agents); have a family history of cancer or a history of other secondary cancers themselves; or have battled particular types of pediatric cancer, including sarcoma.

The authors noted that a history of cancer among first-degree relatives was found in 22% of the sarcoma patients. They also pointed out that patients who were particularly young when first diagnosed with childhood cancer—those under the age of 4—appeared to have the highest risk of developing sarcoma later.

Nearly 80% of the 104 sarcoma patients had received radiation, although researchers could only confirm that 56% of them had radiation targeting the area where secondary sarcoma ultimately developed.

Even those pediatric cancer patients who had never received radiation were still found to have a higher risk for developing sarcoma than the general population.

THEORIES

Henderson suggested that a constellation of factors is probably increasing sarcoma risk among childhood cancer survivors.

"While we confirmed that radiation is a risk and chemo might be as well, it also might be true that these particular patients carry some element of cancer susceptibility and predisposition that we don't understand yet," she said. "Figuring this out is the next phase of research we need to get into."

Henderson stressed that the findings are not cause for undue alarm, as sarcoma remains a relatively rare cancer—even for those at higher risk.

That point was echoed by Dr. Kevin Oeffinger, director of the Program for Adult Survivors of Pediatric Cancer at Memorial Sloan-Kettering Cancer Center in New York City.

"And while radiation was the treatment exposure associated with the highest risk, you have to remember that the majority of people who do have radiation as children will never have a second cancer," Oeffinger added. "And that dose of radiation is often a lifesaving part of that therapy. Clearly, if we're not able to cure the first cancer, then talking about a second cancer is without meaning."

RECOMMENDATIONS

Oeffinger, nevertheless, cautioned that pediatric cancer patients should be diligent about follow-up care.

He noted that his own research, conducted among the same pool of patients, revealed that two of three such survivors will ultimately develop at least one chronic and sometimes life-threatening health problem 20 to 30 years after the cancer diagnosis.

"So, the take-home message is not to be overly concerned at this point, but to know that long-term follow-up care—with a health-care professional that is familiar with their long-term risks—is essential to all pediatric cancer survivors," Oeffinger said.

info For more information on the long-term effects of pediatric cancer treatment, visit the Web site of the American Cancer Society at *www.cancer.org/cancertopics/coping/childhood-cancer-survivor-study.*

Lowdown on the New Cervical Cancer Vaccine

Eileen Dunne, MD, MPH, medical epidemiologist; Lauri Markowitz, MD, medical epidemiologist and director, HPV Vaccine Working Group; and Curtis Allen, spokesman, all with the Centers for Disease Control and Prevention, Atlanta.
Jennifer Wu, MD, obstetrician/gynecologist, Lenox Hill Hospital, New York City.
Susan Weller, PhD, professor, family medicine, University of Texas Medical Branch, Galveston
Journal of the American Medical Association.

The first survey of a broad age range of women finds that more than 25% are infected with the human papillomavirus (HPV), thought to be the cause of most cases of cervical cancer. Experts at the Centers for

Disease Control and Prevention (CDC), which conducted the study, said the numbers support the vaccination of young girls and college-age women with the newly approved HPV vaccine, Gardasil.

The CDC currently recommends that the vaccine be routinely given to girls 11 and 12 years of age to help prevent infection with the sexually transmitted virus. The Advisory Committee on Immunization Practices, a committee of 15 national experts that provides guidance to the CDC, also recommends Gardasil for use in girls beginning at age nine—at the provider's discretion —and in young women up to the age of 26.

The new statistics on prevalence won't change those recommendations, the study's authors said.

"It's important for people to know that this is a highly prevalent infection, that sexually active women are likely to acquire this infection, and that it is important to have regular cervical cancer screenings at this point as currently recommended. There are also [CDC] recommendations for using the HPV vaccine to prevent certain types of HPV," said study lead author Dr. Eileen Dunne, a medical epidemiologist with the CDC.

THE STUDY

Her team's survey of more than 2,000 American women ages 14 to 59 found that 26.8% of the women tested positive for the presence of HPV in the vaginal tract—equivalent to almost 25 million women.

HPV prevalence rose during adolescence and peaked among college-age women (20 to 24 years of age), with almost half (44.8%) of women in this age group testing positive for the virus.

Overall, the rate of infection for females ages 14 to 24 was 33.8%, or about 7.5 million young women. That rate is substantially higher than previous estimates of about 4.6 million HPV infections in this age group, the researchers noted.

Rates dropped off gradually as women got older, the study found.

IMPLICATIONS

Because the body's immune system usually clears HPV from the body within six months, the study results do not reflect a woman's lifetime risk of ever acquiring the virus, the researchers stressed.

"People acquire these infections and then clear them," explained the study's senior author, Dr. Lauri Markowitz, another CDC medical epidemiologist who is director of the agency's HPV Vaccine Working Group.

In other words, a woman might pick up one strain of HPV through sexual contact in her teen years, then eliminate it, only to catch another strain later in life.

"So, this study was just a cross-section [of prevalence] at a point in time," Markowitz explained. "It doesn't explain your lifetime risk."

The study also found that 3.4% of women ages 14 to 59 were infected with one of the four HPV strains covered by the Gardasil vaccine —strains 6, 11, 16 and 18. Strains 16 and 18 are suspected of being especially "oncogenic" (cancer-causing), experts say.

While 3.4% may not seem like a large number, Markowitz again stressed that this figure is reflective of a "point in time" and does not demonstrate a woman's lifetime risk of picking up these particularly dangerous strains. "So, this doesn't change our thinking about our [vaccine] recommendations," she said. "It substantiates the evidence that is already out there."

EXPERT REACTION

Another expert agreed that the new statistics support the widespread vaccination of young girls against HPV. However, efforts to do so have met with opposition from conservative groups and some parents, who worry that vaccination might encourage premarital sexual activity.

"That's more of a political question, of course," said Dr. Jennifer Wu, an obstetrician/gynecologist at Lenox Hill Hospital in New York City. "One thing that we do need to think about, however, is that we already vaccinate [girls] against hepatitis B—it's a universal vaccine for children. And hepatitis B is also a sexually transmitted disease."

VACCINE SIDE EFFECTS

The CDC has received reports of side effects to Gardasil, however, "those side effects have been relatively mild and within the expected range," said CDC spokesman Curtis Allen. Most involved events such as transient dizziness, injection-site swelling, fainting, fever or nausea —common to many injections, Allen said.

And, while there were a few cases of a rare, dangerous condition called Guillain-Barre syndrome, the incidence was similar to that seen in unvaccinated girls. "So, there doesn't seem to be anything that would cause alarm," Allen said.

Wu agreed. "At this point in time, we still think the benefits [of vaccination] outweigh the risks," she said. "We think that with widespread immunization, we could essentially eliminate cervical cancer."

DETECTING CERVICAL CANCER

In the meantime, another expert said it remains important that women of all ages get a regular Pap smear to check for the early signs of cervical cancer—even if they receive the Gardasil vaccine.

Women who are vaccinated for HPV would still need to get Pap smears according to regular clinical guidelines, since there are still some types of HPV not covered by the vaccine that cause cancer, explained Dr. Susan Weller, a professor of family medicine at the University of Texas Medical Branch, Galveston.

According to the American Cancer Society, more than 11,150 new cases of invasive cervical cancer will be diagnosed in US women this year, and about 3,670 women will die of the disease.

Myeloma Drug Works Better at Lower Dose

Len Lichtenfeld, MD, deputy chief medical officer, American Cancer Society, Atlanta.

Howard Streicher, MD, senior investigator, National Cancer Institute, Bethesda, MD.

Proving that less really can be more, government researchers say that a lower dose of chemotherapy raises the survival of patients with the blood cancer multiple myeloma.

In fact, one-year survival rose so dramatically —from 86% to 96%—for patients receiving a lower dose of the steroid *dexamethasone* in a National Cancer Institute (NCI) clinical trial

that the study was prematurely halted so all participants could reap the potential benefit of the lower dose.

Patients were receiving the lower-dose steroid alongside another cancer-fighting drug, *lenalidomide* (Revlimid). Lenalidomide is a newly developed chemical cousin of thalidomide, said Streicher, a senior investigator at the NCI.

"This treatment reduces the risk of side effects and, at the same time, it is more effective, demonstrating that more is not always better," said Dr. Len Lichtenfeld, deputy chief medical officer with the American Cancer Society. He was not involved with the study.

The disease, a malignancy of plasma cells residing in the bone marrow and bloodstream, is diagnosed in almost 20,000 Americans each year, according to the NCI.

BACKGROUND

Beginning in the mid-1990s, scientists began to realize that the drug *thalidomide* might help fight myeloma, primarily through its effect in shrinking the cancer's blood supply.

According to study coresearcher Dr. Howard Streicher, drugs such as thalidomide may also inhibit myeloma by interfering with key signaling molecules called *cytokines*, or by boosting immune responses.

Thalidomide has a checkered past, however, most notably as the cause of devastating birth defects.

"It doesn't seem to cause the same kind of birth defects, it doesn't have the sedative quality, and it is probably more potent and active than thalidomide in myeloma," said Streicher.

Doctors have also long used *dexamethasone* (Decadron) to fight myeloma, because the drug appears to induce cancer cell death.

But dexamethasone has its drawbacks, too— most notably an increase in the risk for *deep vein thrombosis* (DVT) and pulmonary embolisms, potentially life-threatening blood clots.

NEW STUDY

The new trial attempted to see if a lower dose of dexamethasone would work just as well as the higher dose, when combined with the same dose of lenalidomide.

In the trial, Streicher and his colleagues compared survival and toxicity levels in 445 patients with newly diagnosed multiple my-eloma. None of the patients had been on any other form of chemotherapy prior to the trial, which was scheduled to run for two years. Patients were randomly chosen to receive either low- or high-dose dexamethasone treatment plus lenalidomide.

POSITIVE RESULTS

The one-year results have been a pleasant surprise, Streicher said.

"The response rates in terms of survival were very high in both arms, and it was even higher with a lower dose of dexamethasone," he said. "It was higher than anything that we had hoped for."

He said it's unclear why lowering the dose of dexamethasone improved survival, although reduced toxicities probably played a big role. Rates for most side effects—especially danger-ous clotting—associated with the steroid de-creased as the dose got lower, Streicher noted.

PROMISING ACTION

In fact, the results have been so positive that (the study's review board) stopped the trial early so that they would not deny the patients in this trial—and patients in general—to be treated in the safer, more effective way, Lichtenfeld ex-plained. "That's usually a very, very positive in-dicator of a successful trial," Lichtenfeld said.

CAUTIOUS OPTIMISM

Streicher stressed that the findings remain preliminary, however.

"We don't know what it will look like at two years," he said. "It's possible that we'll find out that the benefits continue for a long time, or that some-thing else needs to be done somewhere down the line if patients relapse. Those are important questions that still need to be answered."

Lichtenfeld called the trial's success "all part of the targeted therapy story," which he said is revolutionizing cancer care.

FUNDING NEEDED

But he also warned that current funding shortfalls at public health institutions such as the NCI—which support and organize many of these types of clinical trials—threaten these types of advances.

"We are understanding myeloma better and we are able to apply these drugs," Lichtenfeld said. "But if we do not continue to support these types of activities, we stand a chance of losing our progress."

Tests Show Measles Kill Bone Marrow Cancer

Mayo Clinic news release.

Researchers are launching a Phase I clini-cal trial to test an engineered measles virus against the bone marrow cancer multiple myeloma.

THE STUDY

In this trial, conducted at the Mayo Clinic Cancer Center in Rochester, Minnesota, a spe-cifically genetically engineered measles vaccine will be administered intravenously to adults with relapsed or refractory (meaning patients have failed more than one type of treatment) myeloma. The participants must not have had allogenic (from another person) stem cell trans-plants and must have previously had the measles or been vaccinated against it.

This is the third in a series of Mayo studies testing the potential of measles to kill cancer. The other two studies are looking at the effect of measles on recurrent ovarian cancer and a type of brain tumor called glioblastoma multiforme.

The measles viruses used in the research were engineered by inserting additional genes into the measles vaccine strain. The measles vi-ruses seek out a protein called CD46—which is overexpressed by many cancers—and use it as a receptor to enter the cancer cells.

Once inside the cancer cell, the measles vi-rus spreads and infects nearby tumor cells. This causes tumor cells to fuse together, increasing cancer cell death.

Kitchen Counter Cancer "Cures"

Neal Freedman, PhD, cancer prevention fellow, National Cancer Institute, Bethesda, MD.

Tara Miller, MS, RD, program manager, Center for Corporate Wellness, New York University Medical Center, New York City.

Melanie Polk, RD, nutrition and education adviser, American Institute for Cancer Research, Rockville, MD.

American Association for Cancer Research.

If you want to reduce your risk of several common types of cancer, help may be no farther away than your kitchen. A trio of new studies found that vegetables and fruits help lower your chances of getting head and neck, breast, ovarian and pancreatic cancers.

One of the studies found that just one additional serving of vegetables or fruits could help lower the risk of head and neck cancer. Still, the more fruits and vegetables you can consume, the better.

"Those who ate six servings of fruit and vegetables per 1,000 calories had a 29% decreased risk relative to those who had 1.5 servings," said Dr. Neal Freedman, a Cancer Prevention Fellow in the division of Cancer Prevention at the National Cancer Institute and author of one of the studies.

THE FIRST STUDY

Freedman analyzed the fruit and vegetable intake and the incidence of head and neck cancers in 490,802 adults. During the five-year study period, 787 people were diagnosed with head and neck cancers.

After accounting for smoking and alcohol use —known head and neck cancer risk factors— the researchers found that those who consumed the most fruits and vegetables had the lowest risk for head and neck cancers. Vegetables appeared to offer more cancer prevention than fruits alone did.

Adding just one serving of fruit or vegetables per each 1,000 calories consumed daily resulted in a 6% reduction of risk, Freedman said.

"Quitting smoking and reducing alcohol use protects against head and neck cancer. Our results suggest that increasing consumption of fruits and vegetables may also contribute to reduced head and neck cancer risk, and add

support to current dietary recommendations to increase fruit and vegetable consumption," Freedman noted.

"I think Americans fall pretty short of the recommendations [for fruit and vegetable consumption]," said Tara Miller, program manager for the Center for Corporate Wellness at New York University Medical Center in New York City. "So, it's good news that only an extra serving a day could make a difference."

THE SECOND STUDY

Researchers at the University of California, Los Angeles, conducted lab experiments to determine if broccoli and soy protein offered any protection against aggressive breast and ovarian cancers.

Digesting broccoli and soy together forms a compound called *diindolylmethane* (DIM). In the lab experiments, the researchers found that DIM could affect the motility of breast and ovarian cancer cells, which could help keep cancers from spreading.

Miller said one concern about soy is that it may be a problem for people with estrogen-fueled cancers, because soy acts like estrogen in the body. She said soy is a nutritious, healthy food, but she recommends eating it in moderation.

THE THIRD STUDY

The third study looked at the diets of 183,518 people from California and Hawaii, and compared their intake of flavonols to their risk for pancreatic cancer. Flavonols are protective compounds found in fruits and vegetables, such as onions, apples, berries, kale and broccoli.

Those who had the highest consumption of flavonols reduced their risk of pancreatic cancer by 23%, scientists from the Cancer Research Center of Hawaii found. The benefit was even greater for people who smoked. Smokers with high levels of flavonols reduced their risk for pancreatic cancer by 59%.

RECOMMENDATIONS

"These studies give lots more ammo to what we've been saying—eating a large variety of plant-based foods is one of the best things you can do for your health in terms of cancer prevention," said Melanie Polk, the nutrition education adviser for the American Institute for Cancer Research.

"If you're eating three or four servings daily, don't think that eating one or two additional servings won't make a difference, though working toward a goal of five to nine servings a day makes sense," Polk said.

She suggested visiting farmers' markets or even taking more time to explore the options available in your local grocery store. Additionally, Polk said you should try to find new recipes for vegetables. "There are lots of ways to fix them that really taste good," she said. "Don't just settle for a boiled pot of kale."

Better Prostate Cancer Test May Mean Fewer Biopsies

Robert H. Getzenberg, MD, professor, urology, Johns Hopkins University, Baltimore.
Durado Brooks, MD, director, prostate and colorectal cancers, American Cancer Society, Atlanta.
Dr. Robert H. Getzenberg, professor of urology and director of research at Johns Hopkins University's James Buchanan Brady Urological Institute.
Urology.

A test that focuses on a blood protein produced by prostate cancer cells may improve disease diagnosis, researchers report. Levels of this protein, called prostate cancer antigen-2 (EPCA-2), appear to give an accurate picture of cancer present in the body, experts say.

"We've been able to show that blood levels of it are low in normal individuals and high in prostate cancer, and that it distinguishes between cancers that are confined to the prostate and those that have spread outside the gland," explained study lead researcher Dr. Robert H. Getzenberg, professor of urology and director of research at Johns Hopkins University's James Buchanan Brady Urological Institute, in Baltimore.

Prostate cancer is the most common malignancy in American men. There will be some 218,890 new cases in the US this year and 27,050 deaths linked to the disease, the American Cancer Society estimates. Prostate cancer is highly curable if caught early, however.

THE STUDY

In the new study, Getzenberg's team measured blood levels of EPCA-2 in 330 men. Some of the men had an enlarged but noncancerous prostate gland, some had prostate cancer but displayed normal PSA levels, some had prostate cancer that had spread beyond the gland, and some had other cancers or medical conditions.

A specific level of ECPA-2 identified 90% of the men with cancer confined to the prostate and 98% of those in whom it had spread outside the gland. The test was negative in 97% of the men without prostate cancer, the researchers said.

That's an improvement on the standard PSA test, which provides only a rough guide in many such cases. For example, a high blood level of PSA can sometimes indicate prostate cancer, but often a biopsy reveals no such malignancy.

Conversely, a low PSA level does not necessarily mean that a man is free of prostate cancer, the researchers said.

IMPLICATIONS

"If this test works out, we can avoid a lot of unnecessary biopsies," Getzenberg said. About 1.3 million men in the US will have biopsies this year to find only 200,000 cancers, he noted.

"Clearly, we need further validation," Getzenberg added. "We are doing good-sized validation studies, and we are also testing the ability of the marker to identify aggressive forms of the disease."

Spotting especially life-threatening prostate tumors is "the holy grail" of diagnosis, he said. Current PSA testing cannot distinguish between cancers that will grow so slowly that they pose no danger to life and those that require quick action. The hope is that the ECPA-2 test will identify men whose slow-growing cancers make them candidates for "watchful waiting" rather than immediate surgery or other treatment.

The Hopkins team, working with researchers from the University of Pittsburgh, has licensed the test to a company, Onconome Inc. The ECPA-2 screen is a simple antibody test requiring "no special kind of technology or equipment," Getzenberg noted.

"In general, it does look very promising," Dr. Durado Brooks, director of prostate and colorectal cancers at the American Cancer Society, said of the ECPA-2 test. But much more work must be done, he added.

Brooks said the test seems to be sensitive and accurate for locating prostate cancer. "The challenge is taking it out of this isolated and rigorous setting and seeing how it performs in other laboratories and also in much larger screening-type populations," said Brooks.

info For more information on prostate cancer, go to the Prostate Cancer Foundation Web site at *www.prostatecancerfoundation.com*.

Hormone Therapy for Advanced Prostate Cancer Not for Everyone

Andrew Loblaw, MD, radiation oncologist, Toronto-Sunnybrook Regional Cancer Center, Toronto, Canada.

Howard I. Scher, MD, chief, genitourinary oncology, Memorial Sloan-Kettering Cancer Center, New York City.

Journal of Clinical Oncology.

For men with advanced prostate cancer, starting hormone therapy quickly comes with benefits and risks that may—in some cases—cancel each other out, according to new guidelines issued by the American Society of Clinical Oncology.

WEIGHING THE RISKS

"The message is that immediate use of hormones does reduce the risk of dying of prostate cancer by about 17%," explained the guidelines' lead author, Dr. Andrew Loblaw, a radiation oncologist at Toronto-Sunnybrook Regional Cancer Center in Canada. "But also, early use of hormone therapy increased the risk of dying of something else by about 15%, so there is no survival advantage. This is something that men and their physicians need to discuss," he said.

The guidelines are aimed at about 100,000 of the roughly 250,000 men with prostate cancer in the United States and Canada, Loblaw said. Specifically, they apply to men whose cancer comes back after treatment, those whose cancer progresses after a period of "watchful waiting,"

and those whose cancer has spread beyond the prostate when they are first diagnosed.

OPTIONS

Hormone therapy is standard treatment for those men, since male hormones (mainly testosterone) drive the progression of prostate cancer. Treatment can be in the form of anti-androgens —drugs that block the body's ability to use testosterone and other male sex hormones—or drugs called luteinizing-hormone-releasing hormones (LHRH), which eliminate testosterone from the blood stream. A third treatment, surgical removal of one or both testicles, is another possibility.

Guidelines issued two years ago by ASCO sidestepped the issue of when hormone therapy should be started for these men, because "there was not sufficient evidence to allow us to make a meaningful comment," Loblaw said. However, "there have been two important studies since 2004 that allow us to make a comment on the issue," he said.

The update recommends either surgery or LHRH as initial treatment, with combined androgen blockage that adds nonsteroidal anti-inflammatory drugs (NSAIDs) to be considered in cases where the cancer has advanced or spread outside the prostate.

The new guidelines retain the 2004 statement that there is not enough data to recommend use of intermittent androgen blockage, in which hormone therapy is stopped from time to time, for these men.

THE QUESTION STILL LINGERS

Debate continues among oncologists as to the use of early hormone therapy for prostate cancer, Loblaw said.

"Doctors should discuss with patients the risks and benefits of early androgen deprivation therapy vs. deferred therapy," he said. "If the patient prefers to defer therapy, he should have regular visits with his doctor every three to six months to monitor the disease."

The report marks a shift in thinking about prostate cancer treatment, said Dr. Howard I. Scher, chief of genitourinary oncology at Memorial Sloan-Kettering Cancer Center in New York, another author of the guidelines.

"What this is starting to show is that there are patients in whom hormonal therapy can be used more appropriately, depending on their cancer risk," Scher said. "There is a subset of patients we can identify who need aggressive treatment early. We used to give hormone therapy to everybody. We don't have to do that anymore."

It is important for both patients and doctors to understand "why hormones are being given and what they are expected to do," Scher said. "We have to understand the position of each individual patient. There has to be more negotiation, if you will."

info To learn more about prostate cancer treatment options, visit *familydoctor.org* and search "prostate cancer treatment."

New Research Proves Prostate Surgery Okay for Older Men

Shabbir M.H. Alibhai, MD, assistant professor, departments of health policy management and evaluation, University of Toronto, and scientist, University Health Network and the Toronto Rehabilitation Institute, Ontario, Canada.

Warren A. Jones, MD, distinguished professor, health policy, and professor, family medicine, University of Mississippi, Jackson.

Journal of the National Cancer Institute.

Surgery for prostate cancer can be safe and worthwhile for older men above the traditional cutoff age of 70. That's the conclusion of emerging research that calls into question the traditional view that men should be denied the surgery based on advanced age alone.

Dr. Shabbir M.H. Alibhai, a scientist at University Health Network and the Toronto Rehabilitation Institute in Canada, published a study evaluating the effect of radical prostatectomy—removal of the prostate gland—among more than 11,000 men in Ontario.

The finding: In otherwise healthy older men up to age 79, the risk of death after this surgery is relatively low.

RETHINKING OLD GUIDELINES

Alibhai thinks the study, because it was carefully done and included a large sample size, is beginning to change medical practice.

"We are finding surgeons are less cautious in thinking about this surgery for men over age 70," said Alibhai. "People are being a little bit more scientific about this thing, [saying], 'Let's look at the aggressiveness of the cancer and how healthy the man is.'"

The prostate gland, about the size of a walnut and located just below the bladder and in front of the rectum, helps produce seminal fluid. More than 234,000 men in the United States will learn they have prostate cancer this year, and more than 27,000 will die from the disease. Annual exams should begin at age 50—or earlier for men at high risk, according to the American Cancer Society.

Traditionally, Alibhai said, many surgeons would make their decision to remove the prostate based on age alone, suggesting to men over 70 that they undergo radiation or hormone treatment, instead.

Alibhai hopes his research spurs men to act as their own advocate. He believes many men are now justified to say to their surgeon, "Just because I am over 70 does not mean I am going to have horrible complications."

THE STUDY

For the study, Alibhai and his coresearchers looked at the death and complication rates in 11,010 men who had prostate surgery between 1990 and 1999. The researchers looked at the first 30 days after the procedure.

"Although on a relative level there was an increase in the risk of mortality with each decade of age, the absolute risk was still quite low in older men," Alibhai said.

Overall, 53 men died, and 2,246 had one or more complications within 30 days of surgery. Other factors that increased the risk of 30-day mortality were previous heart disease or stroke, Alibhai said. "If you had either or both those risks, you were at a significantly higher risk of having 30-day mortality than if you didn't have any of those conditions," he said.

The bottom line: The researchers found that what really increases the risk of nearly all complications during the first 30 days after prostate surgery is other medical problems, such as heart problems, rather than age alone.

NEW RECOMMENDATIONS

Alibhai advises men to consider what other health problems they have and how aggressive their cancer is when trying to decide on surgery. "The first thing the person needs to ask is, 'Do I need aggressive therapy? What is the chance this is going to grow and cause me trouble in my remaining days?'

"If a man is older than 70, and the cancer isn't that aggressive, he may want to avoid surgery, especially if he has other health problems. But if he's fit and healthy, and the cancer is more aggressive, surgery might be the best choice," Alibhai said.

Men also need to consider the likelihood of long-term complications from surgery, such as urinary incompetence or sexual dysfunction. Such complications weren't studied in Alibhai's research, and the risks do increase with age.

Another expert, Dr. Warren A. Jones, a distinguished professor of health policy and professor of family medicine at the University of Mississippi, said men should discuss the pros and cons of surgery with their family doctor, ideally one they have seen for many years, so he or she can assess their health status and advise them accordingly.

info For more information on treatment and clinical trials for prostate cancer, visit the Web site of the National Cancer Institute at *www. cancer.gov/cancertopics/types/prostate.*

Gene Test Determines Best Lung Cancer Treatment

Anil Potti, MD, assistant professor, Duke Institute for Genome Sciences, and assistant professor, medicine, Duke University Medical Center, Durham, NC.
Len Horovitz, MD, pulmonary specialist, Lenox Hill Hospital, New York City.
New England Journal of Medicine.

Marking a new era in cancer care, researchers say a genetic test can help predict which patients with early-stage lung cancer will most likely benefit from postoperative chemotherapy to survive and which will have a good prognosis with surgery alone. The test may herald a new approach to disease management, where treatments are tailored to each patient's genetic code.

"This is the tip of the sword. It's the first step and it is definitely personalized medicine at its best," said Dr. Anil Potti, lead author of the study and assistant professor at the Duke Institute for Genome Sciences. "They were looking at a group of genes in a way similar to fingerprinting. Based on that fingerprint, researchers can identify which patients are going to have a recurrence from lung cancer."

The test could theoretically apply to other cancers as well.

The researchers are now embarking on a larger trial involving 1,200 patients at multiple medical centers to validate the results further.

Dr. Len Horovitz, a pulmonary specialist at Lenox Hill Hospital in New York City, added, "It's a very exciting study and I think the clinical trial will bear out what is in this preliminary study."

BACKGROUND

Lung cancer is the leading cause of cancer death for both men and women, killing over 163,000 Americans each year. Non-small cell lung cancer (NSCLC) accounts for about 80% of these deaths.

Chemotherapy is generally reserved for later-stage tumors, while early-stage malignancies are treated with surgery and are generally considered to have high likelihood for cure. Yet even in this group, 30% to 35% of patients will have a recurrence and most likely die. "Chemo is not standard for stage 1 because it's considered curable by surgery," Horovitz said.

The tough question for doctors has been identifying who is most at risk for this type of relapse. "Currently, there is no way to identify who's going to have a recurrence," Potti said.

NEW STUDY

The authors of this study identified gene-expression profiles that predicted who, in a group of 89 patients with early stage NSCLC, had a higher risk for recurrence.

Then they validated the test, called the "Lung Metagene Predictor," in a group of 134 patients. The test scans thousands of genes in individual tumors. It predicted the patients' risk of recurrence with up to 90% accuracy, Potti said.

Of course, "There's no point in identifying high-risk patients if you can't do much about [their prognosis]," Potti said. But with the new test, "You're actually in a position to save lives based on individual profiles," he added.

The test could be widely available after results of the larger clinical trial are in, Horovitz said.

 For more information on lung cancer, visit *lungcancer.org* sponsored by Cancer*Care*.

Test That's Better Than Pap Smears for Cancer Screening

American Association for Cancer Research news release.

Testing for the presence of *human papillomavirus* (HPV) is a more effective cervical cancer screening tool than Pap smear for women ages 40 and older, a Danish study finds. The study of nearly 10,000 women concluded that the Pap smear is still better for screening younger women, however.

HPV infection is the leading cause of cervical cancer.

The researchers said that HPV infection is both frequent and transient in younger women —meaning that they would often test positive for HPV when they had little risk of cervical cancer.

However, in older women, HPV infection is less common and more persistent, which puts them at substantial risk for cancer before changes in cervical cells (which are detected by Pap smears) are obvious, the researchers said.

STUDY FINDINGS

They found that older women who test positive for HPV have a 20% greater risk of developing cervical cancer within 10 years than older women who don't have HPV. Furthermore, most women who test positive for HPV also test negative on a Pap smear done at the same time.

RECOMMENDATION

"Based on these results, we feel that an HPV test would benefit older women, whether or not that test is used in conjunction with Pap smears, or used by itself as an initial screen," said senior author Dr. Susanne Kruger Kjaer, professor and head of the department of virus, hormones and cancer at the Danish Cancer Society.

Don't Take a Shortcut With Your Colonoscopy

Robert L. Barclay, MD, partner, Rockford Gastroenterology Associates, IL.
Durado Brooks, MD, director, prostate and colorectal cancers, American Cancer Society, Atlanta.
New England Journal of Medicine.

Doctors who perform colonoscopies for early detection of colorectal cancer get better results if they spend at least six minutes looking for abnormal growths, a new study shows.

THE STUDY

The study reviewed 7,882 colonoscopies performed by 12 experienced gastroenterologists. Of these procedures, 2,053 were for patients who'd never had a colonoscopy. In 501 of those first-time—or screening—exams, the amount of time spent was less than six minutes.

RESULTS

Cancerous or precancerous growths were detected in 23.5% of all patients examined. But such growths were detected in only 11.8% of exams where the period of examination—called withdrawal time—was six minutes or less.

Growths were detected in 28.3% of exams with a withdrawal time of more than six minutes.

"We think our data suggest that if the goal of colonoscopy is to detect and remove polyps, spending slightly more time in the procedure seems to translate into a better outcome for patients," said study coauthor Dr. Robert

L. Barclay, a partner in Illinois-based Rockford Gastroenterology Associates.

RESULTS IN ACTION

The results of the study have led to a change in the way colonoscopy is done by our medical group, Barclay said.

"We've reviewed these results, and they were so impressive that we now take an extended minimum amount of time," Barclay said.

"We have measured detection rates for a withdrawal time of eight minutes, and we found that with that simple step, there was a dramatic increase in polyp detection among all our physicians."

AMERICAN CANCER SOCIETY RECOMMENDATION

"This basically reinforces and provides evidence for the quality recommendations that have already been made," said Dr. Durado Brooks, director of prostate and colorectal cancers for the American Cancer Society.

Withdrawal time is "a very important measure of the quality of colonoscopy," Brooks said, and the US Multisociety Task Force on Colorectal Cancer has recommended a minimum withdrawal time of six minutes.

"This study clearly shows that six minutes is a critical point, and those patients who had less had a strikingly low rate of adenoma [growth] detection, and there is at least a suspicion that the cancer detection rates would be lower," he said.

EXPERT REACTION

Brooks applauded the report. "I'm not sure that there has been a study as well done as this one showing a marked difference between withdrawal rates less than six minutes and more than six minutes," he said.

info To learn more about colorectal cancer, go to the Centers for Disease Control and Prevention at *http://www.cdc.gov/cancer/colorectal*, or to the Jay Monahan Center at New York-Presbyterian Hospital and Weill Medical College of Cornell University, *www.monahancenter.org*.

The Write Stuff Helps Cancer Patients

Susan Bauer-Wu, instructor in medicine, Harvard University School of Medicine, and director, Cantor Center for Nursing and Patient Care Research, Dana Farber Cancer Institute, Boston.

Robin Fivush, PhD, professor of psychology, Emory University, Atlanta.

It's certainly not the final word on the subject, but researchers say that writing can help cancer patients better deal with the trauma and challenges of their disease.

Research done by Susan Bauer-Wu, director of the Cantor Center for Nursing and Patient Care Research at the Dana Farber Cancer Institute, Boston, suggests that by spending 30 minutes each day writing out their innermost thoughts and feelings, cancer patients can significantly boost their mental and physical health.

"Many people are so surprised at how it really works," says Bauer-Wu. "They'll go through the process and have that 'A-ha' moment. They'll tell us, 'Wow, I never realized this about myself, or about this disease…it just came out onto the paper.'"

THE THEORY

The concept is called "expressive writing therapy." Patients are encouraged to write what is on their mind, letting their hopes and fears flow out in a natural, unrestrained way. It's akin to keeping a journal, but more focused on the things that might be bothering you or triggering stress.

"Don't worry about the punctuation, the words, just go with the process," Bauer-Wu says. "We also encourage them to build on whatever they have written before."

For many patients, such written expression provides a catharsis—a release and articulation of issues bottled up inside—and a healthy coming to terms with issues related to living with cancer.

"It's about stepping back and thinking about things in a different way, making linkages," explains Robin Fivush, a professor of psychology at Emory University who has conducted her own research on expressive writing.

"It's not just about expressing the emotion, because then you'd just ruminate on it," says Fivush. "If you take a close look at those who benefit from it most, you see a lot of them using what we call 'cognitive processing' words—'I realize, I understand, now I see that.'"

Insights like these appear to help patients with cancer or other illnesses cope better, studies suggest. In one review of 140 studies on this subject, the practice of expressive writing "seems very effective," she adds.

THE FINDINGS

Bauer-Wu has conducted three studies, tracking the effects of expressive writing and journal therapy on patients with breast and other cancers. "In my work, we do a four-day intervention, but then repeat it a month later and then a month later again." She adds that some patients benefit from longer-duration writing therapy.

"One of the things that's been found in cancer patients across different studies is what we call 'improvements in health-care utilization,'" she says. "Patients end up going to their doctor or calling nurses less frequently. They need fewer sessions with a mental health counselor. Basically, they are having fewer physical symptoms and coping better."

"There's data that suggest that writing out your emotions eases stress and, in turn, boosts the immune system," adds Fivush.

Patients can write using a pen and paper or computer. "What's most important is that you find that place each day where you can most freely write," Bauer-Wu says.

But this therapy works better for some cancer patient than others. Preadolescent children, especially, will probably not benefit, says Fivush. "We think that they may not have the cognitive or emotional skills [at that age] to work through things on their own."

Bauer-Wu says it's self-care. "People can heal themselves." According to Bauer-Wu, patients who are solitary and private by nature may benefit the most. "There's a lot of hype about support groups, but we know that some people just aren't 'talkers,'" she says. "To me, expressive writing is a wonderful alternative for these people. It gives them a way to express their feelings and process what's going on in their minds."

One key is to not write with an intended audience in mind. In most cases, the researcher says, patients don't even have to read back their own journal entries to benefit. "It's the act of writing that seems to be important," Fivush says.

■ ■ ■ ■

Massage Relieves Cancer Symptoms

It can reduce pain, nausea, fatigue and depression as effectively as drug therapy but without side effects. Insurance coverage varies. Look for a certified massage therapist who has training with cancer patients.

Barrie Cassileth, PhD, chief of integrative medicine at Memorial Sloan-Kettering Cancer Center, New York City, and leader of a study of 1,290 cancer patients receiving massage therapy, reported in *Journal of Pain and Symptom Management.*

5

Diabetes Update

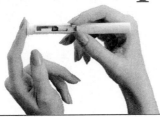

Diabetes Drug Raises Cardiovascular Risk

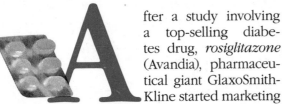

After a study involving a top-selling diabetes drug, *rosiglitazone* (Avandia), pharmaceutical giant GlaxoSmith-Kline started marketing the drug as a medicine to prevent type 2 diabetes in those with prediabetes (impaired glucose tolerance or impaired fasting glucose). But clinical trials can backfire. In this case, rosiglitazone did successfully lower the risk of diabetes, but at the cost of an increased risk of cardiovascular (CV) events.

This is a disturbing finding, notes Steven E. Nissen, MD, chairman of the department of cardiovascular medicine at the Cleveland Clinic and president of the American College of Cardiology. Dr. Nissen says that drugs to prevent and treat diabetes should *decrease* cardiovascular events, not increase them, since 65% of all diabetics die from cardiovascular complications.

THE STUDY

In the trial known as DREAM (*Diabetes REduction Assessment with ramipril and rosiglitazone Medication*), researchers found that rosiglitazone reduced by 62% the number of individuals with prediabetes who developed diabetes. Elevated blood sugar (higher than normal), referred to as prediabetes, has received increasing attention from medical experts in recent years, since it puts people at a higher risk of developing full-blown diabetes. Unfortunately, that benefit was offset, as rosiglitazone also slightly increased the incidence of adverse cardiovascular events—such as heart attacks, stroke and most notably heart failure.

The results were very surprising, given that rosiglitazone is not a new drug, says Dr. Nissen. It has been available for many years and is used by hundreds of thousands of Americans. While the increase in cardiovascular problems overall did not meet the standard for statistical significance

---

Steven E. Nissen, MD, chairman of the department of cardiovascular medicine, Cleveland Clinic, Cleveland, OH, and president of the American College of Cardiology.

(with the exception of heart failure), in Dr. Nissen's view, it still raises serious concerns.

SAFER ALTERNATIVES

Based on his analysis of the DREAM study, use of rosiglitazone to prevent diabetes should not be recommended, says Dr. Nissen. He adds that it should now be used cautiously in diabetics, particularly in those with a CV history. Fortunately, this is not your sole alternative. Dr. Nissen points out those lifestyle alterations (a healthier diet, regular exercise, weight management, etc.) have met with excellent results in preventing or treating type 2 diabetes. And, if necessary, other medications, including *metformin* (Glucophage) have also proven effective in controlling high blood sugar.

Diabetes Hikes Heart Disease Risk 60%

Caroline S. Fox, MD, MPH, medical officer at the National Heart, Lung, and Blood Institute's Framingham Heart Study.

Gregg Fonarow, MD, professor of clinical medicine, University of California, Los Angeles.

Larry Deeb, MD, president, medicine and science, American Diabetes Association, Alexandria, VA.

Circulation.

As the number of Americans with type 2 diabetes has soared over the past 50 years, so, too, has heart disease linked to the blood sugar illness, researchers report.

"The proportion of heart disease due to diabetes has increased about 60% over time," said lead author Dr. Caroline S. Fox, a medical officer at the National Heart, Lung, and Blood Institute's Framingham Heart Study. "Compared with other risk factors for heart disease, diabetes is becoming more of an issue," she said.

"I'm not surprised, but I am frightened," added Dr. Larry Deeb, president for medicine and science at the American Diabetes Association. "If you have diabetes and you have a heart attack, you don't do as well and the death rates are worse."

The only solution is to prevent diabetes, Deeb said. In one major prevention trial, "we showed that with a half-hour of exercise a day and the loss of 10 to 15 pounds, you reduce the new diabetes cases by over 58%," he said.

BACKGROUND

In obesity-linked type 2 diabetes, the body either doesn't produce enough insulin—the hormone that converts blood sugar to energy for cells—or the cells ignore the insulin. Left untreated, the disease can produce complications such as heart disease, blindness, and nerve and kidney damage.

Almost two-thirds (65%) of diabetics will die from heart disease or stroke, according to the American Heart Association.

THE STUDY

In this study, Fox's team collected data on 9,540 people ages 45 to 64, who participated in the Framingham Heart Study, a large population-based study.

The researchers used the data to compare risk factors for heart disease and cardiovascular events such as heart attacks from two different time periods. The first group was examined between 1952 and 1974, and the second group was examined between 1975 and 1998, according to the report.

They found that risk for heart disease attributable to type 2 diabetes was 5.2% between 1952 and 1974. However, that number jumped to 7.8% between 1975 and 1998. The majority of the increased risk occurred among diabetic men.

In addition, Fox's group also found that the prevalence of diabetes among those with heart disease almost doubled between the time periods. The prevalence of obesity also increased over time, they found.

The findings echo those from a study published by the same group. In that study, Fox's team analyzed data on more than 3,400 Americans ages 40 to 55 who were also participating in the Framingham study. Following the participants from the 1970s through to the 1990s, Fox and her colleagues found that rates of diabetes doubled over that period of time.

IMPLICATIONS

"In terms of public health, diabetes needs to be more effectively managed with respect to cardiovascular disease management," Fox concluded. "Ultimately, diabetes needs to be prevented," she said. That includes curbing the obesity epidemic, experts say.

Another expert agreed that more needs to be done. "This is a very important study that highlights the increased risk for cardiovascular disease that patients with diabetes face," added Dr. Gregg Fonarow, a professor of clinical medicine at the University of California, Los Angeles.

"There is an urgent need to aggressively treat all patients with diabetes with cardiovascular protective medications, risk factor control, and lifestyle change as recommended in national guidelines," Fonarow said.

Blood Pressure Drugs Skyrocket Diabetes Risk

William Elliott, MD, PhD, Department of Preventive Medicine, Rush University Medical Center, Chicago.

Stuart Weiss, MD, endocrinologist, New York University Medical Center, and clinical assistant professor, NYU School of Medicine, New York City.

Byron K. Lee MD, assistant professor, medicine, Division of Cardiology, University of California, San Francisco.

The Lancet.

British Medical Journal.

S ome common blood pressure drugs can substantially increase the risk of diabetes, especially among those already at risk for the condition, researchers report. According to the study, beta-blockers and diuretics are the blood pressure drugs most associated with diabetes. Angiotensin-receptor blockers (ARBs) and angiotensin-converting-enzyme (ACE) inhibitors are least associated with the condition, followed by calcium-channel blockers.

"There are differences across the various types of drugs that we use to treat high blood pressure in people who develop diabetes," said study author Dr. William Elliott, from the department of preventive medicine at Rush University Medical Center, Chicago.

THE STUDY

In the study, Elliott and his colleague Peter Meyer looked at 22 clinical trials that included more than 143,000 people. These people had high blood pressure but did not have diabetes at the start of the trials. In each trial, the participants received long-term treatment with each class of blood pressure drugs or placebo.

The traditional medicines used to treat high blood pressure in the US are diuretics and beta-blockers, Elliott said. "It so happens that they are the two drug classes that are most likely to precipitate diabetes. It turns out that two of the new classes of drug—ACE inhibitors and ARBs—are the two that have the least amount of diabetes associated with them. In the middle, we have calcium-channel blockers," he said.

Elliott noted that your risk of getting diabetes while taking diuretics and beta-blockers depends on several factors. These include how long you are on the medication, your weight, your family history of diabetes, whether or not you have recently gained weight, and other risk factors, he said.

IMPLICATIONS

How doctors should be prescribing these drugs in light of these findings isn't clear cut, Elliott said. "In Britain, they have issued new guidelines, where, in fact, the diuretic and beta-blocker combination are not to be used together because of the excess risk of diabetes," he said.

Doctors who take a patient's risk for diabetes into account might be better off prescribing an ACE inhibitor or an ARB, rather than a beta-blocker or a diuretic as first-line treatment, Elliott said.

"However, if you have a patient who has high blood pressure, kidney disease and had a major heart attack recently—there is no question they are going to get the beta-blocker to protect them from another heart attack," he said. "They are also going to get a diuretic, because of the kidney disease. If they get diabetic, you just accept that and move on. You are not going deny them the medicines they need today over the risk of diabetes down the road," he said.

REACTION

One diabetes expert thinks that doctors should take a patient's risk for diabetes into account when prescribing blood pressure medications.

"Individualization of therapy is important," said Dr. Stuart Weiss, an endocrinologist at New York University Medical Center. "With the explosion of diabetes in the country, we need to take that into consideration when providing patients with their initial antihypertensive."

Weiss thinks that those people who are at risk for diabetes should not be started on beta-blockers or diuretics. "With all the data about the long-term use of ACEs and ARBs and their lower risk for diabetes, it's a good thing to get these drugs in early in somebody who is even at modest risk for type 2 diabetes," he said.

A cardiologist agreed that treatment needs to be tailored to individual patient needs.

"Since doctors generally have many drug options to lower blood pressure, it makes sense to tailor the drug choice to the patient who may be at higher risk for certain diseases," said Dr. Byron K. Lee, an assistant professor of medicine, Division of Cardiology, at University of California, San Francisco.

"For example, those at higher risk for diabetes may be given an ACE inhibitor or ARB, whereas those at higher risk for heart attacks may be given a beta-blocker," Lee said.

info For more information on diabetes and heart disease, go to the American Heart Association Web site at *www.s2mw.com/heart ofdiabetes/index.html.*

Diabetes–Parkinson's Link Grows Stronger

Cathy Nonas, MS, RD, CDE, director, diabetes and obesity programs, North General Hospital, and assistant clinical professor, Mount Sinai School of Medicine, New York City.

Gang Hu, MD, PhD, senior researcher, National Public Health Institute, and adjunct professor, University of Helsinki, Finland.

Diabetes Care.

As people with obesity-linked type 2 diabetes age, their risk of getting Parkinson's disease also climbs, a new study warns.

In fact, excess weight may explain why diabetics are at increased risk of getting the neurological disorder, a Finnish study suggests.

"These findings are important from a clinical and public health point of view," said study author Dr. Gang Hu, senior researcher at the National Public Health Institute in Helsinki. "Type 2 diabetes is increasing rapidly in all populations, and its impact on various health outcomes is not fully known or even explored."

His team's study is the first large effort to follow people over time and evaluate the diabetes–Parkinson's link.

BACKGROUND

Parkinson's disease affects about 1.5 million Americans, according to the National Parkinson Foundation. It occurs when certain brain cells or neurons die or become impaired. These cells normally produce a substance called dopamine, which helps regulate coordinated movement. Some symptoms of Parkinson's include tremor, slow movement and difficulties keeping one's balance.

In type 2 diabetes, the body doesn't properly use insulin or doesn't make enough insulin, which is crucial for the body's uptake of glucose for energy. Excess weight is the major risk factor for type 2 diabetes.

THE STUDY

Hu's team's study included more than 51,000 Finnish men and women between the ages of 25 and 74 with no prior history of Parkinson's.

During the 18 years of follow-up, 324 men and 309 women developed Parkinson's disease.

When Hu and his team evaluated the subjects' medical histories, they found that people with type 2 diabetes were 83% more likely to get Parkinson's.

The increased risk was still present even after the researchers took into account body mass index (BMI), alcohol intake, coffee/tea intake, smoking and physical activity.

THEORY

So, what's behind the association? "It could be hypothesized that diabetes might increase the risk of Parkinson's disease partly through excess body weight," Hu said. "The positive association between body weight and the risk of Parkinson's disease has been found in our previous studies."

Cathy Nonas, director of diabetes and obesity programs at North General Hospital and an assistant clinical professor at Mount Sinai School of Medicine, New York City, said the association does make sense. "I could theorize—just theorize—that because it takes a lot of energy for brain cells to use glucose, that insulin resistance in type 2 diabetes might affect carbohydrate metabolism in dopaminergic neurons, causing some sort of dysfunction and rendering them unable to defend against cell damage," she said.

FUTURE RESEARCH

In fact, Nonas is studying the effects of very low-protein, very low-carbohydrate diets on Parkinson's patients. The theory is that when you deplete the body of carbs, it makes more *ketones*—substances produced when the body breaks down fat for energy. According to Nonas, ketones may be an easier fuel than glucose for the brain to use, perhaps improving some Parkinson's symptoms.

ADVICE

But that research is in its infancy. For now, Nonas said, the best advice is for anyone with type 2 diabetes to keep it under control and see their doctor regularly. If they develop new symptoms, such as difficulty walking or tremors, they should make their doctor aware of them, she added.

info To learn more about Parkinson's disease, visit the Web site of the National Parkinson Foundation at *www.parkinson.org*.

No Memory Problems From Low Blood Sugar

Alan Jacobson, MD, professor, psychiatry, Harvard Medical School, and director, behavioral and mental health research program, Joslin Diabetes Center, Boston.

Maria Ramos-Ramon, MD, assistant professor, internal medicine, University of Texas Southwestern Medical Center at Dallas.

New England Journal of Medicine.

People with type 1 diabetes don't need to worry that they may have brain function problems in the future if they've had a bout or two of severe hypoglycemia (low blood sugar), a new study suggests.

Researchers found that while serious hypoglycemic episodes did sometimes occur as a result of aggressive diabetes control, those low blood sugar events didn't have any effect on cognitive function.

"Hypoglycemia did not seem to predict the advent of worsening cognitive function," said the study's lead author, Dr. Alan Jacobson, director of the behavioral and mental health research program at the Joslin Diabetes Center in Boston.

"Of course, it goes without saying that hypoglycemia can be a serious problem," he added. "But, if you've had a more severe hypoglycemia event, at least it appears that you don't have to worry that 10 years later you may have trouble doing your job or thinking," he said.

BACKGROUND

People with type 1 diabetes—the inherited form of the disease, which affects about 5% of diabetics—have to maintain a difficult balancing act. They have to try to get their blood sugar to as near-normal levels as possible, but they can't go too low, or they'll have problems with hypoglycemia.

Adding to that difficulty is that while people without diabetes experience clear warning symptoms that their blood sugar is dropping too low, such as shakiness, dizziness or sweating, some people with type 1 diabetes eventually stop receiving those warning signs from their bodies. *Hypoglycemia unawareness* occurs when a diabetic does not know that their blood sugar is too low until it's so dangerously low that it results in a seizure or coma. This condition is one of the reasons people with type 1 diabetes are advised to monitor their blood sugar levels often throughout the day.

Experts have been concerned that repeated episodes of severe hypoglycemia might affect cognitive function, because it can cause nerve cell death.

NEW STUDY

To assess whether or not several bouts of severe hypoglycemia could have any effect on long-term cognition, Jacobson and his colleagues tested the cognitive abilities of 1,144 people with type 1 diabetes.

The team measured the participants' cognitive performance at the start of the study and then again an average of 18 years later.

Those participating in this study were between the ages of 13 and 39 years old at the start of the study, which commenced in the mid- to late 1980s.

The trial randomized participants into one of two treatment options. The first were sent to "standard" diabetes treatment, with no long-term blood sugar goal provided. The second group was part of an "intensive management" regimen that the researchers hoped would reduce the risk for long-term diabetes complications, such as blindness, kidney failure and cardiovascular disease.

Those in the intensive management part of the trial were asked to try to attain a near-normal A1C level—a measure of long-term blood sugar—of less than 6%.

THE RESULTS

During the six-and-a-half-year trial, those in the intensive management portion lowered their A1C to 7.1%, while those in the standard management group kept their blood sugar at 9.0%.

By the end of the whole study period—18 years—there were a total of 1,355 episodes of coma or seizure due to hypoglycemia. Three of the more than 1,100 people in the trial also died during the study period due to hypoglycemia. Not surprisingly, there were more incidences of low blood sugar in those in the intensive management portion of the trial.

BLOOD SUGAR AND COGNITIVE FUNCTION

The good news from this study is that those occasional hypoglycemic events didn't appear to have any effect on long-term cognition.

However, the researchers did note that the opposite might be true—higher average blood sugars might also negatively affect cognition.

The study found a small, subtle *decrease* in certain measures of cognitive function for those who failed to manage their diabetes well, as defined by an A1C above 8.8%.

REACTION

On the whole, the study results are "reassuring for people with type 1 diabetes," said Dr. Maria Ramos-Ramon, a diabetes specialist and an assistant professor of internal medicine at the University of Texas Southwestern Medical Center at Dallas.

But, she said, it's important for people with type 1 diabetes to know that their care must be individualized. Not everyone can safely reach a goal of an A1C under 6%.

"We have to individualize care and set a goal of glycemic control on a patient by patient basis," said Ramos-Ramon.

info To learn more about hypoglycemia, visit the Web site of the American Diabetes Association at *www.diabetes.org/type-1-diabetes/hypoglycemia.jsp*.

Depression May Trigger Diabetes

Mercedes R. Carnethon, PhD, assistant professor, preventive medicine, Feinberg School of Medicine, Northwestern University, Chicago.

Lana Watkins, PhD, associate professor, department of psychiatry, Duke University Medical Center, Durham, NC.
Archives of Internal Medicine.

D epression may trigger diabetes in older people, researchers report, after many years of studying adults over 65.

"Older adults who report high levels of depressive symptoms are more likely to develop diabetes over time than older adults who have lower depressive symptoms," said lead researcher Dr. Mercedes R. Carnethon, assistant professor of preventive medicine, at the Feinberg School of Medicine at Northwestern University.

"We need to carefully evaluate older adults for depressive symptoms, and they need to be taken seriously because of the potential impact," she added.

However, whether treating depression reduces the risk for developing diabetes isn't known, Carnethon said.

THE STUDY

Carnethon's group collected data on nearly 4,700 people age 65 and older who were not diabetic when the study began in 1989.

Over the following 10 years, participants were evaluated for symptoms of depression related to changes in mood, irritability, calorie intake, concentration and sleep.

The researchers scored symptoms of depression on a scale of zero to 30, with a score of eight or higher indicating high levels of symptoms. When the study began, the average symptom score was 4.5. In addition, one-fifth of the people had a score of eight or higher.

During the 10 years of follow-up, half the people saw their scores increase by at least five points. In all, 234 study participants developed diabetes. The rate of diabetes was higher among those with a score of eight or more compared with those whose scores were below eight, Carnethon's team found.

CAUSES

Carnethon believes the link between depression and diabetes has several causes.

"One is behavioral," she said. "Individuals who are depressed may be less likely to engage in healthy physical activities that would protect against the development of diabetes. They may be less likely to sleep well, have healthy diets, all of which are risk factors for developing diabetes," she said.

There also could be biological factors at play. These include increased levels of blood markers of inflammation, such as C-reactive protein, which have been linked to both diabetes and depression, Carnethon said.

EXPERT REACTION

"This paper extends earlier findings of a relationship between depressive symptoms and increased risk of developing diabetes, by demonstrating that individuals with worsening depression or with persistent depression are also at increased risk of developing diabetes," said Dr. Lana Watkins, an associate professor in the department of psychiatry at Duke University Medical Center in Durham, North Carolina.

Watkins believes that further research is needed to confirm the finding.

"In order to identify conclusively whether depression increases diabetes risk through excessive caloric consumption and/or through sedentary behavior, better measures of these two factors are needed," Watkins said.

info For more information on diabetes and depression, go to the Web site of the American Diabetes Association at *www.diabetes.org/type-2-diabetes/depression.jsp.*

Diabetes Drug May Not Be Worth Risk

Center for the Advancement of Health news release.

It's unclear whether the health benefits outweigh the risks of the widely prescribed diabetes drug *pioglitazone* (Actos), say the authors of a review that examined 22 studies of the drug involving 6,200 type 2 diabetes patients.

THE STUDY RESULTS

"Our results showed that published scientific studies of at least 24 weeks of pioglitazone treatment in people with type 2 diabetes mellitus did not provide convincing evidence that patient-oriented outcomes like mortality, morbidity, adverse effects and health-related quality of life are positively influenced by this drug," said lead author Dr. Bernd Richter.

Not only were he and his colleagues unable to identify any definite benefit from taking pioglitazone, they also found that patients taking the drug had increased rates of edema (fluid buildup and swelling) and heart failure.

They also concluded that the drug may cause dangerous drops in blood glucose in people taking pioglitazone in combination with another class of drugs called *sulfonylureas,* which include medications such as *tolbutamide* (Orinase), *glipizide* (Glucotrol) and *glimepiride* (Amaryl), among others.

RECOMMENDATIONS

"Until new evidence becomes available, the benefit-risk ratio of pioglitazone therapy in type 2 diabetes mellitus remains unclear," said Richter, an assistant professor in the department of endocrinology, diabetes and rheumatology at Heinrich-Heine University in Germany.

Richter said pioglitazone treatment should be restricted to patients who show real benefits —fewer diabetic complications and improved health-related quality of life—from taking the drug.

Pioglitazone belongs to a family of drugs called *thiazolidinediones*. These drugs are designed to increase the body's sensitivity to naturally produced insulin to foster better intake of glucose into cells and lower blood-glucose levels.

"The kernel from this review is that pioglitazone is effective in glucose-lowering, has some other beneficial and potentially harmful associated features, and just has not been evaluated in the right way to prove that it will help people lead longer and more productive lives," said Dr. John Buse, director of the Diabetes Care Center at the University of North Carolina School of Medicine at Chapel Hill.

Caution: In August 2007, the FDA announced that the manufacturers of Actos is required to add a severe warning box to all product labels, cautioning that Actos may cause heart failure.

How to Stop Diabetes in Its Tracks

Robert Rizza, MD, professor of medicine at Mayo Clinic College of Medicine in Rochester, MN. He is also president of the American Diabetes Association, *www. diabetes.org.*

The epidemic of type 2 diabetes is alarming—and more dangerous than many people ever imagine. The disease, which affects 20 million Americans, increases the risk for heart attack and stroke. Complications include blindness, kidney failure, impotence and poor wound healing that can lead to amputation.

Until recently, doctors diagnosed diabetes only when a patient had full-blown symptoms, which typically develop gradually over a period of years.

Now: You can stop diabetes in its tracks if you recognize and take action against "prediabetes," which affects more than 40 million people ages 40 to 74. *Here's how…*

WHEN SUGAR ISN'T SWEET

Glucose, a simple sugar molecule that is metabolized from the food you eat, is basic fuel for your body. It's broken down in cells of all kinds to produce energy that powers your muscles, lets you think and keeps your heart pumping and your lungs breathing.

The hormone insulin, which is produced by your pancreas, plays a key role, escorting glucose from the bloodstream into the cells. When there isn't enough insulin to do the job or the insulin is not effective, sugar builds up in the blood. That's when the trouble begins.

To diagnose diabetes, doctors order blood tests that measure the amount of glucose in your bloodstream. One test, fasting plasma glucose (FPG), checks the level first thing in the morning, before you've eaten anything. A normal glucose level is less than 100 milligrams per deciliter (mg/dl).

The oral glucose tolerance test (OGTT) is a bit more complicated—after fasting all night, you're asked to drink a sugary liquid, and your glucose level is tested two hours later (normal is less than 140 mg/dl).

If your FPG is 126 mg/dl or higher…or the two-hour OGTT is above 200 mg/dl, you likely have diabetes. Your pancreas no longer secretes enough insulin for proper glucose metabolism. This means that your chance of developing complications, such as heart disease, kidney failure or vision loss, has more than doubled.

AN EARLIER DIAGNOSIS

There's also an intermediate condition. Fasting blood sugar of 100 mg/dl to 125 mg/dl is called impaired fasting glucose. If the two-hour OGTT is 140 mg/dl to 200 mg/dl, it is known as impaired glucose tolerance.

Nowadays, these conditions are called prediabetes. With prediabetes, your insulin activity has already started to fall short of the amount your body needs. And if something isn't done, there's a good chance you'll go on to develop full-blown diabetes.

What are the odds? Fasting blood sugar between 100 mg/dl and 110 mg/dl means you have a 20% chance of developing diabetes within five to 10 years. If it's above 110, it's a 40% chance. If both the fasting blood sugar and two-hour glucose tolerance tests are elevated, the odds increase even more.

At the prediabetes level, excess blood sugar already has started to take its toll, researchers have discovered. For example, the risk for heart disease is one-and-one-half times higher than that of people with normal blood sugar.

DO YOU HAVE PREDIABETES?

To determine whether you have prediabetes, ask your doctor for a fasting glucose test—especially if you are at increased risk due to...

• **Excess body weight** (defined below).

• **Family history of diabetes** (parent, brother or sister).

• **Diabetes during pregnancy** (gestational diabetes).

• **Asian, African-American or Hispanic ethnicity.**

If any of these risk factors applies to you, have your blood sugar checked at your next physical—after age 45, do it at least every three years. Given the high rates of diabetes today, everyone over age 45 should consider getting tested.

TREATMENT FOR PREDIABETES

Slightly elevated blood sugar doesn't mean you're destined to get diabetes. With fairly moderate lifestyle changes, you can reduce that risk by more than 50%.

Obesity increases diabetes risk. If you are overweight, bring your weight down by 5% to 10% (an achievable goal for most people). Ideally, your weight should be brought down to the normal range, which means a body mass index (a ratio of weight to height), or BMI, of 18.5 to 24.9. To find your BMI, use the free calculator at the National Heart, Lung and Blood Institute Web site at *http://nhlbisupport.com/bmi*. Or use the formula (weight in pounds × 703) ÷ height in inches squared.

Important finding: A Finnish study of 522 middle-aged, overweight people with prediabetes found that diabetes risk among those who participated in a diet and exercise program for three years was reduced by 58% compared with a control group, who experienced no reduction.

HOW TO STOP PREDIABETES

• **Diet wisely.** Consuming fewer calories than you burn is the key to weight loss. Some research also suggests that reducing saturated fat (most beef and some dairy products), and the resulting weight loss that can occur, helps reverse prediabetes, allowing your body to use insulin more efficiently. A diet rich in complex carbohydrates, such as fruits, vegetables and whole grains, will meet these goals—and is best for everyone's general health.

• **Exercise regularly.** Physical activity helps control your weight and improves your body's ability to use insulin. Aim for at least 30 minutes five or more days a week. The type of exercise doesn't seem to matter, as long as it requires modest exertion—brisk walking, swimming, riding a bike, etc.

• **Forgo medication.** Blood sugar in people with prediabetes can be reduced with prescription diabetes medication such as *metformin* (Glucophage). However, research on prediabetes suggests that this drug is not as effective as diet and exercise in preventing diabetes.

Important finding: In a *New England Journal of Medicine* study, 3,234 men and women with prediabetes were randomly assigned to a lifestyle program or the drug metformin. Weight loss and exercise reduced diabetes incidence nearly twice as much as drug treatment over the next three years (a reduction of 58% versus 31%).

Surprising Causes of Fungal Infections

John R. Perfect, MD, an infectious disease specialist and professor of medicine at Duke University School of Medicine in Durham, NC. A medical mycologist, he specializes in the diagnosis and treatment of invasive fungal diseases.

Most people blame viruses or bacteria when they get an infection. But there's another—often-overlooked—possibility, that is fungi. Fungal infection is more common than most people realize.

Example: Candida, a fungus that causes yeast infections, is the fourth most common microorganism found in the blood of hospitalized patients. Candida can infect the mouth, causing white, painful patches on the tongue and inside the cheeks (thrush). In the hospital or during serious illnesses, these mild fungal infections can develop into potentially fatal ones, which can affect the heart or brain.

Fungi are normally present on the skin and in the intestinal tract. Local fungal infections, such as athlete's foot, are common and relatively easy to treat. Mild infections also can occur in the other places that fungi normally inhabit, such as the vagina, mouth, groin area or in fingernails or toenails.

It's rare for someone who's healthy to get a serious fungal infection. Those at greatest risk include people with compromised immune systems, such as hospitalized patients and individuals with diabetes, lung disease, kidney failure, cancer, human immuno-deficiency virus (HIV) or some other chronic illness…as well as anyone who has undergone an organ or bone-marrow transplant.

To learn more, John R. Perfect, MD, a renowned specialist in fungal infections answered the following questions…

How difficult is it to diagnose a fungal infection?

Infections of the skin usually can be diagnosed just by looking at them. Dermatophytosis (ringworm), for example, usually appears as scaly, red ring-shaped patches. Systemic infections (that have spread into several organs) usually require taking a sample of body fluid, such as sputum from the lungs or blood, and culturing it in a laboratory and/or examining specimens under a microscope for fungal forms.

Caution: Fungal infection in the lungs can be mistaken for cancer on an X-ray. The only way to distinguish the two is by taking a biopsy.

Are fungal infections contagious?

Some fungal infections of the skin, such as ringworm, can be passed from one person to another by sharing towels or clothing or having direct contact with a rash. Most other fungal infections occur when microscopic spores in the air come in contact with the skin or are inhaled. Many fungi reproduce and spread through these microscopic spores.

Is there any way to protect yourself from developing a fungal infection?

We live in a virtual "sea of fungi," so it is impossible to avoid them. The vast majority cannot cause disease. The best prevention is for your doctor to be aware of these infections and for you to get treatment early if one develops.

Does a skin/nail infection indicate that there's a more serious underlying problem?

Usually not. It's possible that someone with a serious, underlying illness will get a nail or skin fungal infection—but it's unlikely that the infection would be the first sign. The most dangerous fungal infections, such as aspergillosis and cryptococcosis, tend to occur in patients who are already sick and perhaps undergoing extensive medical treatments. Both of these infections primarily affect the lungs but occasionally spread to other areas of the body.

Someone with cancer or diabetes might be more likely to develop a severe Candida infection because he/she may be in a hospital receiving intravenous antibiotics or chemotherapy, which may allow fungi to proliferate in the body. Although Candida most often causes yeast infections, in more serious cases, it can invade the bloodstream or certain organs.

Some fungal infections may be important warning signs. Therefore, anyone who's getting fungal infections more than twice a year or has an infection that doesn't respond to treatments needs to consider the possibility that his/her immune system isn't working well—and see his doctor right away.

Aren't fungal infections difficult to treat?

Fungi are very hard to kill. Like humans, fungi are eukaryotes (single-celled or multicellular organisms whose cells contain a distinct membrane-bound nucleus). This means that we share the same kinds of "cellular machinery." It's difficult to develop drugs that will kill a fungus without killing human cells at the same time. Fungi grow slowly and protect themselves inside host cells. Despite this, there has been great improvement in the drugs we have for invasive fungal infections. However, some antifungal medications can be costly—up to $250 for a month's treatment.

Latest development: The newest class of antifungal drugs, known as candins, include *caspofungin* (Cancidas), *micafungin* (Mycamine) and *anidulafungin* (Eraxis), which are used to treat aspergillosis and serious Candida infections. These medications inhibit a component that fungi require to create cell walls. Since human cells don't have that component, they aren't affected by these drugs. Because of this, the candins are less likely to cause toxicity and/or side effects than older antifungal agents, such as polyene drugs, including *amphotericin B* (Fungizone).

Topical antifungal drugs are effective, but they don't necessarily work quickly. It's common for patients with athlete's foot to apply the creams for weeks or months. Treating a nail fungus may require oral antifungal drugs.

What happens if a fungal infection goes untreated?

That depends on the severity of the infection. Mild skin fungal infections sometimes clear up on their own—and even if they don't, they may require minimal treatment. A patient with a nail fungus, for example, might choose to ignore it, since the only symptom—usually yellow, green or brown nail discoloration—is cosmetic.

Athlete's foot, jock itch and vaginal yeast infections, on the other hand, can be itchy and uncomfortable. They respond well to over-the-counter topical agents, such as *clotrimazole* (Gyne-Lotrimin or Mycelex) or *miconazole* (Monistat).

An invasive fungal infection, which usually begins in the lungs or bloodstream, can spread rapidly to other parts of the body and always requires treatment. The drugs may be given orally or intravenously. In the highest-risk patients, such as those getting chemotherapy, an antifungal drug can be given prophylactically—that is, to prevent an infection from occurring.

■ ■ ■ ■

The Latest Drug Research

New diabetes drug *Januvia* blocks an enzyme that suppresses the release of insulin after blood sugar rises—for instance, after a meal, says Carol Levy, MD. This lets the body release insulin longer. Januvia—chemical name *sitagliptin phosphate*—works like the injected drug *exenatide* (Byetta), but Januvia is taken by mouth. It is best for people with type 2 diabetes who cannot keep their blood sugar levels low enough with older diabetes medications, such as *metformin*.

Carol Levy, MD, a diabetes specialist, is an assistant attending physician at NewYork–Presbyterian Hospital/Weill-Cornell Medical Center, New York City.

How You Can Beat Prediabetes

Sandra Woodruff, RD, a Tallahassee, Florida–based licensed dietitian/nutritionist and author of numerous books on healthful eating. She is also coauthor, with Christopher Saudek, MD, of *The Complete Diabetes Prevention Plan*. Avery. Her Web site is *www.eatsmarttoday.com*.

Underlying today's epidemic of type 2 diabetes is a larger epidemic—prediabetes, meaning blood sugar levels that are higher than normal but not high enough to be called diabetes. A diagnosis of prediabetes doesn't mean that you're destined for diabetes. Prediabetes can be reversed—and diabetes prevented—simply by making some basic lifestyle changes.

Almost everyone who develops type 2 diabetes has passed through the earlier phase of prediabetes. The number of Americans with prediabetes is now about 41 million. If left untreated, prediabetes almost always turns into diabetes within 10 years. Even if it's not high enough to be labeled diabetes, high blood sugar can still significantly harm your body. It can cause high blood pressure and damage to small blood vessels, including those in your kidneys and eyes.

WHO'S AT RISK

If your fasting blood sugar level (after not eating or drinking anything but water for at least eight hours) is between 100 and 125 milligrams per deciliter (mg/dL), you already have prediabetes. Your doctor can do a simple blood test to find this figure. You're at greater risk of prediabetes now and diabetes later if you…

•**Are age 45 or older.** Prediabetes risk increases with age.

•**Have a family history of diabetes.**

•**Had gestational diabetes** (high blood sugar during pregnancy) or gave birth to a baby weighing over nine pounds.

•**Are overweight,** with a body mass index (BMI) of 25 or more. (To find your BMI, divide your weight in kilograms by your height squared in meters—or check the calculator at *www.nhlbisupport.com/bmi*.) The heavier you are, the greater your risk. If overweight, you're at greater risk if your excess weight is around your waist (in other words, you're shaped like an apple) than if it's carried in your hips and thighs (you're shaped like a pear).

• **Have low HDL** ("good") cholesterol and high triglycerides (tiny fat particles in the blood).

• **Have high blood pressure** (129/90 or higher).

• **Have a sedentary lifestyle.**

African-Americans, Asian-Americans and Native Americans are at the highest risk, but anyone with one or more risk factors can develop prediabetes and diabetes. The more risk factors you have, the greater the likelihood that you'll become diabetic.

STEPS TO TAKE

You *can* prevent or reverse prediabetes and keep diabetes from developing. How? *With three small but consistent lifestyle changes...*

1. Lose weight. If you are overweight, losing just 5% of your body weight can make a big difference, but even just holding your weight steady and stopping weight gain will help. If you weigh 180 pounds, for example, you would need to lose only nine pounds to see improvement. Cutting just 100 calories a day (the equivalent of a couple cookies) and adding 30 minutes of walking a day, which burns about 100 calories, will lead to slow, safe, steady weight loss.

2. Eat better. Cut back on high-calorie, low-nutrition food, such as cookies and chips.

3. Get moving. Do moderate exercise (walking, for instance) for 30 minutes every day.

Can this plan really prevent diabetes? Yes. A major study called the Diabetes Prevention Program proved it in 2002. Overall, the study participants who followed all three steps cut their risk of diabetes by nearly 60%. Among those over age 60, the improvement was even greater —they cut their risk by more than 70%.

BETTER FOOD CHOICES

• **Eat good carbohydrates** (food made from whole grains without added sugars). Take an inventory of the carbohydrates you regularly eat. If you're eating bread, make it whole grain. If you're eating sugary breakfast cereal, make it unsweetened whole grain. Instead of ordinary pasta, try whole-wheat pasta—today there are many excellent whole-wheat and other whole-grain pastas. Instead of white rice, switch to brown. Substitute other whole grains, such as barley, for white potatoes. Instead of cookies and snack foods, go for fresh fruit or a handful of dry-roasted nuts.

• **Get rid of bad fats.** Choose lean meats and low-fat dairy products. Avoid dangerous trans fats (partially hydrogenated vegetable oil) that are found in processed foods and margarine. Use healthy oils, such as canola and olive oils, when cooking or in salad dressing.

• **Enjoy dessert, but in moderation.** The first few bites of a dessert taste the best, so go ahead and have them—just don't have any beyond that. If you keep your portion small to begin with, you won't be tempted to eat more.

At home, put portions on small plates. When eating out, ask for a half portion or split an order with someone else. When making desserts yourself, cut back on the sugar and use whole-grain flours. Make an apple crumble with oatmeal, nuts and a small amount of brown sugar instead of using the standard recipe.

You can even continue to enjoy between-meal snacks. We've come to think that a snack has to come from a package and be highly processed, but snacks should be real food as often as possible—think of a snack as a mini-meal. Try fresh fruit, low-fat yogurt, vegetables with hummus, low-fat popcorn, baked corn chips with bean dip, string cheese, some salad, half a sandwich or a small bowl of soup.

THE ACTIVE INGREDIENT

Exercise is a very powerful tool for preventing diabetes. Just a half hour a day of moderate exercise acts on your body very much like an insulin-sensitizing drug. Think of exercise as your daily dose of antidiabetes medication—a medication that's free and has no side effects. Exercise makes your cells more responsive to insulin, and that helps lower your blood sugar. In addition, regular exercise helps with weight loss.

Does Pollution Cause Diabetes?

Duk-Hee Lee, MD, PhD, an associate professor in the Department of Preventive Medicine and Health Promotion Research Center, School of Medicine, Kyungpook National University in South Korea. She is a medical doctor and epidemiologist who has written extensively about the relationship of persistent organic pollutants (POPs) and diabetes.

Scientists know that elements in the environment often interact with elements of our own physiology to cause serious problems. And new research is emerging that suggests we may be seeing this phenomenon with diabetes.

We've long known that obesity is a major risk factor for diabetes. But now it appears that exposure to pollutants can seriously aggravate the risk, and—in combination with obesity—may be associated with the increased risk of becoming diabetic. A recent study in the journal *Diabetes Care* looked at the connection between six persistent organic pollutants (known as POPs) and diabetes...and what they found was dramatic.

THE STUDY

Lead researcher Duk-Hee Lee, MD, PhD, and her team divided the 2,016 subjects into groups based on five levels of pollutants. Group 1 had the lowest levels and group 5 had the highest levels. The results showed that the prevalence of diabetes increased by 14- to 38-fold as the concentrations of the sum of the six POPs increased, irrespective of participants' weight.

Compared with group 1 (which had a .4% incidence of diabetes), group 2 had a 6.7% incidence of diabetes, while group 5 had an astonishing 25.6% incidence of the disease (groups 3 and 4 ranged in between). Dr. Lee says that while obesity remains a risk factor for type 2 diabetes, the obese and overweight people with very low concentrations of POPs had a much lower incidence of diabetes. Could obesity and pollutants interact to cause diabetes?

RESEARCHERS' THEORIES

"It's our hypothesis that obesity might be only weakly associated with diabetes among people with very low serum concentrations of POPs," said Dr. Lee. She explained that while her research concentrated on only six specific pollutants out of about 50 POPs identified in the National Health and Examination Survey, there was a striking connection between the blood concentrations of these six toxins and the prevalence of diabetes.

This is not the first time that such a connection has been demonstrated. Earlier research from Sweden also found that exposure to POPs may contribute to the development of type 2 diabetes. Prior research also demonstrated that exposure to at least one toxin—a dioxin called TCDD—increases the risk of diabetes and insulin resistance. It's believed that these toxins may interfere with glucose metabolism.

POLLUTANTS EVERYWHERE

Persistent organic pollutants (POPs) include certain chemical byproducts, PCBs and certain insecticides. They have been linked to cancer, neurobehavioral impairment, endocrine problems and reproductive disorders. Previous researchers looked at groups who are occupationally or accidentally exposed to high levels of these pollutants, for example, Vietnam veterans. (The US Department of Veterans Affairs includes type 2 diabetes in its list of presumptive diseases associated with exposure to the dioxin-containing Agent Orange.)

Dr. Lee's study is the first to examine the cumulative effect of most commonly detected POPs among a random low-level exposure in the general population. The six toxins in the study are found in the environment, and they move through the air and water to accumulate in the environment.

Caution: Dr. Lee was careful not to say that pollutants by themselves necessarily cause diabetes, and she expressed the usual researcher's caution about jumping to strong conclusions based on one or two studies. "Plenty of people have exposure to these pollutants and don't get diabetes," she explained. "But the strong connection between high levels and increased incidence is very hard to ignore, as is the fact that there are such low levels of diabetes among those with low levels of exposure, even among the overweight and obese." Could genes be a factor? "It's prudent to act as if everyone is at risk, regardless of genetic makeup," she said.

HOW TO LIMIT EXPOSURE

How do we get exposed to these chemicals in the first place? "Exposure to POPs comes mostly from animal fatty food consumption," says Dr. Lee.

Her recommendation: "A low intake of animal food and a higher intake of plant food may be beneficial. And, aside from trying to avoid POPs, preventing obesity is still very important because the toxicity of POPs appeared to synergistically increase the risk of type 2 diabetes among obese persons."

■ ■ ■ ■

Saturated Fat Can Raise Diabetes Risk

Saturated fat increases insulin resistance, the first step in developing the most common form of diabetes. Insulin resistance involves overproduction of insulin, which also has been linked to fertility problems and increased risk of certain cancers.

Self-defense: Limit saturated-fat intake to no more than 10% of calories, the equivalent of about 20 grams per day for the average adult. Most Americans get 12% of calories from saturated fat. The main sources of saturated fat are high-fat meats (regular ground beef, sausage, ribs and well-marbled steaks) and high-fat dairy products (whole milk, regular cheese, ice cream). Limiting portions of these foods and choosing lean/low-fat versions make the saturated fat goals easily attainable.

Karen Collins, RD, a registered dietitian and nutrition adviser to the American Institute for Cancer Research (AICR) in Washington, DC. She is the author of *Planning Meals That Lower Cancer Risk,* AICR, available at many college libraries, and "Nutrition Notes" and "Nutrition-Wise," weekly columns syndicated to more than 700 newspapers nationwide. She maintains a private practice in Jamestown, NY.

6

Drug News

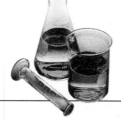

Breakthrough Drugs

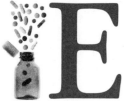

Each year, the FDA approves a variety of new prescription drugs. Most are "me too" drugs—that is, they are very similar to medications that are already available.

However: Some new drugs do represent significant breakthroughs. These medications treat diseases in entirely new ways or are the only available treatment for a given condition. *Important new treatments of the past year...*

CONSTIPATION

•**Lubiprostone (Amitiza).** It's one of the first prescription drugs, aside from laxatives, for treating chronic constipation in adults—specifically, idiopathic constipation, in which the cause is unknown.

Why it's important: Most patients with constipation can get significant relief with lifestyle changes, such as eating high-fiber foods, getting regular exercise, drinking more water, etc.

However, some patients don't always improve with these approaches.

Taken orally, lubiprostone relieves constipation by increasing the secretion of intestinal fluids, which eases stool passage.

Side effects or complications: About 31% of patients taking lubiprostone have experienced nausea, while 13% reported headaches or diarrhea.

Dose: Take 24 micrograms (mcg) twice daily, with food. If side effects occur, the dosage can be reduced to once daily. Patients should ask their doctors how long they should take lubiprostone.

COUGH

•**Tdap (Adacel).** Whooping cough, a highly contagious respiratory disease characterized by severe cough, has long been known to affect children, but this bacterial infection, also known as pertussis, strikes adults, too.

Gianna Zuccotti, MD, deputy editor of *The Medical Letter on Drugs and Therapeutics, www.medletter.com,* based in New Rochelle, NY. It is an independent, nonprofit organization that provides drug-prescribing recommendations to health-care providers.

According to the Centers for Disease Control and Prevention (CDC), the number of people infected with pertussis has reached the highest level in 30 years. Nearly 26,000 cases were reported in the US in 2004, although the actual number may be as high as 600,000 cases annually among adults, according to the CDC. This is partly because only children—not adults—are routinely vaccinated against pertussis.

A new vaccine, called Tdap, provides protection against pertussis as well as tetanus and diphtheria—and it's approved for use by anyone ages 11 to 64. Additional research is needed before it can be approved for people age 65 or older.

Why it's important: Adults infected with pertussis can transmit it to infants and children, who are at a high risk for complications, such as pneumonia, encephalitis (inflammation of the brain), seizures and even death. Older adults also can experience severe complications.

CDC advisory committee recommendation: If it's been 10 years since your last tetanus/diphtheria booster, ask for the Tdap vaccine the next time you see your doctor. Get it as soon as two years after your last booster if you spend time with children.

Side effects or complications: Fever and pain or swelling at the injection site.

Dose: The shot should provide protection for several years, but the exact duration is unknown.

DIABETES

•**Insulin human (rDNA origin) inhalation powder (Exubera).** Most people with diabetes who require insulin give themselves injections three or more times daily. The injections are inconvenient and sometimes uncomfortable.

Exubera is a dry, powdered form of insulin that is administered before each meal via a device similar to an asthma inhaler. It works as quickly as regular injected insulin and appears to be as effective in controlling blood sugar.

Why it's important: Inhaled insulin gives patients another treatment option to maintain optimal glucose control—and it's easier to use than injections.

Side effects or complications: A mild to moderate cough. Some people have a temporary decrease in lung function in the first few weeks after starting treatment.

Important: Pulmonary testing is required before starting inhaled insulin. The tests are repeated at six months, then annually. If lung function declines by more than 20%, the drug should be discontinued and insulin injections resumed.

Caution: Inhaled insulin is not recommended for smokers, people with asthma, chronic obstructive pulmonary disease (COPD) or other lung diseases.

Dose: One or more inhalations taken before meals. The amount varies, depending on an individual's weight and needs.

HEART DISEASE

•**Omega-3-acid ethyl esters (Omacor).** Studies indicate that fish oil, from eating fish or taking supplements, can reduce the risk for cardiovascular death by up to 45%. Fish oil works, in part, by lowering triglycerides, blood fats that are harmful when elevated.

Omacor, a new prescription fish oil, has been found to reduce mortality in patients who have had a recent acute coronary event, such as a heart attack, by 29% after two years. At high doses, it can lower triglycerides by as much as 50%.

Why it's important: Fish oil supplements are sold over-the-counter (OTC), so they aren't monitored by the FDA. Therefore, it's impossible to know if all fish oil products actually contain the amount of omega-3s (the beneficial oils in fish) listed on the label...or if the dose is standard in different products—or even the same from pill to pill. As a prescription drug, Omacor is monitored by the FDA—and is tested to ensure that it meets quality standards.

Note: The US Pharmacopeia (USP), which sets official standards for supplements and drugs, has verified the content and purity of some OTC fish oil products. For a list of several fish oil supplements that have received USP certification, go to the USP Web site, *www.usp.org*.

Side effects or complications: Like fish oil supplements, Omacor may cause belching and/or a fishy aftertaste and can prolong bleeding time in patients taking high doses.

Important: If you take a blood-thinning drug, such as *warfarin* (Coumadin), consult your doctor before taking Omacor.

Dose: 1 g daily for patients who have had a heart attack…and 2 g to 4 g daily for those with elevated triglycerides.

SMOKING

•**Varenicline (Chantix).** It's a non-nicotine drug that appears to work better than other treatments at helping smokers quit.

Why it's important: Varenicline binds to nicotine receptors in the brain and reduces cravings. Studies indicate that it's more effective than nicotine patches or gums or *bupropion* (Zyban), which curbs cravings by altering the brain's chemistry in a way that is not precisely understood. In one 12-week study, the quit rate in smokers taking a placebo was 18%…30% in those taking bupropion…and 44% with varenicline.

Side effects or complications: Nausea or vomiting. It can't be taken by pregnant women because of a risk for birth defects.

Dose: 1 mg to 2 mg daily, divided into two doses.

Dangerous Side Effects Of Common Drugs

Jack E. Fincham, PhD, RPh, A.W. Jowdy professor of pharmacy care, department of clinical and administrative pharmacy at the College of Pharmacy and adjunct professor of public health, Institute of Gerontology Faculty at the University of Georgia in Athens. He is also editor of the *Journal of Public Health Pharmacy* and associate editor of *The American Journal of Pharmaceutical Education*.

Anyone who has ever waded through the fine print on the package insert of a prescription drug knows that the list of potential side effects can be long and alarming —and difficult to understand.

Recent development: The FDA is updating the design used for prescription drug package inserts to make them easier to read. The redesigned package inserts are required for prescription drugs approved on or after June 30, 2006. For drugs approved in the five-year period prior to that date, the new format will be gradually phased in. Inserts for drugs older than that will be revised by manufacturers on a voluntary basis.

However, this good news does not change the fact that all drugs can cause side effects. Depending on the medication, there are literally hundreds of side effects that can occur, potentially affecting every organ system and bodily function.

Gastrointestinal side effects are among the most common. Dozens of drugs, including the antibiotics *ciprofloxacin* (Cipro) and *erythromycin* (E-Mycin), commonly prescribed for urinary tract, respiratory and skin infections, can cause upset stomach, diarrhea and/or abdominal pain.

Other examples: The antibiotic *amoxicillin* (Amoxil) can cause nausea…*digoxin* (Lanoxin), a heart medication, can cause vomiting…narcotic pain medications can cause constipation.

Hives and/or rashes also are common side effects. These skin conditions, which often are the first sign of an allergic reaction to a medication, can occur with aspirin, antibiotics and *atorvastatin* (Lipitor), a cholesterol-lowering drug.

Anaphylactic shock, a potentially fatal type of allergic reaction in which the breathing passages are constricted and blood pressure drops precipitously, may not occur the first time a drug is taken but rather after a third or fourth dose. Swelling (especially around the face and throat) and/or difficulty swallowing are red flags that you may be suffering from a serious allergic reaction.

Important: Each person responds differently to medication—side effects may occur in some people but not in others. It's crucial to understand the potential side effects of the medications you are taking so that you can report any adverse reactions to your doctor and/or pharmacist.

Spend the 10 to 15 minutes it typically requires to carefully read the package insert. Use reading glasses or a magnifying glass, if necessary. Checking a drug reference book (preferably one with large print) also is helpful. When picking up a prescription, ask to speak to the pharmacist about potential side effects. And of course, discuss potential side effects with your doctor when medication is prescribed.

Once you're taking a prescription drug, it's not always easy to identify side effects, because they can mimic the condition that is being treated. Usually the only way to distinguish between the two possibilities is to stop taking the drug—with your doctor's approval—to see if the side effects stop.

Side effects that are often missed by patients—and doctors…

COGNITIVE PROBLEMS

Prescription drugs that affect the central nervous system can impair thinking, memory, alertness and judgment. These include barbiturates, such as *phenobarbital* (Bellatal), prescribed for epilepsy or insomnia…anticholinergics, such as *atropine* (Sal-Tropine) and *scopolamine* (Scopace), prescribed to slow stomach motility (movement of food through the digestive system)…antispasmodics, such as *propantheline* (Pro-Banthine) and *dicyclomine* (Bentyl), for bowel spasms or cramping…muscle relaxants, such as *chlorzoxazone* (Paraflex) and carisoprodol (Soma), for muscle stiffness or back spasms…and antidepressants, such as *paroxetine* (Paxil) and *fluoxetine* (Prozac). Central nervous system stimulants, such as *methylphenidate* (Ritalin), also can affect cognition. Stimulant drugs are often used for attention deficit hyperactivity disorder (ADHD).

What you may not know: Certain blood pressure medications, such as *methyldopa* (Aldomet) and *clonidine* (Catapres), may affect heart rate and/or cardiac output (the pumping efficiency of the heart), which can lead to disorientation.

Cognitive symptoms to watch for: Cognitive changes, such as forgetting simple things that you normally remember, are worth noting. If family members and/or friends tell you that they see a change in your cognitive function, consult your doctor and/or pharmacist. Your doctor may be able to adjust the dosage, or it may help to take the drug at night. As an alternative, your doctor may prescribe an equally effective drug that won't trigger side effects in you.

SEXUAL DYSFUNCTION

Antidepressants, including the widely prescribed selective serotonin reuptake inhibitors (SSRIs), such as *fluoxetine* (Prozac) and *escitalopram* (Lexapro), are known to cause sexual dysfunction, including changes in libido, inability to reach orgasm and/or difficulty achieving an erection. Diuretics, such as furosemide (Lasix) and hydrochlorothiazide, can lead to male impotence. Some drugs that are used to treat benign prostatic hypertrophy (a condition in which the prostate gland is enlarged), such as *finasteride* (Proscar) or *dutasteride* (Avodart), also can affect sexual functioning, as can antianxiety agents, including *alprazolam* (Xanax), *lorazepam* (Ativan) and *diazepam* (Valium).

What you may not know: Older types of drugs used to treat acid reflux and ulcers, including H2 antagonist drugs, such as *cimetidine* (Tagamet), block androgen receptors, which are necessary for male sex hormone activity. These drugs also can decrease testosterone synthesis, leading to impotence and breast enlargement in some men. Newer H2 antagonist drugs, such as *famotidine* (Pepcid) and *nizatidine* (Axid), and some of the proton pump inhibitors, including *omeprazole* (Prilosec) and *esomeprazole* (Nexium), don't have this effect.

Sexual dysfunction symptoms to watch for: Report any changes in sexual function, including inability to have or maintain an erection, change in libido and inability to reach orgasm, to your doctor and/or pharmacist as soon as possible. Your doctor may adjust the drug dosage, prescribe an alternative medication in the same class or suggest alternative dosing schedules, such as taking the drug in the early morning.

WEIGHT GAIN

Some newer drugs, including the antipsychotic agents *olanzapine* (Zyprexa) and *quetiapine* (Seroquel), which are used to treat severe mental disorders, such as schizophrenia, may cause weight gain. The antidepressant *bupropion* (Wellbutrin), which is often used instead of an SSRI because it typically does not cause sexual side effects, also can trigger weight gain.

What you may not know: Some diabetes drugs, such as *glyburide* (DiaBeta) and *chlorpropamide* (Diabinese), can lead to weight gain.

Weight gain symptoms to watch for: If you gain more than five pounds in any four- to six-week period that you are taking a drug, speak to your pharmacist and/or doctor. Consider weighing yourself daily if you are prescribed a drug that can cause weight gain. Meanwhile, try reducing daily calories and/or exercising more to control any weight gain.

■ **More from Dr. Fincham…**

Best Ways to Avoid Side Effects

To help guard against potentially dangerous side effects, follow these steps when your doctor prescribes medication…

•**Review the dosage.** Drug dosages are usually determined by studies based on young, healthy volunteers or patients with uncomplicated diseases. People who have less body mass (under 120 pounds) don't need the same dose as someone who tops 200 pounds.

What to do: Ask your doctor if he/she is prescribing the lowest possible dose for a person your weight.

•**Mention your age.** As we age, our kidneys and liver are less efficient at metabolizing drugs.

What to do: Ask your doctor whether he is prescribing the lowest possible dose for a person your age.

■ ■ ■ ■

Nicotine Drugs to Quit Smoking

Smokers who use nicotine-replacement medications are twice as likely to kick the habit as people who try to quit cold turkey. These medications deliver small, steady doses of nicotine to ease withdrawal symptoms without the toxic substances contained in cigarettes. Always consult your physician before trying a nicotine-replacement drug.

Over-the-counter and prescription options available…

•**Nicotine patch.** People who smoke a pack or more a day should start with the patch, a full-strength replacement medication. Available over-the-counter and by prescription.

Nicotine gum should be chewed and held in the mouth for about 30 minutes every hour or two. Not for people with dentures. Over-the-counter only.

•**Nicotine inhaler.** Good for smokers who like the hand-to-mouth feeling. People trying to quit smoking can take a puff of the inhaler several hundred times a day. Prescription only.

•**Nicotine lozenges.** Less conspicuous to use than gum, inhalers or spray, lozenges last 20 to 30 minutes. People can use up to 20 a day. Over-the-counter only.

•**Nicotine nasal spray.** This product can be used once or twice an hour. Not for people with asthma. Prescription only.

Michael Fiore, MD, MPH, professor of medicine and director of the Center for Tobacco Research and Intervention, University of Wisconsin, Madison.

Is There an 'Exercise' Pill?

Ronald M. Evans, PhD, investigator and Howard Hughes Medical Institute professor, Salk Institute, San Diego.

Leah Whigham, PhD, research scientist, University of Wisconsin, Madison.

A pill might one day achieve the same calorie-burning effects that vigorous exercise does.

It's possible, according to Ronald M. Evans, a scientist at the Salk Institute in San Diego who has developed a potential weight-loss drug that revved up cellular metabolism in mice.

EXCITING RESEARCH

In the study, the drug "protected the mice who were on high-fat and high-caloric diets and prevented them from gaining weight," he said. "We're very excited to see if the drug will work for people, too."

At stake is a medical solution for people who want to lose weight but who either don't diet and exercise properly or who just can't lose enough. Diet pills have existed for decades, but they have significant side effects and aren't always effective.

One possible solution is to increase the body's metabolism, the process that turns food into energy. That's where Evans's drug enters the picture.

HOW IT WORKS

The drug uses chemicals to turn on a genetic switch in the body known as PPAR-d.

When given the drug in the form of a liquid or powder, the bodies of mice appear to act as if they are exercising even when they aren't, causing their metabolism to speed up, Evans explained. "You then have lower fatty acid levels in the blood, lower triglyceride levels and lower sugar levels," he said. "They all appear to be linked."

Mice who received the drug were also able to exercise twice as long, turning into what researchers call "marathon mice."

COULD IT WORK ON HUMANS?

According to Evans, the drug could indeed become a "fat pill," although "anything like this would be more effective if it were part of a regimen of a healthy diet and exercise. If you only took the drug, weight loss will always be somewhat of a challenge."

Several companies are testing drugs that target the genetic switch in people, Evans said.

While an effective weight-loss pill is the "holy grail" of obesity research, there are plenty of reasons to be cautious about the new finding, said Leah Whigham, a research scientist who studies nutrition at the University of Wisconsin in Madison.

"The most obvious caution is that this research was conducted on mice, which are very different from humans and have different energy expenditure mechanisms. It remains to be seen if this research can translate into something useful for humans," she said.

There is also less diversity in mice than in humans. "Something that works in all mice of a given strain might not be as effective across a population of humans who have different genetic, ethnic, cultural and environmental backgrounds," she explained.

Still, Whigham said, "that doesn't mean this research isn't very exciting. It is just very preliminary at this point."

info To learn more about obesity from NAASO, the Obesity Society, visit their Web site at *www.obesity.org*.

Popular Drugs That Steal Nutrients

Frederic Vagnini, MD, medical director of the Heart, Diabetes and Weight-Loss Centers of New York and an assistant clinical professor of surgery at Weill Cornell Medical College, both in New York City. Dr. Vagnini is coauthor of *The Side Effects Bible: The Dietary Solution to Unwanted Side Effects of Common Medications*. Broadway.

Depletion of nutrients is among the most common—and overlooked—side effects of both over-the-counter (OTC) and prescription drugs, according to Frederic Vagnini of Weill Cornell Medical College.

Here's what happens: Medications can cause improper absorption of vitamins and minerals—or they can accelerate the elimination of nutrients from the body. The consequences may range from bothersome symptoms, such as fatigue or stomach upset, to serious heart, muscle or nerve damage.

Most doctors are aware of some minerals that are depleted through the use of diuretics (water-excreting drugs). However, few doctors are aware of the dangers of nutrient depletion caused by many other types of medication, because the problem is not widely reported.

Popular drugs that deplete the body of nutrients...

ANTIBIOTICS

The most commonly prescribed antibiotics include *azithromycin* (Zithromax), *amoxicillin* (Amoxil), *ampicillin* (Omnipen), *ciprofloxacin* (Cipro), *ofloxacin* (Floxin) and *erythromycin* (Eryc).

Nutrients depleted...

• **B vitamins.** The B vitamins are essential for normal metabolism as well as immune and nervous system functioning.

• **Vitamin K.** This vitamin is critical for blood clotting and bone strength.

• **"Friendly" intestinal bacteria** known as *Bifidobacterium bifidum* and *Lactobacillus acidophilus*. Antibiotics kill not only harmful bacteria but also "good" bacteria that promote gastrointestinal health and help balance immune response.

If you are prescribed an antibiotic: Ask your doctor about also taking a B-complex vitamin—50 mg...vitamin K supplement—60 micrograms (mcg) to 80 mcg...and probiotic supplements providing 15 billion live B. bifidum and 15 billion live L. acidophilus organisms daily.*

In addition, eat more vitamin B–rich foods, such as beef liver, chicken, pork, fortified breads and cereals, whole-grain pastas, legumes, nuts and dark, leafy greens.

To increase your intake of vitamin K, eat kale ...collard, turnip or mustard greens...spinach... broccoli...and Swiss chard.

Caution: Do not take vitamin K supplements or eat excessive amounts of vitamin K–rich foods if you take *warfarin* (Coumadin) or another blood-thinning drug.

For additional B. bifidum, eat more asparagus, garlic and/or onions, which stimulate growth of this friendly bacteria. For L. acidophilus, yogurt containing live cultures is your best food source.

HIGH-CHOLESTEROL DRUGS

The most widely prescribed cholesterol-lowering "statins" include *atorvastatin* (Lipitor), *simvastatin* (Zocor), *fluvastatin* (Lescol), *lovastatin* (Mevacor) and *pravastatin* (Pravachol).

Nutrient depleted...

•**Coenzyme Q10 (CoQ10).** All cells require CoQ10 for the proper function of mitochondria (tiny energy-producing structures within the cells). The more energy a cell must produce, the more it depends on CoQ10. That's why cells of the heart, in particular—because it is constantly beating—require an abundance of CoQ10.

Unfortunately, statin drugs, which effectively block the production of harmful cholesterol, also prevent CoQ10 production.

Some doctors worry that long-term use of statins may worsen heart failure. Studies have found that patients with chronic heart failure have lower CoQ10 levels, and that CoQ10 supplements may improve their heart condition. Signs of CoQ10 deficiency include fatigue and muscle weakness.

If you are prescribed a statin: Ask your doctor about taking 30 mg to 100 mg of a CoQ10

*If you're taking any medications, consult your doctor before changing your diet or beginning a supplement. In rare cases, increasing a nutrient may interfere with a drug's potency or worsen your condition.

supplement daily. This nutrient also is available in some foods, including beef, chicken, salmon, oranges and broccoli.

PAINKILLERS

Millions of Americans take a nonsteroidal anti-inflammatory drug (NSAID), such as *ibuprofen* (Motrin, Advil), *naproxen* (Aleve), *celecoxib* (Celebrex) and *nabumetone* (Relafen), to help relieve arthritis and other inflammatory pain.

Nutrient depleted...

•**Folic acid.** Your body needs this water-soluble B vitamin to produce new cells and DNA and to synthesize and utilize proteins.

Several large epidemiological studies have linked low folic acid levels to increased risk for colon, breast and pancreatic cancers.

Heart health is also affected by folic acid. As folic acid levels decline, levels of the amino acid homocysteine rise. Studies suggest that elevated homocysteine can raise the risks for blood clots, heart attack and stroke.

Low folic acid levels may cause loss of appetite, irritability, weakness, shortness of breath, diarrhea, anemia, headaches, heart palpitations and a sore tongue.

If you take an NSAID regularly (daily for at least one to two weeks): Talk to your physician about also taking 400 mcg to 800 mcg of folic acid daily.

You also can get more folic acid by consuming fortified breakfast cereals, orange juice, spinach and other leafy greens, peas and beans.

BETA-BLOCKERS

Beta-blockers, such as *propranolol* (Inderal), *atenolol* (Tenormin), *betaxolol* (Betoptic S), *carteolol* (Cartrol) and *labetalol* (Normodyne), are commonly prescribed for high blood pressure or glaucoma.

Nutrients depleted...

•**CoQ10.** Not only does CoQ10 appear to improve cardiac function in patients with chronic heart failure, studies suggest that it also may prevent second heart attacks and possibly protect against Parkinson's disease.

•**Melatonin.** The hormone melatonin is essential for healthy sleep-wake cycles, and there's some early evidence that it may slow aging.

If you take a beta-blocker: Ask your physician about taking 30 mg to 100 mg of CoQ10 daily...and 1 mg to 3 mg of melatonin nightly, just before bed, if you have trouble sleeping.

ACE INHIBITORS

Angiotensin-converting enzyme (ACE) inhibitors, such as *enalapril* (Vasotec), *benazepril* (Lotensin) and *ramipril* (Altace), as well as angiotensin II receptor blockers (ARBs), including *candesartan* (Atacand) and *irbesartan* (Avapro), are prescribed for high blood pressure and heart failure, and to help prevent heart attacks in high-risk patients.

Nutrient depleted...

•**Zinc.** Zinc boosts immunity, and some studies have shown that it reduces the duration of cold symptoms.

Zinc also is necessary for wound healing, strong bones and male potency, and it may help slow the progression of age-related macular degeneration (AMD).

In a recent six-year National Eye Institute study involving 3,600 people with AMD, zinc and antioxidant supplements reduced the risk of developing advanced AMD by 25%.

If you take an ACE inhibitor or ARB: Ask your doctor about taking 50 mg to 100 mg of zinc daily and eating more zinc-rich foods, such as oysters, beef, dark-meat chicken, pork tenderloin, yogurt, milk, peas, beans and nuts. If you continue to take zinc indefinitely, do not exceed 50 mg daily.

Important: Many medications combine an ACE inhibitor or ARB with a diuretic—for example, enalapril and *hydrochlorothiazide* (Vaseretic) is an ACE inhibitor plus a diuretic...*candesartan* and *hydrochlorothiazide* (Atacand HCT) is an ARB plus a diuretic.

If you're taking a combination drug, you'll need to compensate not only for zinc, but also for the electrolytes and nutrients excreted by the diuretic, including potassium, magnesium, *thiamine* (B-1) and calcium. Ask your doctor for advice.

DIABETES DRUGS

People with type 2 diabetes are often prescribed *tolazamide* (Tolinase), *acetohexamide* (Dymelor), *glimepiride* (Amaryl) or *glipizide* (Glucotrol)—all sulfonylurea drugs. These medications stimulate the pancreas to produce more insulin, which lowers blood sugar.

Nutrient depleted...

•**CoQ10.** Diabetes more than doubles your chances of dying from heart disease or stroke—and low CoQ10 levels exacerbate those risks.

If you're taking a sulfonylurea drug: Ask your doctor about supplementing with 30 mg to 100 mg of CoQ10 daily.

REFLUX DRUGS

Proton pump inhibitors, such as *esomeprazole* (Nexium), *lansoprazole* (Prevacid), *omeprazole* (Prilosec) and *rabeprazole* (Acip-Hex), are prescribed for chronic heartburn—also known as gastroesophageal reflux disease (GERD)—and ulcers.

Nutrients depleted...

•**Vitamin B-12.** Vitamin B-12 is essential for producing red blood cells and maintaining a healthy nervous system. Deficits may cause fatigue, dizziness, shortness of breath, diarrhea, tingling in the hands or feet, unsteady gait, nervousness, cognitive changes and even dementia.

Vitamin B-12 is found in red meat, fish, eggs and dairy foods, but our bodies require stomach acid to release the vitamin from these foods. Proton pump inhibitors reduce the production of stomach acid, inhibiting the release and absorption of vitamin B-12.

•**Iron.** Low iron reduces the amount of oxygen your red blood cells can transport to body tissues, leaving you feeling weak and fatigued. A serious iron deficiency results in anemia.

If you take a proton pump inhibitor: Ask your doctor about taking 500 mcg to 1,000 mcg of vitamin B-12 daily and for advice on the best way to increase your iron intake.

Caution: Never take an iron supplement without consulting your physician—excess iron can accumulate in your major organs and cause severe damage. Most people, however, can safely eat more iron-rich foods, including liver, beef, dark-meat chicken or turkey, legumes and fortified cereals.

■ ■ ■ ■

Melatonin May Improve Symptoms of Tinnitus

About 15 million Americans have severe tinnitus, the sensation of a ringing, roaring or humming sound. Sleep disturbance is common among tinnitus sufferers.

Recent study: Researchers gave people with tinnitus 3 milligrams (mg) of melatonin every night for one month to help them sleep, then tracked them for a second month when they did not take the supplement. By the end of the study, tinnitus symptoms had been reduced by nearly 30%. Participants slept best while taking melatonin, but the improvement in their sleep and tinnitus symptoms continued through the month when they were not taking it. Patients with the greatest sleep disturbances improved the most.

Jay F. Piccirillo, MD, professor, otolaryngology–head and neck surgery, Washington University School of Medicine, St. Louis, and lead author of a study of tinnitus sufferers, published in *Otolaryngology—Head and Neck Surgery*.

Study Questions Antibiotic Guideline for Treatment of Pneumonia

Jesse M. Pines, MD, attending physician, department of emergency medicine, Hospital of the University of Pennsylvania, Philadelphia.

Tareg Bey, MD, professor, emergency medicine, and director, International Emergency Medicine, department of emergency medicine, University of California, Irvine.

Annals of Emergency Medicine.

Many patients arriving at US hospital emergency rooms who receive antibiotics based on a federal guideline to treat pneumonia don't need the drugs, a new study contends.

That means the guideline may not be feasible and may be contributing to the growing problem of antibiotic resistance, the study authors said.

The researchers were studying a 2004 guideline that stipulates that emergency-room doctors administer antibiotics within four hours to adult patients displaying symptoms of pneumonia.

The Centers for Medicare and Medicaid Services (CMS) and the Joint Commission on Accreditation of Healthcare Organizations (JCAHO) established the guideline as a core measure of hospital performance. Earlier studies had shown that administering antibiotics within this time window was associated with a small decrease in death rates.

The University HealthSystem Consortium, an alliance representing almost 90% of the nation's nonprofit academic medical centers, has a goal of achieving 90% compliance with the guideline. At the University of California, San Francisco, where the study was done, nonphysician staff bonuses are dependent upon this performance.

ABOUT THE STUDY

The study followed a group of 152 emergency room patients who met eligibility criteria for receiving antibiotics. Of this group, 65.1% received antibiotics within four hours of arriving at the hospital. The remaining 34.9% were identified as "outliers," and more than half (58.5%) of the outliers did not have a final diagnosis of pneumonia. And 43% of the outliers had an abnormal chest X-ray, compared with 95% of those who received antibiotics.

"It was not possible in many of the cases to actually have given them antibiotics because a lot of them didn't actually have pneumonia or got a diagnosis later," said Dr. Jesse Pines, an attending physician in the department of emergency medicine at the Hospital of the University of Pennsylvania in Philadelphia. He supports the study findings.

The authors concluded that it may not be feasible to identify 90% of emergency department patients admitted with pneumonia using the current JCAHO/CMS case definitions. Either the goal or the case definitions need to be changed, the researchers said.

Pneumonia is the leading cause of visits to an emergency room, Pines said.

TIME FOR A CHANGE

Many experts are critical of the guideline and the studies on which they were based.

"I think it is extremely problematic and controversial when CMS and Joint Commission create national performance standards based on retrospective, clinically nonvalidated retrospective studies," said Dr. Tareg Bey, professor of emergency medicine and director of international emergency medicine at the University of California, Irvine. "I could easily imagine that this program would increase antibiotic-resistance of pneumonia bacteria just because physicians prescribe antibiotics earlier and more often to meet the goals of the CMS program.

"Performance-based medicine is principally a good thing, but it has to be based on very powerful scientific data," Bey added. "Retrospective studies alone, and not recognizing the complex interdependencies of our extremely stressed health-care delivery system, are not good enough to link a four-hour rule to a performance for payment program."

THE REAL PROBLEM

Pines said the guideline may not even address the main underlying problem, which is emergency-room crowding.

"Because emergency rooms are so crowded, getting a chest X-ray and doing all the things that go into getting a rapid diagnosis of pneumonia is not possible," he said. "What's happening with the performance measure is that patients with suspected pneumonia end up getting antibiotics before they have a diagnosis in order to meet the government-mandated standard."

info For advice on when antibiotic use is appropriate, visit the American Academy of Family Physicians at *http://familydoctor.org*.

Constipation Drug Pulled From Market

Roshini Rajapaksa, MD, gastroenterologist, New York University Medical Center and assistant professor at the NYU School of Medicine, New York City.

John K. Jenkins, MD, director, Office of New Drugs, Center for Drug Evaluation and Research, US Food and Drug Administration.

Z elnorm, a drug that is used to treat constipation associated with irritable bowel syndrome (IBS), has been taken off the market because of an increased risk of heart attack, stroke and death, US health officials said recently.

People who suffer from IBS have bowels that do not function properly and may experience symptoms such as abdominal pain or discomfort (often reported as cramping, bloating, gas, diarrhea, and/or constipation).

"Novartis, the maker of Zelnorm, has voluntarily agreed to stop marketing the drug in the United States," said Dr. John K. Jenkins, director of the Office of New Drugs, Center for Drug Evaluation and Research at the US Food and Drug Administration (FDA).

Zelnorm (generic name *tegaserod maleate*) was first approved by the FDA in 2002 for the short-term treatment of women with irritable bowel syndrome whose primary symptom was constipation. Two years later, the drug was approved for the treatment of chronic constipation in men and women under age 65, Jenkins said.

The withdrawal was prompted by a recent review of 29 studies. The review was undertaken by Novartis at the request of a Swiss health agency. The FDA reviewed that data and decided that the risk-to-benefit profile of Zelnorm was no longer favorable, Jenkins said.

WHAT THE REVIEW FOUND

It was discovered that 13 out of 11,614 patients taking the drug had a cardiac event, including one death, compared with one case among 7,031 patients who took a placebo.

"While the absolute risk was small, the relative risk was significantly greater," Jenkins said.

The FDA is advising patients who take the drug to see their doctor to discuss alternative treatments, Jenkins said. "There may be some patients with severe symptoms that do not have other effective treatment options," he said.

The agency has agreed that Novartis can make a new drug application to allow patients with no other treatment options to get Zelnorm, Jenkins said. "For these patients, the benefits may outweigh the risks," he said.

The FDA has also agreed to consider a reintroduction of Zelnorm, provided there is data that indicate that, for some patients, the benefits of the drug outweigh the risks, Jenkins said.

PATIENTS DON'T HAVE MANY OPTIONS

Dr. Roshini Rajapaksa, a gastroenterologist at New York University Medical Center and assistant professor at the NYU School of Medicine, said, "This is very big and disturbing news, because Zelnorm was really the only effective and approved drug available for irritable bowel syndrome with constipation.

"IBS is the most commonly diagnosed gastrointestinal condition and is second only to the common cold as a cause of absence from work," he added. "People, mostly women, really suffer from this condition, and Zelnorm offered real relief to many. I think patients are going to be very reluctant to give up the Zelnorm, but strokes and heart attacks are much more deadly than IBS, so it is appropriate to pull the drug."

info For more information on IBS, visit the US National Digestive Diseases Information Clearinghouse at *http://digestive.niddk.nih.gov.*

Drugs Work as Well as Angioplasty

William E. Boden, MD, professor of medicine and public health, University at Buffalo School of Medicine and Biomedical Sciences, NY.
Judith S. Hochman, MD, professor of cardiology, New York University School of Medicine, New York City.
American College of Cardiology annual meeting, New Orleans.
New England Journal of Medicine.

Aggressive drug therapy appears to be just as good as angioplasty for patients with stable heart disease, a new study finds.

"This is really good news for patients," said study lead author Dr. William E. Boden, a professor of medicine and public health at the University at Buffalo School of Medicine and Biomedical Sciences. "We have more treatment options for patients than we thought we did."

EXCITING NEW RESEARCH

There has been a belief that patients with chronic stable heart disease need to have either an angioplasty or heart bypass surgery, Boden said. "There has been an unproven assumption that patients must proceed to some type of revascularization procedure," he said.

Patients with stable heart disease make up about three-quarters of all the patients who undergo angioplasty and receive stents in the United States, Boden noted. Angioplasty is a medical procedure that uses a balloon to open narrowed or clogged blood vessels of the heart. Usually, during the procedure a stent—a wire mesh tube—is placed in the vessel to keep it open.

"What the Clinical Outcomes Utilizing Revascularization and Aggressive Drug Evaluation (COURAGE) trial tells us is that optimal medical [drug] therapy, when combined with lifestyle changes, appears to be the equal of angioplasty and optimal medical therapy combined," Boden said.

THE STUDY

For the study, the COURAGE group randomly assigned almost 2,300 patients with stable but significant heart disease to one of two treatment regimens at 50 United States and Canadian treatment centers. The first group received drug therapy alone, while the second group received the drug therapy plus angioplasty. In the latter group, 94% received at least one stent.

During a follow-up from two to seven years, the researchers looked for incidence of heart attack or death. They found that 211 people (19%) in the angioplasty group had died or had a heart attack, compared with 202 people (18.5%) in the group that only received drug treatment.

There were also no significant differences between patients who had angioplasty and those who had drug therapy alone in rates of death, heart attack, stroke or hospitalization for acute coronary syndrome (20% vs. 19.5%) or heart attack alone (13.2% vs. 12.3%).

The only benefit of angioplasty, according to Boden's team, was that it reduced chest pain over the long-term compared with drug therapy alone.

SOMETIMES ADDITIONAL HELP REQUIRED

About 30% of the patients who received drug therapy alone did eventually undergo angioplasty because their symptoms couldn't be managed with drugs alone. In addition, about 21% of the patients who received stents needed to have another procedure, Boden said.

Based on these findings, Boden believes that drug therapy for patients with stable heart disease should be tried as first-line treatment. "I am hopeful that physicians will have the courage to consider medical therapy as a viable option," he said.

However, Boden doesn't think initial use of drug therapy alone will reduce the number of angioplasties being performed. "What it may do is delay the timing of when angioplasty gets done," he said.

"As an initial strategy, medical therapy is a defendable approach," Boden added. "We should no longer consider it to be putting patients in harm's way, or thinking of it as an inferior treatment strategy."

The COURAGE trial was sponsored by the US Department of Veterans Affairs Office of Research and Development and the Canadian Institutes of Health Research, and research grants from a number of top pharmaceutical companies.

STENT TYPE QUESTIONED

The makers of stents and physicians who support their use were critical of the study, saying its design left it "doomed to fail," according to published reports.

Addressing some of the critics' concerns, including the fact that the trial didn't include drug-coated stents, Boden said that these stents were not available at the start of the trial.

"We would have loved to use them," he said. "But there is not a shred of scientific evidence to support the fact that drug-eluting stents are superior to bare-metal stents, in terms of reducing death and heart attack. Using drug-eluting stents would have no difference in the primary endpoint. It might have resulted in fewer revascularizations."

VIABLE INITIAL OPTION?

One expert agrees that drug therapy is a viable initial option for most patients with stable heart disease.

"Intensive medical therapy to dramatically reduce risk factors, such as reducing bad cholesterol and raising the good cholesterol, was associated with outcomes that were similar when that same therapy was used and angioplasty was added," said Dr. Judith S. Hochman, a professor of cardiology at New York University School of Medicine.

"There was no additional benefit from angioplasty, beyond what has evolved to be excellent medical therapy," she added.

Hochman said it was striking that many patients had reductions in chest pain on drug therapy alone. "Many patients became angina-free," she said. "Although angioplasty was better at relieving symptoms, it wasn't better in preventing death or heart attack."

Hochman noted, however, that if a person is having a heart attack, angioplasty remains the appropriate treatment. "If you are having a high-risk unstable syndrome, angioplasty is very effective at reducing the chance of dying," she said.

But, for patients with stable heart disease, Hochman believes the first approach to care should be medications. "A trial of intensive medical therapy without angioplasty, to see how the symptoms respond, is what's indicated," she said.

Angioplasty should be reserved for patients who have continuing symptoms, Hochman said. "If you have too much angina to do the activities you want to do, despite a trial of intensive medical therapy, then angioplasty is a good option," she said.

info To learn more about heart disease, visit the US National Library of Medicine at *www.nlm.nih.gov/medlineplus/heartdiseases.html*.

Are Doctors Paid to Prescribe These Dangerous Drugs?

Len Lichtenfeld, MD, deputy chief medical officer, American Cancer Society, Atlanta.

Ajay Singh, MD, clinical chief, renal division, director, dialysis, Brigham and Women's Hospital, and associate professor, medicine, Harvard Medical School, Boston.

The New York Times.
Bloomberg.

A US Food and Drug Administration advisory panel recently called for new warnings and additional safety studies on anemia drugs commonly used to treat patients undergoing kidney dialysis or chemotherapy.

These medications have been the subject of controversy since some of their dangerous side effects—including the risk of heart attacks and stroke—came to light earlier this year. In March, the FDA issued stronger label warnings for the popular drugs.

Two months later, the agency's advisory panel of experts voted 15-2 in favor of new prescribing restrictions and 17-0 for new clinical trials to prove the safety of Amgen's Aranesp and Johnson & Johnson's Procrit, *Bloomberg* reported.

FURTHER EXAMINATION NEEDED

"Many of us on the committee are concerned and have a lot of questions," said advisory panel chairwoman Gail Eckhardt, an oncologist at the University of Colorado in Aurora, according to *Bloomberg.*

Eckhardt said the questions concerned the design of the trials, why regulators have limited access to results from company studies, and why the drugs have been marketed for improving quality of life if there isn't sufficient evidence for the claim.

Amgen, of Thousand Oaks, California, claims that 4 million patients have taken the medicines since they were introduced in 1989, and more than 9,000 people have been studied in clinical trials with cancer patients, the *Bloomberg* report said.

"We want to consider the totality of the evidence and consider what's best for patients," Roger Perlmutter, Amgen's head of research and development, told the panel. The anemia drugs don't shorten patients' life spans or make tumors spread more rapidly, based on the findings of 55 studies, he added.

The FDA isn't required to follow the recommendations of its advisory panels but typically does.

DANGEROUS SIDE EFFECTS

The drugs *darbepoetin* (Aranesp) and *epoetin alfa* (Epogen and Procrit) are genetically engineered versions of a natural protein, erythropoietin, that boosts red blood cell counts to combat anemia. The recent research has shown that they can lead to blood clots, strokes, heart attacks and death in patients with chronic kidney failure who receive them at higher-than-recommended doses, a practice that is becoming increasingly common. Other studies have discovered that higher doses might produce more rapid tumor growth in patients with head and neck cancer.

"There has clearly been an issue raised about the efficacy, the effectiveness and safety of these drugs when used to treat anemia from cancer," said Dr. Len Lichtenfeld, deputy chief medical officer at the American Cancer Society, before the panel voted.

Another expert said he thinks the FDA needs to carefully define when and for whom these drugs should be used.

"The FDA needs to provide a strong message and guidelines about under what circumstances, and for what populations, patients need to be treated with these drugs," said Dr. Ajay Singh, clinical chief of the renal division and director of dialysis at Brigham and Women's Hospital in Boston.

"In addition, we need updated and independent guidelines that advise doctors how to use these drugs that support what the FDA is recommending," Singh said.

Anemia is a common side effect with certain forms of kidney disease, especially for patients undergoing dialysis, and for cancer patients undergoing chemotherapy. The three drugs are approved to treat anemia in patients with chronic kidney failure and in patients with cancer whose anemia is caused by chemotherapy. Epogen and Procrit are also approved for patients scheduled for major surgery to reduce potential blood transfusions and for the treatment of anemia due to zidovudine therapy in HIV patients, the FDA said.

Lichtenfeld noted that, when used properly, these medications are effective. They are really for patients undergoing chemotherapy or radiation, not for patients who have completed their treatment, he said.

"These drugs are valuable, and they do play a significant role in helping patients during chemotherapy," Lichtenfeld said. "They help people get through treatment and help reduce the need for transfusion."

ARE KICKBACKS INVOLVED?

Singh thinks there have been financial incentives that promote the off-label use of these drugs, which, in this case, involves increasing the patient's hemoglobin level above that recommended on the label.

"We need to have [Medicare] reimbursement guidelines that remove some of the incentives for off-label use of these drugs," Singh said.

Lichtenfeld noted these drugs make up the majority of medications reimbursed by Medicare for treating cancer patients. "And their use has been going up every year," he added.

"There appears to be a substantial off-label use of these drugs," Singh said. "Physicians need to be cognizant of the label, because it is put into place in a deliberate and thoughtful manner. The off-label use needs to be curtailed."

The New York Times reported that Amgen and Johnson & Johnson paid doctors millions of dollars in rebates to use these drugs.

"Such payments—to cancer doctors and the other big users of the drugs, like kidney dialysis centers—total hundreds of millions of dollars a year and are an important source of profit for doctors and the centers. The payments have risen over the last several years, as the makers of the drugs, Amgen and Johnson & Johnson, compete for market share and try to expand the overall business," the *Times* reported.

Doctors quoted in the article said their use of the drugs was influenced by the amount of money they could make and the belief that the drugs were useful.

info For more information on these anemia drugs, visit the US Food and Drug Administration at *www.fda.gov.*

Wake Up to the Dangerous Side Effects Of Sleeping Pills

Gregg Jacobs, PhD, insomnia specialist, Sleep Disorders Center, Beth Israel Deaconess Medical Center, and assistant professor, psychiatry, Harvard Medical School, Boston.

Russell Katz, MD, director, US Food and Drug Administration, division of neurology, Office of Drug Evaluation I, Center for Drug Evaluation and Research, Washington, DC.

Prescription sleeping pills, including such popular brands as Ambien and Lunesta, can cause strange and potentially dangerous side effects, the US Food and Drug Administration warned recently.

Those side effects can include dangerous allergic reactions and bizarre behaviors such as "sleep-driving," in which a person will drive a car while not fully awake and have no memory of doing so.

NEW FDA REQUESTS

The FDA is asking makers of the sleep aids, called sedative-hypnotic drugs, to strengthen product labels to include stronger warnings about the potential risks. In addition to "sleep-driving," the agency said it has received reports of consumers walking or eating while not fully awake, and not remembering it later.

"Because these drugs are designed to put people to sleep, they might not know that they are having a side effect," said Dr. Russell Katz, director of the FDA's division of neurology in the Office of Drug Evaluation I, Center for Drug Evaluation and Research in Washington, DC.

Sleep-driving and other strange behaviors might occur if consumers take a higher-than-recommended dose of the drug, or drink alcohol or consume other similar drugs, Katz said. "We believe that all the drugs in the class can produce these effects," he said.

Katz said it's not possible to know how many cases of these side effects have occurred because the system for reporting adverse effects is voluntary. "We believe these are rare occurrences," he said. "But we don't know the actual number of cases."

The 13 drugs involved are: Ambien and Ambien CR, made by Sanofi Aventis; Butisol Sodium, made by Medpointe Pharm HLC; Carbrital, made by Parke-Davis; Dalmane, made by Valeant Pharm; Doral, made by Questcor Pharms; Halcion, made by Pharmacia & Upjohn; Lunesta, made by Sepracor; Placidyl and Prosom, made by Abbott; Restoril, made by Tyco Healthcare; Rozerem, made by Takeda; Seconal, made by Lilly; and Sonata, made by King Pharmaceuticals.

At the end of last year, the FDA sent letters to the drug makers, asking them to revise their product labels to include warnings about the potential for severe allergic reactions—called anaphylaxis—and severe facial swelling—called angioedema.

At that time, the FDA also asked the manufacturers to add warnings about complex sleep-related behaviors, including sleep-driving, making phone calls, and preparing and eating food or having sex while asleep, Katz said.

In addition to these label changes, the FDA is asking the manufacturers to send letters to health-care providers notifying them about the new warnings.

The FDA has also asked the drug manufacturers to develop "Patient Medication Guides" to inform people about the risks associated with these drugs and precautions they can take. These guides will be given to patients when one of these drugs is prescribed. There is no deadline for the availability of these guides, Katz said.

HOW TO MINIMIZE RISKS

Katz said people can minimize their risk of side effects by taking only the prescribed dose and not mixing the drugs with alcohol or other medicines that have similar effects.

Since little is known about these drugs and their potential side effects, the FDA has recommended that the drug makers carry out clinical studies to find out which medications are most associated with sleep-driving and other odd sleep behaviors.

"So far, no drug company has agreed to do these studies," Katz said.

One insomnia expert thinks the labeling changes for these drugs are long overdue, but don't go far enough.

"It's about time," said Gregg Jacobs, an insomnia specialist at the Sleep Disorders Center at the Beth Israel Deaconess Medical Center and an assistant professor of psychiatry at Harvard Medical School, both in Boston. "It's been demonstrated that pharmaceutical companies exaggerate the benefits of medication and minimize the side effects."

LONG-TERM STUDIES NEEDED

Since little is known about the long-term side effects of these sleep medications, the FDA should make the drug companies do long-term studies on the potential risks, Jacobs said.

"The side effects that the drug companies have studied are based only on short-term studies," he said. "The typical study on sleeping pills averages seven days, but the majority of people who take sleeping pills take them, on average, for 24 months, and a third use them for five years."

Jacobs also said he thinks the number of people who experience sleep-behavior side effects is underreported "because many people don't remember having them.

"In my practice, 10% of people who take sleeping pills have reported some kind of side effects that involve amnesia. The only way they know it is that a family member tells them about it," he said. "If somebody lives on his own, he won't know it.

More than 20 million Americans suffer from chronic insomnia, which is defined as poor sleep every night or most nights for more than six months, according to the American Insomnia Association.

According to *Consumer Reports,* pharmacists filled 43 million prescriptions for sleep drugs in 2005, a 32% increase from 2001. Prescription insomnia medications brought pharmaceutical companies more than $2.7 billion in 2005.

info For more information on sleep disorders, visit the National Sleep Foundation Web site at *www.sleepfoundation.org.*

Multiple Sclerosis Drug Combats Vision Loss

Laura J. Balcer, MD, associate professor of neurology, University of Pennsylvania School of Medicine, Philadelphia.

Nicholas LaRocca, PhD, director of health care delivery and policy research, National Multiple Sclerosis Society, New York City.

Anne H. Cross, MD, professor, neurology, Washington University School of Medicine, St. Louis.

Neurology.

The controversial multiple sclerosis drug Tysabri also reduces vision loss associated with the disease by 47%, a new study found.

EXCITING RESEARCH

"Vision loss is probably one of the most disabling things that happens to people with MS," said lead researcher Dr. Laura J. Balcer, an associate professor of neurology at the University of Pennsylvania School of Medicine in Philadelphia. "The first exciting thing about the study is that we have now developed an eye-chart test that can pick up vision loss and it can show if treatments are helping vision. Secondly, this particular drug appears to actually help prevent vision loss."

In the study, Balcer's group looked at the results of two trials—called AFFIRM and SENTINEL—that included 2,138 people with relapsing MS. More than half the patients received Tysabri (generic name *natalizumab*) every four weeks for two years.

NEW VISION TEST

To evaluate eyesight, the researchers used a specially developed eye chart of low-contrast letters. They found vision loss was reduced by as much as 47% among the people taking Tysabri, compared with those taking a placebo.

Balcer thinks that other MS drugs may have similar effects on vision, and there is now a test that can be included in trials to evaluate this. "Now, we can get to see how these other medications may help vision," she said.

"Vision is one more dimension of MS that the drug helps," Balcer said. "It has already been shown that the drug reduces the rates of relapses and disability."

NEVER AN EASY PATH

Tysabri's history has been marked by some controversy.

It received US Food and Drug Administration approval in November 2004, only to be pulled from the market three months later after several patients in clinical trials developed a rare but deadly viral infection of the brain called progressive multifocal leukoencephalopathy. In June 2006, the FDA allowed the drug to return to the market, but with strict conditions. According to the new guidelines, Tysabri can only be administered by approved doctors, infusion sites and pharmacies that register and comply with a patient-safety program designed by Biogen-IDEC, the maker of Tysabri, and approved by the FDA.

Caution: One expert thinks that despite the vision benefit, Tysabri should be reserved for patients with aggressive MS or for those who used other medications unsuccessfully.

"This study confirms the benefits of this particular MS drug in relapsing MS patients," said Dr. Anne H. Cross, a professor of neurology at Washington University School of Medicine, in St. Louis. "In addition, it validates the use of a new vision test which is relevant to MS."

But the benefit to vision doesn't negate the risks associated with the drug, Cross said. "I don't think I will change my prescribing habits based upon this paper," she said. "I will probably continue to use it in the same type of patients I have been using it in in the past."

NEW INFORMATION ALWAYS WELCOME

However, Nicholas LaRocca, the director of health care delivery and policy research at the National Multiple Sclerosis Society in New York City, said the new study provides additional insight into the benefits of the drug and may influence the decision whether to start using it or not.

"For patients who are on natalizumab or are considering it, this gives them another piece of information to consider as they are trying to make their decision," he said.

■ ■ ■ ■

What Is Multiple Sclerosis?

According to the US National Institutes of Health, multiple sclerosis is an unpredictable disease of the central nervous system that can range from relatively benign to somewhat disabling to devastating, as communication between the brain and other parts of the body is disrupted. Many researchers believe MS to be an autoimmune disease—one in which the body, through its immune system, launches a defensive attack against its own tissues. In the case of MS, it is the nerve-insulating myelin that comes under assault.

info For more information about multiple sclerosis, contact the National Multiple Sclerosis Society at *www.nationalmssociety.org.*

Drug Shows Promise as New Treatment for MS

American Academy of Neurology news release.

The drug *rituximab* reduces disease activity in people with the relapsing-remitting form of multiple sclerosis (MS), according to two new studies.

Rituximab selectively targets and depletes a subset of immune cells called B-cells by targeting a specific protein on the cell surface. It's the first drug designed to target B-cells and may offer a new treatment for relapsing-remitting MS.

THE STUDIES

In one study, researchers from the University of California, San Francisco, gave two infusions of rituximab, delivered two weeks apart, to 69 patients, while 35 other patients received a placebo.

During the following six months, the patients who received rituximab had 90% fewer brain lesions and 58% fewer drug relapses than the patients who received the placebo (14.5% vs. 34.3%).

In the second study, researchers at McGill University in Montreal gave 26 patients two infusions of rituximab two weeks apart (one course of treatment) and then gave them another course of treatment six months later. The patients were followed for at least a year.

The patients showed a 90% reduction in brain lesions, and the relapse rate went from an average of at least one per patient per year to only a few for the entire group of patients during the year of treatment.

Both studies were supported by Genentech Inc., and Biogen Idec., the companies marketing the drug in the United States, where it is currently approved for treating certain types of lymphoma and for a moderate to severe form of rheumatoid arthritis. Rituximab is not approved for treatment of MS.

FINDINGS ARE PROMISING

"While these are early-stage clinical trials, the results are exciting because the current drugs available for MS are only partially effective in reducing disease activity and preventing exacerbations," Dr. Stephen Hauser, author of the California study, said in a prepared statement.

"New and more effective treatments for MS are sorely needed, especially for people who do not adequately respond to current available medications. These data are also important because they demonstrate that B-cells, which are the precursors of antibody-producing cells, play an essential role in mediating relapses of MS," Hauser said.

info For more information about Multiple Sclerosis, contact the American Medical Association at *www.ama-assn.org*.

Skin Patch Approved for Early Parkinson's

US Food and Drug Administration.

The Neupro patch (*rotigotine* transdermal system) has been approved by the US Food and Drug Administration (FDA) as the first skin patch to treat symptoms of early Parkinson's disease.

The active drug, rotigotine, hadn't been approved previously in the United States. It is a member of the dopamine agonist class of drugs, which activates body processes that mimic the effects of the neurotransmitter dopamine. Parkinson's is caused by a loss of dopamine-producing brain cells.

During clinical testing involving more than 1,100 people, side effects for the Neupro patch included skin reactions, dizziness, nausea, vomiting, drowsiness and insomnia. The FDA cited other "potential safety concerns" including the possibility of falling asleep while driving and a sudden drop in blood pressure upon standing up.

The agency cited statistics from the Parkinson's Action Network that revealed that more than 1 million Americans live with the disease and 60,000 new cases are diagnosed annually. Symptoms include trembling of the arms, legs, jaw and face; impaired balance; and stiffness of the limbs and trunk.

The Neupro patch is produced by Schwarz Bioscience of Research Triangle Park, North Carolina.

 For more information about this approval, contact the FDA at *www.fda.gov*.

Many MS Patients Miss Out on Effective Drugs

Wake Forest University news release.

Many multiple sclerosis (MS) patients in the United States are not taking or being prescribed immunomodulatory agents (IMAs) to treat the disease, even though the drugs reduce the frequency of relapse and slow disease progression.

There are six types of IMAs approved for sale in the United States.

Researchers from the Wake Forest University Baptist Medical Center reviewed more than 6.7 million visits by MS patients to family doctors and neurologists between 1998 and 2004.

The study found that about 62% of patients seen by neurologists and 92% of patients seen by family doctors were not taking IMAs.

"When we looked at patients who are being seen by family practitioners and by neurologists, we were surprised at the number of people who are not benefiting from drugs proven to help reduce the side effects of MS," neurologist and study coauthor Dr. Cormac O'Donovan said in a prepared statement.

PUZZLING

"Our study could not determine exactly why these FDA-approved drugs were not being prescribed for the treatment of MS," O'Donovan added.

"Some individuals may have mild symptoms at first and decide to defer treatment. Other factors may be that physicians are not as familiar with the newer drugs on the market and the risk-to-benefit ratio," he said. "Some patients may not even be aware of the pros and cons of IMAs or were advised by their physician that they did not meet the criteria for taking the drug. The increased use of IMAs by neurologists probably reflects greater awareness of the drugs' availability and their use by specialists who more often treat patients with MS. We need to spend time looking further into the issue."

 For more information on multiple sclerosis, visit the National Institute of Neurological Disorders and Stroke at *www.ninds. nih.gov/disorders*.

Nearly 80% of Hospitalized Kids Get 'Adult-Only' Drugs

Samir S. Shah, MD, attending physician in pediatric infectious diseases, Children's Hospital of Philadelphia, and assistant professor of pediatrics and epidemiology and senior scholar, Center for Clinical Epidemiology and Biostatistics, University of Pennsylvania School of Medicine, both in Philadelphia.
Archives of Pediatrics and Adolescent Medicine.

Almost 80% of children hospitalized in the United States are given drugs that have been approved only for adult patients, a new study found.

Although the study didn't look at safety issues, the practice is potentially problematic, experts said.

OFF-LABEL USE WORRISOME

"Any time you prescribe a medication, you ideally think the benefits outweigh the risks," said Dr. Samir S. Shah, lead author of the study and an attending physician in pediatric infectious diseases at the Children's Hospital of Philadelphia. "The problem when you're using a drug off-label is, oftentimes, that there may not be enough evidence to help you make that decision in an informed way. We think the benefits outweigh the risks, but we don't have enough evidence."

Using drugs "off-label" for conditions other than their original approval is perfectly legal but causes concern among some experts. A 2001 US government report concluded that, overall, about 21% of prescribed drug use was for conditions not indicated on the label.

The practice is particularly prevalent with children. Few medications are studied in children or specifically approved for that age group, and evidence varies.

"Some of the drugs we currently use have been studied quite well and haven't received FDA [US Food and Drug Administration] approval, and others have not been studied very well at all," Shah explained. "This is the first step in a series of steps to try to get a better grasp on this problem."

Previous studies in the United States had not looked at hospitalized children.

THE STUDY

For this study, the researchers analyzed patient records from 31 children's hospitals over the course of one year, 2004. Patients had to be 18 years old or younger to be included in the study.

Medications approved for use on the central or autonomic nervous system, as well as nutrients and gastrointestinal medications, were most likely to be used off-label. More than one quarter (28%) of patients in the database were given morphine, for example, even though it has not been approved for use in children.

Cancer drugs were the least likely to be used off-label, possibly because many of these drugs have been tested and are approved for use in pediatric patients.

The children most likely to receive drugs off-label had undergone surgery, were more than 28 days old, and suffered more critical conditions, suggesting that, perhaps, other therapies had failed.

At least one drug was used off-label in 297,592 —78.7%—of 355,409 patients, the study found.

STUNNING NEWS

Off-label use accounted for $270 million, or 40.5% of the total dollars spent on medications for hospitalized children. Although the frequency of off-label prescribing was not particularly surprising, the dollars involved were.

"We were a little shocked by that number," Shah said. "That's a good chunk of health-care costs."

Post-marketing surveillance (seeing how a drug is performing after it has been approved) might help define this uncharted territory.

"Once a drug is on the market, it really behooves the drug companies and the FDA to mandate post-marketing surveillance to figure out exactly what's going on with the drugs," Shah said. "Knowing the risks of drugs puts drug use in a more appropriate context, and that's the whole goal of safe medical practice. A lot of medications simply do not have enough information to make the informed decisions that we need to be making and that patients and parents expect us to be making."

info To read more about off-label drugs and their dispensation, go to *www.medical newstoday.com.*

20% of High-Risk Patients Don't Get Critical Drugs

Gregg C. Fonarow, MD, professor, cardiology, University of California, San Francisco.

Alan Kadish, MD, associate director, Bluhm Cardiovascular Institute, Northwestern University Feinberg School of Medicine, Chicago.

American Heart Association's Annual Scientific Forum, Washington, DC.

Although well-known medicines can curb a dangerous cardiovascular condition called atherothrombosis, at least 20% of people who could benefit from the drugs are still not getting them, a new study finds.

Atherothrombosis occurs when blood collects in the arteries, raising clotting risks. The condition can be well-managed with a range of drugs that include statins, antiplatelets, beta-blockers and angiotensin-converting enzyme (ACE) inhibitors.

THE STUDY

For the study, Gregg C. Fonarow, MD, a professor of cardiology at the University of California in San Francisco, and his colleagues studied data from 26,000 US patients enrolled in the Reduction of Atherothrombosis for Continued Health (REACH) trial, an ongoing international study of more than 68,000 patients with atherothrombosis who are managed in primary-care offices in 45 countries.

Depending upon a patient's condition, doctors can prescribe drugs—along with a healthy lifestyle and diet—to significantly reduce the risk of recurrence or onset of atherothrombosis-linked events, such as stroke and cardiovascular disease.

But Fonarow and his colleagues found that only three-quarters of such patients across the country were taking antiplatelets, which prevent blood clots, or statins, which reduce cholesterol. Approximately half were taking beta-blockers and ACE inhibitors, which reduce blood pressure and lessen heart disease risk.

Doctors from the University of California, San Francisco, say that hospital outpatient facilities aren't keeping track of patients who need the preventive medicines.

"There is a need to implement systems which would improve care in outpatient practice," said Dr. Fonarow. "A large number of patients have stroke and cardiovascular deaths that could have been prevented."

VARIES BY REGION

Getting the right medications may also depend on where you live in the United States, Fonarow added. Patients in the Northeast received more of the clot-preventing drugs than those living in other parts of the country, despite the existence of clear guidelines supporting their use. Fifty-five percent of the patients in that region were taking at least three of the four drugs recommended for managing their diseases, compared with 52% in the Midwest, 51% in the West and 50% in the South.

"The extent of regional variations is surprising," Fonarow commented. "The current thinking is that the guidelines are distributed widely and that doctors in all regions would be treating patients in a similar fashion."

These regional percentage differences may seem relatively small, Fonarow explained, but they represent hundreds of thousands of patients. "Even small differences [in percentages] have important consequences," he said.

ADDITIONAL FINDING

The study also discovered that patients who exhibited symptoms were 50% more likely to receive preventive care than patients who had risk factors but showed no symptoms of atherothrombosis.

There are many possible reasons why these patients weren't getting the drugs they needed, Fonarow said, including changing physicians, prescription changes, or the introduction of new drugs that patients didn't know about.

"Half to three-quarters of patients are getting treatment, but there is still room for improvement," he said, "and this type of data is helpful for identifying the fact that there is an issue with gaps in treating the outpatient population."

Dr. Alan Kadish, associate director of the Bluhm Cardiovascular Institute at Northwestern University Medical Center in Chicago, said he was disappointed by what the study found.

"In a registry like this the numbers will never be 100%, but we have to do a better job of translating new medical advances into everyday practical use, like putting better drugs into practice," he said.

info For more information about how to prevent strokes, contact the American Stroke Association at *www.strokeassociation.org*.

Sleeping Pill Wakes Woman After Two Years in Coma

James Grisolia, MD, neurologist, Scripps Mercy Hospital, San Diego.

Tetsuo Ashizawa, MD, professor and chairman, department of neurology, University of Texas Medical Branch, Galveston.

Annals of Neurology.

A dose of the prescription sleep aid Ambien had the opposite effect on one French woman, awakening her from a two-year coma.

The 48-year-old woman suffered from akinetic mutism—a sort of persistent coma in which the patient is alert but can neither speak nor move. She had lain in this state after sustaining damage to the frontal lobe of her brain due to a lack of oxygen caused by an attempted suicide by hanging.

But one day she was given *zolpidem* (Ambien) to treat ongoing insomnia.

"Twenty minutes later, her family noticed surprising signs of enhanced arousal," the study authors wrote. "She became able to communicate to her family, to eat without (swallowing) troubles, and to move alone in her bed. These effects started 20 minutes after drug administration and lasted for two to three hours."

After treatment, the patient could walk for short periods, and to speak if prompted, though not spontaneously. "This phenomenon was so reproducible that caregivers used to give her up to three tablets each day without sleepiness as a 'side effect,'" the researchers wrote.

INCREASED BLOOD FLOW

Using positron emission tomography (PET) scans, the researchers found that the drug treatment caused the woman's frontal lobes to become "way more active," noted Dr. James Grisolia, a neurologist at Scripps Mercy Hospital in San Diego. He was not involved in the research, which was led by Dr. Christine Brefel-Courbon, of the University Hospital in Toulouse, France.

Speaking of the case, Grisolia said that "it is a function of drugs like this that, besides from putting you to sleep, that they can also increase blood flow. And that activity apparently trumped the sleepiness caused by the medication in this one patient.

"This is a clinical mini-miracle that may give more insight into how the brain works," Grisolia added. "In the long run, it might help us to help other people that are in unresponsive or semi-coma states."

According to Grisolia, other case reports have shown coma patients "awakening" through stimulant medications, but never from a medication like zolpidem. How the drug worked its magic in this case remains unknown. "It needs case reports and further study in the lab to get a handle on this," he said.

CAUTION ADVISED

Dr. Tetsuo Ashizawa, professor and chairman of the department of neurology at the University of Texas Medical Branch, Galveston, called the report "interesting." But he cautioned against using such a single-patient study as a basis for treating other, seemingly similar cases.

"I understand the desire of the family member to give Ambien to patients" as a result of this study, he said, "but I would not tell them that they should expect improvement. As a physician, I would say this worked in this lady but it may not work in your father or mother, so they should not have unreal expectations. If it works, OK, but if it doesn't, don't be disappointed."

Still, Grisolia said he expects more reports on the effect of zolpidem in akinetic mutism will be published as a result of this study.

"I'm sure that anyone who has a relative in a long-term coma is going to be interested in having the doctor try Ambien and see if it makes a difference. So we may get more case reports very quickly," he said.

A spokeswoman for Sanofi-Aventis, the pharmaceutical company that manufactures Ambien, declined to comment on the study.

info For more information on zolpidem, visit the US National Library of Medicine at *www.nlm.nih.gov/medlineplus/druginformation.html.*

New Epilepsy Drug Helps Reduce Seizure Frequency

Roger J. Porter, MD, University of Pennsylvania, Philadelphia.
American Academy of Neurology news release.

An epilepsy drug with a new method of action is safe and effective, according to a new study.

Retigabine works by opening potassium channels and is being developed to treat people with partial-onset seizures whose seizures are not fully controlled by other drugs.

The finding may be good news for people with epilepsy who don't respond well to current available medications, said study author Dr. Roger J. Porter, of the University of Pennsylvania in Philadelphia. When the study was conducted, Porter worked for Wyeth Pharmaceuticals, which developed retigabine. The study was sponsored and conducted by Wyeth.

ABOUT THE STUDY

The study included 399 patients who were divided into four groups: three groups received different doses of retigabine for 16 weeks, and one group received a placebo. At the start of the study, all of the patients were having an average of eight to 10 seizures a month and were also taking one to two other epilepsy drugs.

Patients who took the highest dose of retigabine had an average of 35% fewer seizures during the study, compared with 13% for patients who took the placebo. The study also found that 33% of the patients who took the highest dose of the drug had a 50% or greater reduction in seizure frequency.

Drowsiness, dizziness, confusion, tremor, amnesia and speech disorders were among the side effects experienced by patients who took retigabine.

info For more information about epilepsy, contact the Epilepsy Foundation at *www.epilepsyfoundation.org*.

Could Viagra Put the Brakes on Jet Lag?

Robert Vorona, MD, associate professor, division of sleep medicine, department of internal medicine, Eastern Virginia Medical School, Norfolk.

Diego Golombek, MD, researcher, Universidad Nacional de Quilmes, Buenos Aires, Argentina.

Proceedings of the National Academy of Sciences.

Worried about jet lag? Researchers think they might have just the ticket to perk you up: Viagra. While it's too early to know if it will work in humans, Argentinean researchers are reporting that *sildenafil* (Viagra) appears to reduce symptoms of jet lag in hamsters.

"We do need more effective therapies for jet lag and for sleep difficulties that occur as a consequence of shift work," said Dr. Robert Vorona, an associate professor in the Division of Sleep Medicine at Eastern Virginia Medical School.

THE STUDY

In the study, researchers administered small doses of sildenafil to hamsters before adjusting the cycles of light and dark they lived in. This reset their body clocks as if they'd taken a six-hour plane trip to the east.

The hamsters recovered 25% to 50% more quickly from the equivalent of human jet lag, needing less time to synchronize themselves to the new schedule, said Dr. Diego Golombek, a researcher with the Universidad Nacional de Quilmes in Buenos Aires. He said sildenafil worked at least as well as melatonin, a jet-lag treatment.

But the drug didn't help hamsters who underwent a simulation of westward jet travel.

THEORY

The popular erectile-dysfunction drug, originally developed to treat high blood pressure and angina, might alleviate jet lag by interfering with a molecule that sends signals to the brain's body clock mechanism, Golombek said.

PRECAUTIONS

But the potential impact on humans isn't clear, and Golombek said people shouldn't rush out to prevent jet lag with doses of Viagra. For one thing, Viagra can cause side effects such as low blood pressure.

As for the next step, Golombek said "a full-scale clinical trial has to be performed in humans, which is indeed quite expensive and time-consuming. Jet-lag trials might involve laboratory simulations, but we also need 'the real thing,' which means testing pharmacological treatments on long-haul air travel."

info For more information on jet lag, visit the Web site of the National Sleep Foundation at *www.sleepfoundation.org*.

Promising News! Prozac Fights Osteoporosis

Ricardo Battaglino, PhD, assistant member, department of cytokine biology, The Forsyth Institute, Boston.

Grant Mitchell, MD, chief, psychiatry, Northern Westchester Hospital Center, Mount Kisco, NY.

Journal of Cellular Biochemistry.

Could a widely used treatment for depression be a remedy for osteoporosis? Researchers have discovered that the drug *fluoxetine* (Prozac) also increases bone mass, at least in mice. Prozac is a member of a group of antidepressants called "selective serotonin reuptake inhibitors" (SSRIs) that act on this receptor.

"Treating animals for six weeks with Prozac resulted in an increase in *trabecular* bone mass," said study lead author Ricardo Battaglino, assistant member of the staff in the department of cytokine biology at The Forsyth Institute in Boston. "It was a pretty significant 60% increase."

Trabecular bone, one of two main types of bone in the body, has a spongy, honeycomb-like structure and makes up the inner layer of bone.

Although it's way too early to advocate popping Prozac to reverse or stop bone loss, experts say it's a tantalizing lead for future research.

"For several reasons, people need to be cautious because fluoxetine has central nervous system effects," said Dr. Grant Mitchell, chief of psychiatry at Northern Westchester Hospital Center in Mount Kisco, New York. "But it is interesting that current treatments for bone loss in osteoporosis do not take this approach, so the idea that we could at some point have another approach to reducing bone loss or even rebuilding new bone is actually exciting. Having more options would be great."

THE STUDY

For this study, laboratory mice were treated with Prozac for six weeks.

The drug was administered both systemically (like taking a pill) and locally (directly to the bone), and the effects were observed with both delivery methods, the researchers reported.

Prozac both spurred the formation of new bone under normal conditions and reversed overall bone loss triggered by inflammation.

However, Prozac was not effective in female mice without circulating estrogen (i.e., after their ovaries had been removed). In those cases, Prozac "did not prevent bone loss associated with estrogen deficiency," Mitchell said. "It looks like, to be effective in relation to bone loss, Prozac needs to be in the presence of estrogen." This has implications for women moving into menopause who lose estrogen and have an increased risk of osteoporosis, he said.

An earlier study, however, with Prozac found that the drug actually *hindered* bone growth. The discrepancy may have been due to the way bone mass or density was measured and also to the fact that it involved children, not adults, Battaglino said.

IMPLICATIONS

The new findings need to be replicated and tried in humans, but given the number of people taking Prozac, the implications could be enormous.

"Fluoxetine is one of the most widely prescribed psychoactive drugs in this country and most likely the world, and it's been like that for at least 15 or 20 years," Battaglino said. "From the public health point of view, this would be pretty relevant."

It is not known whether other SSRIs—such as Celexa, Paxil and Zoloft—might have the same effect on bone, Battaglino added, since similar tests on those drugs haven't yet been performed.

info To find out more about bone loss, visit the Web site of the National Osteoporosis Foundation at *www.nof.org*.

Late Afternoon Surgeries Could Be Deadly

Melanie Wright, PhD, assistant professor of anesthesiology, Duke University Medical Center, Durham, NC.

David Birnbach, MD, director of the Center for Patient Safety, University of Miami.

James S. Hicks, MD, associate professor, anesthesiology and perioperative medicine, Oregon Health and Science University, Portland, and chairman, American Society of Anesthesiologists Committee on Quality Management and Departmental Administration.

Quality & Safety in Health Care.

New research suggests that unexpected adverse events related to anesthesia are more likely to occur when surgery starts in the late afternoon than when started early in the morning.

According to the study, which analyzed data from 90,000 surgeries, adverse events were most common for operations starting between 3 p.m. and 4 p.m., as compared with 7 a.m. The lowest probability of having an adverse event (1%) was at 9 a.m. and the highest (4.2%) at 4 p.m.

But these problems, say researchers, are mostly minor ones. "We're mainly dealing with an increase in nausea and pain," says Dr. James S. Hicks of Oregon Health and Science University in Portland, and chairman of the American Society of Anesthesiologists Committee on Quality Management and Departmental Administration.

THE STUDY

For this study, researchers analyzed more than 90,000 surgeries performed at Duke Hospital from 2000 to 2004, and categorized them according to type or severity of the adverse event. The categories were then cross-referenced with the time of the surgery.

Scientists had hypothesized that the time of day surgery took place would influence the number of adverse events related to anesthesia.

In other professions, past research shows impaired performance with lack of sleep, long work hours, and disruption in circadian rhythms. But those problems typically occur during nighttime work, not in the afternoon.

The two most common types of problems were pain management and postoperative nausea and vomiting. Patients also experienced more "administrative delays," such as waiting for test results, doctors running late and rooms not ready, during the late afternoon. This could also contribute to adverse events.

THE THEORIES

In this study, researchers didn't look specifically at why more anesthesia-related problems occurred in afternoon surgeries. But possible explanations include doctors are busier and more fatigued as the day progresses, there are more communication problems in the afternoon, or even patients' circadian rhythms.

"Patients might be more susceptible to pain in the afternoon," notes study author Melanie Wright, assistant professor of anesthesiology at Duke University Medical Center.

The late-afternoon period also coincides with natural lows in the circadian rhythm, or the body's internal clock. Anesthesia care teams usually change at about 7 a.m. and again between 4 p.m. and 6 p.m. This could be colliding with circadian low points and end-of-day fatigue.

A new concept called "chronobiology" might even be at fault. "It is possible that people react to drugs differently at different times of the day," says Dr. David Birnbach, director of the University of Miami's Center for Patient Safety. "People are now looking at the effect on drugs of circadian rhythms, how long since the last cup of coffee, how many visitors, was it a quiet time or busy time."

Another theory: Too much work, too few bodies. "We have fewer guys watching more cases. We've got tired folks handing off patients, and there's lots of room for communication problems," says Wright.

Still, experts say it's not accurate to suggest that anyone forego surgeries later in the day. "You can't overgeneralize," says Birnbach. "You can't say, 'Don't have surgery in the afternoon.'"

info The National Patient Safety Foundation offers resources on anesthesia at *www.npsf.org*. Click on "Resource Center."

7

Emotional Well-Being

Stress Kills Brain Cells

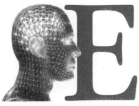 **E**veryone knows that stress can contribute to weight gain, diabetes and many other ailments, but few people realize just how harmful stress can be for your brain.

Latest development: Although chronic stress has long been known to trigger the release of excessive amounts of stress hormones, such as cortisol and adrenaline, recent studies show that both hormones actually kill brain cells and interfere with the production of new ones.

Fortunately, new research on the brain suggests that there may be ways to minimize, slow down and perhaps even reverse this damage. Here Richard O'Connor, PhD, a renowned psychotherapist who has extensively studied the harmful effects of stress, gives his advice on the most effective brain-protection strategies.

Why has stress become such a serious health threat in recent years?

It's a long-term historical trend that involves culture and economics. Before the Industrial Revolution (in the late 18th century), people tended to awaken in the morning when it became light and to go to bed when it turned dark. They also had a great deal of leisure time. That's been changing—and just in the past 25 years, it has changed dramatically. We're working 25% longer and harder to attain the same standard of living we did a quarter of a century ago. In fact, Americans now work as many hours as anyone in the world, including the Japanese, who are known for working incredibly long hours.

Doesn't a certain amount of stress make people more productive?

Yes, people are more productive when their work provides enough of a challenge to help them grow. But when the work is too difficult or

---

Richard O'Connor, PhD, a psychotherapist with offices in Canaan, CT, and New York City. He is also the author of *Undoing Perpetual Stress: The Missing Connection Between Depression, Anxiety, and 21st Century Illness* (Berkley), *Undoing Depression: What Therapy Doesn't Teach You and Medication Can't Give You* (Berkley) and *Active Treatment of Depression* (Norton).

the hours are too long, or our home life provides no relief, then stress becomes chronic. Research has consistently shown that chronic stress disrupts the functions of the immune, endocrine and digestive systems. This can result in a variety of health problems, such as asthma, heart disease and immune system deficiencies.

During the last 15 years, advances in technology have given scientists an opportunity to examine the human brain in great detail. For example, imaging studies have allowed researchers to visualize the significant loss of gray matter (the brain's information-processing center) that can result from years of stress-related conditions, such as depression and anxiety. Unfortunately, no one knows for sure whether these effects are permanent.

Are most people aware of the degree to which they are suffering from stress?

By no means. We have an interest in denying the effects of stress. Our society admires people who show grace under pressure, and we all want to believe we can handle whatever life dishes out.

Given the nature of our lives today, is it really possible to avoid stress?

Yes, absolutely. The first step is to believe that you have some degree of control over your own life. Many people feel out of control—as if events are driving them rather than the other way around. Many people think that they must work 60 hours a week, but that's simply not so. If your job requires long, stressful hours, consider changing professions or finding a job in your profession that has shorter hours.

The stakes are high. People who can't reduce chronic stress live shorter lives, suffer more illness and disability, have less satisfying relationships and often are plagued by anxiety and/or depression.

What if it's not practical to make such a drastic change?

Changing our thought patterns helps. This can allow us to prevent and even reverse some of the adverse changes, such as loss of gray matter, that occur in our brain's neural circuitry as a result of chronic stress. Meditation is an effective stress-reducing strategy. Research has shown that people who spend just 20 minutes a day focusing on their breath or on calming thoughts achieve such benefits as lower blood pressure, less anxiety and reduced chronic pain.

What can be done in addition to meditation?

As we all know, exercise also is an excellent stress fighter. However, few people appreciate the importance of intimate communication. When we feel like we have a partner or are part of a group, we feel safer and more secure. As a result, the stress hormone cascade is reduced. Feeling that we have a purpose in life—having a child or pet to care for, a cause that's meaningful to us, people who need us—these are good stress fighters.

In one landmark study, residents of a nursing home were split into two groups. Half of the residents were told that they were responsible for taking care of a plant. The other half were told not to worry about the plant. After one year, the people who were caring for a plant were healthier and had fewer illnesses. They also lived longer.

How can we improve the way we communicate with others?

Communication always occurs on two levels. It's not only about the content of what's being said, but also the nature of the relationship between the people. Content communication is usually conveyed through words...relationship communication comes through tone, face and body language. It's perfectly possible to say the words "I love you" but contradict the words through a dismissive tone or a frown. Content communication should be consistent with relationship communication.

What if these strategies aren't effective?

For some people, self-help practices are not enough. Some of the newer antidepressants, such as selective serotonin reuptake inhibitors (SSRIs), appear to reverse stress-related brain damage and help people regain the ability to grow new brain cells.

We have evidence that psychotherapy can do the same thing. Cognitive behavior therapy, which trains patients to see how their psychological problems are the result of faulty thought patterns, has been around for more than 40 years—and it works to fight the effects of stress.

To find a cognitive behavior therapist in your area, consult the Academy of Cognitive Therapy, *www.academyofct.org*, 610-664-1273.

Common Trauma Drug May Be Useless —Even Harmful

Thomas Neylan, MD, medical director, PTSD treatment program, San Francisco VA Medical Center, and associate professor, psychiatry, University of California, San Francisco.

Randall Marshall, MD, director, Trauma Studies and Services, New York State Psychiatric Institute, New York City.

American Journal of Psychiatry.

A drug long used to treat post-traumatic stress disorder (PTSD) appears to have done patients no good and may even have done some harm. In the first-ever randomized, placebo-controlled trial of *guanfacine* (Tenex) for the alleviation of PTSD, "we found that it really offered patients no benefits of any symptoms, and we looked at a lot of symptoms," said lead researcher Dr. Thomas Neylan, medical director of the PTSD treatment program at the San Francisco VA Medical Center.

"We looked at whether people were feeling less anxious, whether they were sleeping better, whether they startled less, whether they were having fewer intrusive memories," said Neylan, who is also an associate professor of psychiatry at the University of California, San Francisco. "But in anything that we looked at, we found there was no benefit for the drug over placebo."

The study results may come as a surprise to psychiatrists and patients, since guanfacine and a related drug, *clonidine* (Catapres), have been used for years to treat PTSD.

"They are commonly used, but what we hope now is that people shy away from using clonidine and guanfacine," Neylan said.

One expert said he was taken aback by the findings.

"I was so shocked that I had to think about it for two days. I was trying to find a hole in the science and I can't—this is a state-of-the-art clinical trial," said Dr. Randall Marshall, director of Trauma Studies and Services at New York State Psychiatric Institute. "There's no hint of a benefit."

Guanfacine's rise and apparent fall as a PTSD treatment may be an object lesson in why randomized, controlled trials—such as the one Neylan's group conducted—are so important to assessing a drug's worth, he said.

BACKGROUND

But no one had ever put this idea to the test in a randomized, controlled trial.

THE STUDY

In its eight-week study, Neylan's group compared the effects of guanfacine and an identical-looking placebo pill in 63 male and female veterans diagnosed with PTSD. Twenty-nine participants were randomly picked to take guanfacine while the other 34 took the dummy pill.

By the end of the study, the researchers found no net difference between the two groups in terms of changes in symptoms.

"But the one thing that did clearly come out was that there were more side effects with guanfacine," Neylan said. "There was more sedation, feeling fatigued, dry mouth."

POSSIBLE EXPLANATION

Why did a pill that should have worked so well in theory fall flat in practice? Neylan offered one possible answer. "[Too much] norepinephrine can be a bad thing," he noted, "but you also need it for your brain to work well. So, lowering the whole pool of norepinephrine did not seem to be an effective strategy."

He said the relatively small sample size in the study means he can't be absolutely certain that alpha-2 agonists have no benefit, "but we did get a zero effect size. That means that even if we had five or six times this sample, the probability of showing a meaningful difference is really, really low."

IMPLICATIONS

Marshall agreed that the methodology is sound, and the findings conclusive. "I think this pretty much answers the question of whether, in this population, guanfacine should be considered as either a primary or an adjunctive treatment. The answer is no—it's a big surprise," he said.

The finding will change the way he and psychiatrists everywhere treat PTSD patients, said Marshall, who is also associate director of the Anxiety Disorders Clinic and an associate professor of clinical psychiatry at the Columbia University College of Physicians and Surgeons.

ALTERNATIVE TREATMENTS

Neylan said a newer drug that works on norepinephrine receptors, but in a different way, might still succeed where guanfacine has failed.

That drug, called *prazosin* (Minipress), blocks one receptor, the alpha-1 receptor, but does not lower norepinephrine release in the brain. "There have been a few trials to show that prazosin does have some promise, and I know the VA is gearing up to do a large multi-site study. It is becoming more popular."

In the meantime, he said, it's important to remember that the first-line therapy for most people with PTSD is antidepressants and/or psychotherapy, especially "exposure therapy," where patients are gently confronted with reminders of the traumatic event itself.

"Most people feel that PTSD benefits most from a combination of pharmacologic treatment and psychotherapy," Neylan said.

info To learn more about PTSD, go to the Web site of the National Institute of Mental Health at *www.nimh.nih.gov/healthinformation/ ptsdmenu.cfm.*

Is It Depression or Bipolar Disorder?

Jim Phelps, MD, a psychiatrist in private practice in Corvallis, OR. He is the author of *Why Am I Still Depressed: Recognizing and Managing the Ups and Downs of Bipolar II and Soft Bipolar Disorder.* McGraw-Hill. To learn more about bipolar disorder, go to Dr. Phelps' Web site at *www.psycheducation.org.*

Until recently, bipolar disorder has been associated only with extreme mood swings—suicidal depressions alternating with manic periods of irrational and even dangerous behavior.

Now: A "soft" form of bipolar disorder has been identified and is estimated to affect 1% to 2% of the American population.

IS IT BIPOLAR DISORDER?

Depression associated with bipolar disorder has the same symptoms as common, or "unipolar," depression—sadness, lack of energy, sleep and appetite problems, loss of interest in life, etc. However, doctors can't always tell one disorder from the other. Psychiatrists are typically best suited to make the diagnosis, but they also can miss the telltale symptoms.

If you experience symptoms of depression in repeated, brief episodes, bipolar disorder should be suspected. Even though bipolar disorder is technically defined by "hypomania" (marked by phases of increased energy and activity), in the softer forms, hypomania can be accompanied by irritability and agitation—not just euphoria and grandiosity, the typical hallmarks.

Another red flag: People with bipolar disorder tend to eat and/or sleep more than usual, not less, when they're depressed.

THE RIGHT TREATMENT

For unipolar depression, standard antidepressants—such as *sertraline* (Zoloft), *fluoxetine* (Prozac), *bupropion* (Wellbutrin) or *venlafaxine* (Effexor)—usually reduce symptoms within days to several weeks. With bipolar disorder, an antidepressant alone can change a person's mood too dramatically—like flicking a switch from depression to mania.

The prescription drugs that work best for bipolar depression are designed to not only ease the depression but also even out the mood swings. These drugs often are combined with an antidepressant to increase the effectiveness of both medications.

Most effective mood-stabilizing drugs...

•**Lithium** is the oldest and, according to many doctors, the best mood-stabilizing drug. Side effects include tremor, diarrhea and confusion.

•**Lamotrigine** (Lamictal) is one of the newest mood-stabilizing drugs. In rare cases, it can cause a potentially fatal allergic reaction, marked by a rash.

• **Olanzapine** (Zyprexa) often reduces symptoms within hours. In some cases, it can cause major weight gain and even diabetes.

• **Valproate** (Depakote) is another tried-and-true mood-stabilizing drug. Side effects include sedation and weight gain.

A HEALTHFUL LIFESTYLE

To maximize the benefits of medication, it helps to adopt a healthful lifestyle. If your symptoms aren't too serious—for example, you're still able to work and maintain close relationships—this approach may stabilize your moods without the use of drugs. *Recommended…*

• **Exercise regularly.** Studies have shown that regular aerobic exercise can relieve depression as effectively as some prescription antidepressant medications.

To get started, try this simple strategy: Walk just seven-and-a-half minutes in one direction, then return. Do this every day. Gradually increase the duration if you can.

• **Consume omega-3 fatty acids.** Fish oil, the best source of these essential fatty acids, has been shown to improve depression and reduce mood swings. Try 1 g daily of *eicosapentaenoic acid* (EPA) from fish oil capsules or liquid. Right now, it's not known if the amount of *docosahexaenoic acid* (DHA) found in fish oil is significant for bipolar disorder.

Caution: Fish oil can have a blood-thinning effect, so check with your doctor if you use blood-thinning medication, such as *warfarin* (Coumadin).

• **Limit alcohol.** For many people, alcohol makes their moods more unstable. If you drink alcohol, abstain for several weeks and monitor your moods. Then slowly reintroduce it—begin with one or two drinks per week and track whether it affects you negatively.

LIGHT/DARK THERAPIES

Maintaining regular sleep habits and frequent light and dark exposure can help stabilize moods and reduce depression.

• **Light therapy** acts like an antidepressant, possibly by affecting levels of the neurotransmitter serotonin.

What to do: Expose yourself to light for 30 minutes or more per day.

Best approach: Use a light box, which can be purchased for about $175 to $300 at Costco or several Web sites, including *www.lighttherapyproducts.com.*

Warning: If you experience hypomania symptoms such as agitation, irritability or crowded thoughts, discontinue light therapy.

• **Dark therapy** acts like a mood stabilizer and is involved in regulating the biological clock.

What to do: Go to bed at the same time each night, keep your room as dark as possible and get up at the same time each morning. In addition, control your exposure to light. Even if you don't sit in complete darkness, keep lights low after 9 p.m.…don't watch TV or use the computer. Use a dawn simulator, a device that wakes you naturally by slowly turning up the lights each morning. For information about where to buy dawn simulators, check my Web site, *www.copsych.com.*

• **Blue light** is the wavelength that is believed to regulate the sleep-wake rhythm.

What to do: If it's past 9 p.m. and you want to use your computer or read without disrupting the cycle, wearing yellow-lensed sunglasses that block blue light may help, though this is still being researched. Yellow-lensed sunglasses are available at *www.lowbluelights.com.*

Eating and exercising at the same time each day also helps stabilize moods.

PSYCHOTHERAPY

Cognitive behavioral therapy (CBT), which helps identify and change thinking and behavior patterns that influence moods, has been shown to be as effective as antidepressants. When adapted for bipolar disorder, it may include strategies to help you maintain a healthful lifestyle, reduce stress and identify characteristic unhealthful thoughts.

info To find a CBT practitioner near you, consult the Depression and Bipolar Support Alliance, 800-826-3632, *www.dbsalliance.org.*

Stressed Out? Hold Your Hubby's Hand

James A. Coan, PhD, assistant professor of psychology and neuroscience, University of Virginia, Charlottesville.

Charles Goodstein, MD, psychoanalyst, New York University Medical Center, clinical professor of psychiatry, New York University School of Medicine, New York City, and past president of the Psychoanalytic Association of New York.

Psychological Science.

If you're a woman stressed out from work, holiday shopping, the kids or even too much traffic, grab your husband's hand for instant relief. Even for women who are single, holding any man's hand is better than none, say the researchers.

"Hand-holding is second nature for kids" when they're under stress, said Dr. James A. Coan, assistant professor of psychology and neuroscience at the University of Virginia, who led the study. "This can also work for adults."

The happier the marriage, the greater the stress-reducing benefit, Coan found. But even a stranger's hand can help reduce stress, he said.

THE STUDY

For the study, Coan recruited 16 married women who scored high on his marriage satisfaction quiz and gave them magnetic resonance imaging (MRI) scans of their brain when confronted with stress. He subjected them to a very mild electric shock in three situations: by themselves not holding anyone's hand; holding their husband's hand; and holding the hand of a male stranger.

"First, we wanted to know what the brain is doing when the women were completely alone," he said. "We got a baseline of how the brain responds to stress."

Then, the researchers looked at the MRI images of the brain when the women held their husband's hand or the stranger's hand. "When your brain is under stress, it has to work hard, it has all these different problems to solve," Coan said.

RESULTS

"We found when you are holding a hand, any hand, the parts of your brain responsible for mobilizing your body into action calm down," Coan said. "It doesn't matter whose hand it is."

But a husband's hand provided the greatest benefits. "Both hands calmed the bodily reaction to stress," Coan said, "but only the spousal hand can calm the mind, only a husband's hand calmed down the region of the brain that keeps your emotions in check."

And the happier the marriage, the greater the benefits. Among couples in the study who scored the highest on marital satisfaction—pairs that Coan termed "super couples"—the women got even more benefit from spousal hand-holding than did the other women.

Coan found that the region of the brain thought to be associated with experience of pain quieted down even more in those women. "If you are in a 'super couple,' hand-holding serves as a kind of analgesic," he said.

Whatever the amount of benefit, Coan said he believes "the brain works a lot less hard when there is someone else helping us cope. One of my students said, 'It's like the brain is contracting out some of the work,' keeping our brain less stressed."

REACTION

Dr. Charles Goodstein, a psychoanalyst at New York University Medical Center and a clinical professor of psychiatry at New York University School of Medicine, said the study gives scientific credence to long-time observations. "Interaction between members of a species can have a momentous impact on emotion, and emotion can have a profound impact on bodily functioning," he said.

Often, Goodstein noted, medications are used to provide relief from anxiety and anticipated anxiety. "This study shows that there is a better way."

info To learn more about social support and its health effects, visit the Web site of the American Psychological Association at *www.apa.org.*

How to Tell What Men and Women Are Really Saying

Marianne Legato, MD, FACP, a physician and professor of clinical medicine at Columbia University, New York City, and founder of Columbia's Partnership for Gender-Specific Medicine. She is author of several books, including *Why Men Never Remember and Women Never Forget*. Rodale.

Neither men nor women can claim that their brains are "better." While men's brains are 10% larger on average, women's brains have more elaborate connections that make them more efficient. Male and female brains unquestionably are different, in terms of both structure and chemistry, and that can cause problems when we try to communicate with one another.

Most of us speak to our spouses just as we would speak to members of our own sex—then wonder why they don't seem to understand.

Here's how to communicate more effectively with the opposite sex...

NONVERBAL CUES

The female brain is good at decoding nonverbal signals, including facial expressions and tone of voice, perhaps because mothers must understand the needs of children too young to speak. When women send nonverbal signals to men, women are often dismayed to find that these signals are ignored.

Women don't realize that the typical male brain is not skilled at interpreting nonverbal communications. Men are particularly bad at identifying signs of sadness in women—though men are pretty good at spotting signs of anger and aggression.

Women: Tell him verbally when something is bothering you. A sad expression or the silent treatment won't get you anywhere. It's not that he is ignoring your feelings—he is just unaware of them.

If a man asks you what he can do to make you feel better, tell him. If you say "nothing," he'll assume that you mean nothing and he'll do nothing. He isn't trying to hurt you—men's brains just work in a more linear, literal manner. Because men often like to be left alone when they're upset, he might conclude that he is doing you a favor by giving you some space.

Men: Search for clues beyond her words when she seems unusually quiet or terse. She might be sending signals that you're not picking up. If you can't figure out the signals and she won't tell you what she needs, remind her that you really want to help, but it's hard for you to pick up her nonverbal cues.

LISTENING

The female brain seems to be better at listening than the male brain—women have more nerve cells in the areas known to process language and put a larger percentage of their brains to work when they hear someone speak.

The more elaborate wiring of the female brain also makes women better multitaskers than men. Evolution likely made women this way so that mothers could keep an eye on the children and still get other things done. Evolution shaped the male brain to focus on one very difficult task at a time. Tiger hunts were more successful when the hunters could focus all their attention on the tiger.

Add men's inferior listening ability to their superior focus, and the result is a phenomenon most wives know well. Tell a man something important while he's watching a ball game, and he might not remember a word of it. He isn't purposely ignoring you—his brain simply isn't wired to hear what you said.

Women: Put him on alert that what you're about to say is important. If it's particularly vital information, begin with a gentle "I need you to look me in the eyes." If there are too many distractions in your present location, ask him to go with you for a walk or out to a quiet restaurant.

Men: Don't be insulted if she doesn't stop what she is doing when you want to talk. Chances are that she can pay attention to you even if she's occupied. If you want her undivided attention, ask for it.

PROBLEM SOLVING

The structure of the male brain makes men straight-ahead thinkers—when they see a problem, their instinct is to try to solve it.

Women are more likely to ruminate over decisions. They'll verbalize a problem and talk though all the implications and issues before they proceed. When women try to talk through their problems with men, they're often dismayed and insulted that the men try to tell them what to do. This confuses the men, who thought they were being asked for a solution.

Women: Tell a man the specific type of response you want before you share a problem. Are you asking the man for a solution, or do you just want to talk through the issue so it's clear in your mind? If you don't specifically tell him that it's the latter, he'll assume it's the former. If he tries to solve your problem anyway, understand that this is just how his brain responds.

As for how to respond to a man's problems, this rarely comes up. Men tend not to share their problems with anyone.

Men: Understand that women like to verbalize their thinking and don't always want you to solve their problems.

Instead, wait for a question before providing an answer. Ask what you can do to help rather than assume you know. And if your wife starts crying, holding her quietly works better than telling her she's being too emotional.

DIFFERENT INTERESTS

Women tend to expect their male partners to be interested in every subject they wish to discuss. That isn't fair. A woman wouldn't expect her female friends to chat about a subject that she knows bores them.

Women: Tailor your conversation to your partner's interests. (Men should do this, too, but because men talk less, it isn't as often an issue.) Find other conversation partners for topics that don't interest him.

Men: Encourage your partner to spend time with female friends so there's another outlet for the conversations that don't interest you. Don't get upset if she's busy with friends when you want to see her.

BETTER ARGUMENTS

During an argument, women are more likely to bring up past events. Estrogen increases the amount of *cortisol*, a memory-boosting hormone, released by the adrenal glands during stressful moments. Because the female brain

has more estrogen, memories of old fights remain fresher in a woman's mind. The male brain finds it easier to forget emotional situations and move on. Maybe forgetting a close call on a tiger hunt made it easier for men of the past to continue to hunt.

Women: Use simple, declarative sentences, and state what you want in outline form when imparting important information to men. Leave out anecdotes and unnecessary adjectives. Take advantage of your ability to read his emotions to spot the signs of boredom. When you see them, sum up your argument with a closing statement and end the conversation. Try not to rehash old arguments.

Men: Try to keep women focused on the point under discussion. If during an argument she brings up a fight you had five years ago, tell her, "We've discussed that already and it isn't going to help to go over it again. Let's focus on the current problem."

Depressed? Manage Your Mood with Marriage

Kristi Williams, PhD, assistant professor, sociology, Ohio State University, Columbus.

Charles Goodstein, MD, psychoanalyst, New York University Medical Center, and clinical professor, psychiatry, New York University School of Medicine, and past president, Psychoanalytic Association of New York.

American Sociological Association annual meeting, Montreal.

With apologies to about 10,000 stand-up comedians, marriage may be the cure for depression, rather than the cause of it. In fact, researchers say, people who experience depression before they get married are the most likely to get emotional health benefits from marriage.

Using a depression scale whose scores ranged from zero to 84, the researchers found that the scores of depressed people went down by almost eight points after marriage, while those who weren't depressed had just under a two-point drop after marriage.

Even the study authors were surprised by their findings. "We thought people who were depressed would be less likely to benefit from marriage than others," said study coauthor Kristi Williams, an assistant professor of sociology at Ohio State University in Columbus. "We thought depression would put a strain on the marriage."

This research comes on the heels of another study that found that people who never marry had a greater chance of dying early than people who were married. In fact, people who'd never married had an even higher risk of early death than people who were divorced, separated or widowed, suggesting that marriage confers some sort of health benefit, even if it doesn't work out.

THE STUDY

Using data from the National Survey of Families and Households, the Ohio State researchers gathered information on more than 3,000 people who were single at the start of the study in 1987–88. The survey participants were interviewed again sometime between 1992 and 1994.

To assess whether or not people were depressed, they were asked 12 questions, such as how many days in the past week they "felt like they could not shake off the blues," "felt lonely," or "slept restlessly."

About 29% were depressed at the start of the study, according to Williams.

During the second part of the study, they gathered information on who had gotten married and reassessed depression.

Williams said at that time, 30% of those who remained unmarried were depressed, while only 26% of those who got married were depressed.

The researchers found that those who were depressed seemed to gain the most mental health benefits from getting married, with depressed people enjoying nearly a six-point higher reduction in their depression scores after marriage than nondepressed people.

"We actually found the opposite of what we expected. We thought depressed people would be less likely to benefit from marriage because the depression of one spouse can put a strain on the marriage and undermine marital quality," said study coauthor, Adrianne Frech, a doctoral student at Ohio State.

IMPLICATIONS

As to why depressed people may enjoy more benefits from matrimony, Williams theorized, "We think that depressed people may have more to gain from the emotional support and close intimate ties that come with marriage."

That doesn't mean people who aren't depressed won't have happy marriages, Williams quickly added: "If you start out happy, you don't have as far to go."

The findings don't mean that depressed people should substitute marriage for depression treatment either, she said.

"This was just an average association," said Williams. "We're not saying that depressed individuals should run out and get married."

REACTION

"Clearly, one should not look upon these results as recommending that depressed people should get married," said Dr. Charles Goodstein, a clinical professor of psychiatry at the New York University School of Medicine in New York City. "The likelihood is strong that such a marriage might fall apart."

But, he added, these study results suggest that depressed people stand to gain more from marriage. "At the very least, the depressed person gets the sense that there's someone who cares about them."

However, Goodstein also pointed out that this particular survey may not accurately assess depression.

"Depression is a much more complicated matter than can be diagnosed on a survey. There is such a wide range of what we call depression, and many people can pass through society without being seen as depressed," he said.

Williams agreed that the survey used in this study can't be used to diagnose individual depression, but said it was designed to give an estimate of depression in a community population.

MORE INFORMATION

info To learn more about depression, visit the Web site of the National Institute of Mental Health at *www.nimb.nih.gov/publicat/depression.cfm.*

Natural Ways to Much Better Sex

Chris D. Meletis, ND, associate professor of natural pharmacology at National College of Naturopathic Medicine, Portland, and a physician at Beaverton Naturopathic Medicine, Beaverton, OR. He is author of *Better Sex Naturally*. Chrysalis.

It's true that drugs can help with the mechanics of sex. A man with erectile dysfunction (ED) may have better erections when he takes Viagra. A woman with low libido may benefit from testosterone cream. Medications are only a temporary solution. They don't solve the underlying problems. Natural remedies often can.

CAUSES

Millions of men and women have impaired circulation, which can reduce the ability to have erections and diminish sexual sensation. Chronic stress dampens libido and sexual performance. Insomnia and low energy can make people too tired to enjoy sex.

Certain herbs and other natural products address these problems and have been used safely and successfully for hundreds of years. Natural remedies, taken alone or in combination, can improve all aspects of sexual energy and performance. They promote better blood flow, increase libido and make erections stronger.

Start with one supplement. Take it for a week or two. If you don't notice a difference, add a second or third supplement that works in slightly different ways.

Example: Combine ginkgo biloba (which enhances blood flow) with ginseng (which improves overall energy). Always check with your doctor before taking any supplement.

Best choices…

GINKGO BILOBA

Function: Dilates blood vessels and improves circulation to the penis or vagina and clitoris. Impaired circulation is the most common cause of ED in men. In women, reduced blood flow can result in diminished sexual sensation and responsiveness. Ginkgo biloba is a very effective vasodilator, which means it opens (dilates) blood vessels. In one study, more than 70% of men with ED who took ginkgo improved their ability to have erections.

Anyone who is taking a selective serotonin reuptake inhibitor (SSRI) antidepressant, such as Prozac, should consider taking ginkgo. It offsets the libido-dampening side effect that often occurs in people taking these drugs.

Suggested dose: 40 mg three times daily. It usually takes one to three weeks to start working.

Caution: Ginkgo reduces the ability of blood to clot. Do not use ginkgo if you are taking *coumadin* (Warfarin) or other blood-thinning drugs. Patients taking daily aspirin, which also inhibits clotting, should be sure to talk to their doctors before using ginkgo.

ARGININE

Function: Increases pelvic circulation…improves erections…boosts libido and clitoral sensation. Arginine is an amino acid that is used by the body to produce *nitric oxide*, a chemical that relaxes blood vessels and promotes better circulation.

Suggested dose: 1,000 mg to 2,000 mg twice daily. People who take arginine typically notice the effects within a few days.

Caution: Patients with heart problems who are taking *nitroglycerin* should not take arginine. The combination could result in excessive vasodilation.

Also: Don't take arginine if you get cold sores from the herpes virus or have genital herpes. Arginine promotes viral replication and can increase flare-ups.

GINSENG

Function: Supports the adrenal glands, which produce hormones that affect genital circulation and the ability to have erections… modulates emotional stress…increases overall energy and libido. Ginseng safely increases levels of testosterone, the hormone that stimulates sexual response in men and women.

Suggested dose: 10 mg twice daily. People who take ginseng usually notice an increase in energy after about one week.

Caution: Ginseng is a mild stimulant that can increase blood pressure. Don't take it if you have been diagnosed with hypertension or heart disease.

YOHIMBE

Function: Improves libido and sexual response in women…promotes firmer erections in men.

Yohimbe is the only herb approved by the Food and Drug Administration for treating low libido and sexual dysfunction in men. It stimulates the release of *norepinephrine* from the adrenal glands, improving genital circulation and the ability to have erections. Women who take yohimbe experience greater sexual arousal.

Suggested dose: Follow directions on the label. Yohimbe works more rapidly than most natural products, so take it one to two hours before sex.

Caution: Yohimbe can cause sharp rises in blood pressure in some patients. It also can cause headaches and nausea. Use yohimbe only under medical supervision.

DHEA

Function: Increases sexual arousal in women…improves erections in men.

Dehydroepiandrosterone (DHEA) is a naturally occurring hormone that is converted to testosterone in the body. Testosterone and other androgens stimulate libido and sexual performance in men and women. The body's production of DHEA declines by about 1% annually after age 30, which can result in diminished sexual desire, performance and satisfaction.

Suggested dose: 5 mg daily for no more than three days a month.

Caution: Patients should take DHEA only if blood tests show that they have lower-than-normal levels. An excessive amount increases risk of side effects, such as acne, facial hair growth in women and sometimes heart palpitations. It also increases risk of tumors in the prostate gland. Men with a history of prostate cancer should not take DHEA.

WATER

Function: Increases blood volume…improves erections in men and sexual responsiveness in women.

How can good old water be an aphrodisiac? Because millions of Americans are chronically dehydrated—they don't drink enough water or they consume excessive amounts of caffeine, a diuretic that removes water from the body. Dehydration can result in diminished blood flow to the pelvis and genitals. Adequate hydration improves blood flow and makes it easier for men to have erections. Women who stay hydrated experience greater sexual comfort and satisfaction.

Suggested dose: Drink at least eight full glasses of water daily. Limit coffee and other caffeinated beverages to one or two servings daily.

Postpartum Depression Hits Dads, Too

James F. Paulson, PhD, assistant professor, pediatrics, psychology and behavioral sciences, Eastern Virginia Medical School Center for Pediatric Research, Norfolk.

William Coleman, MD, professor, pediatrics, University of North Carolina, Chapel Hill.

Pediatrics.

Almost as many new fathers as mothers suffer depression after the birth of a child, a new study shows. About 14% of mothers and 10% of fathers showed signs of moderate or severe postpartum depression, according to the study, which followed more than 5,000 members of two-parent families.

"There have been a few small studies in the last two years showing this, but nothing has been known on a national basis," said study leader Dr. James F. Paulson, an assistant professor of pediatrics and psychology and behavioral sciences at the Eastern Virginia Medical School Center for Pediatric Research.

THE STUDY

New parents who participated in the study filled out questionnaires and were interviewed to determine whether they showed symptoms of depression. Their relationships with their children were determined by questioning such practices as breast-feeding, putting the child to bed on his or her back, and whether the parents read to, played peek-a-boo with or sang to the child.

"What we found in this study is that basic day-to-day interactions were impaired in fathers, just as they were in mothers," Paulson said. "Also, basic activities were impaired."

RISK FACTORS

Fathers usually feel elation after a birth, but that feeling of "engrossment" can fade away, depending on family circumstances, said Dr. William Coleman, a professor of pediatrics at the University of North Carolina and chairman of the American Academy of Pediatrics committee on the psychosocial aspects of child and family health.

That can happen "if the mother is very, very controlling and wants the baby all to herself," Coleman said. "Also, fathers can experience frustration, sexual and emotional, if they forget to remember that the wife is not interested in sex at that time. If the wife is very motherly and maternal, he might feel kind of useless, on the periphery."

Depression in a father leads to a well-known pattern of behavior, Coleman said. "He tends to work longer, to watch sports more, to drink more and be solitary," he said.

DIAGNOSIS

Pediatricians should make a greater effort to identify postpartum depression in both mothers and fathers, Paulson said. "Pediatricians, in general, may be in the best position to catch depression, but they don't often do it," he said, adding he's now doing a study to look at patterns of screening for postpartum depression.

"Physicians do a very poor job asking about or detecting postpartum blues in the mother, and they may not even see the father," he said. "They might detect the mother's feelings, but may not even ask the father."

One problem in detecting postpartum depression in fathers is that "pediatricians are not told to inquire about adult issues," Coleman said. "It is a silent game."

Yet, it's important to detect postpartum depression in a father for the sake of the child's long-term outlook, Paulson said. "Based on what we know of mothers' postpartum depression, it is associated with health problems later on, not only emotional problems and difficulties adjusting to school but also basic health problems," he said.

info For more information on postpartum depression, visit the Web site of the National Library of Medicine at *www.nlm.nih.gov/med lineplus/postpartumdepression.html.*

Surprising Ways to Fight Fatigue! Boost Mood! Prevent Stroke! More!

Pierce J. Howard, PhD, a leading cognitive science researcher and cofounder and director of research at the Center for Applied Cognitive Studies in Charlotte, NC. He is adjunct professor of organizational psychology at University of North Carolina, Chapel Hill, and author of *The Owner's Manual for the Brain.* Bard.

Though many of the brain's inner workings remain a mystery, scientists make new discoveries about this powerful organ almost weekly. Recent brain research has revealed ways to significantly improve memory and mental ability along with practical ways to prevent stroke and other brain diseases, including Alzheimer's.

Highlights…

BOOST PERFORMANCE WITH STRESS

Scientists used to view stress as a detriment to mental performance. They advised people who were trying to improve learning and memory skills to minimize stress—with regular meditation, yoga, etc.

Finding: People learn more efficiently when they maintain an optimal level of stress. A principle called the Yerkes-Dodson Law has shown that a certain amount of stress (arousal) motivates people to try harder.

Balance is the key. People who experience very little stress—when taking a test or writing a paper, for example—tend to make errors of *omission*, such as forgetting to complete all the answers. People who experience too much stress make errors of *commission*, such as hitting the wrong computer keys.

What to do: If you find you're making more errors than usual in completing a task, you're probably experiencing too much stress. If you're bored, your stress levels are too low. For optimal mental performance, it is best to be in between these two extremes.

How to achieve stress balance: Too much stress is typically caused by one of two factors—having too few personal resources in a demanding situation or feeling that you have no options.

In the first case, increase your resources (practice, learn new skills, find helpers) or decrease the demands made on you (change to a less demanding task, simplify the task in some way).

In the second case, talk with your associates or with a counselor or doctor to identify ways to gain more control over the situation.

Too little stress is caused by having too many resources in a situation that is not very demanding—you are overqualified for the task at hand. Address this by handicapping or otherwise limiting yourself.

Example: When my daughter was younger and I played tennis with her, I would hit to her singles court, while she hit to my doubles lanes—so the tennis became more interesting for me. Or you can increase the level of difficulty or complexity of what you are doing. For example, if you are bored writing something, try doing it without using the verb "to be."

REDUCE STROKE RISK WITH CHOCOLATE

People who consume moderate amounts of chocolate have better brain circulation and can reduce their risk of stroke. Cocoa beans—the main ingredient in chocolate—contain natural antioxidants called cocoa flavonoids. The flavonoids in chocolate are more powerful than vitamin C at limiting fatty deposits (plaque) in arteries in the brain and heart. Buildups of plaque can impair mental performance and are the main cause of strokes.

Chemical compounds in chocolate also increase the levels of *nitric oxide*, a critical compound in the blood that relaxes the inner walls of blood vessels and promotes better blood flow and lower blood pressure. A study of 470 healthy men in the Netherlands found that those who ate the most cocoa beans—in the form of chocolate bars, pudding, hot cocoa, etc.—had lower blood

pressure and half the risk of dying during the study period than those who ate the least.

What to do: Have one to two cups of cocoa or two small squares of a bar of chocolate daily. The darker the chocolate, the better. According to the ORAC scale—a measure of the antioxidant levels in foods—dark chocolate has double the amount of antioxidants of milk chocolate.

FIGHT AFTERNOON FATIGUE

Nearly everyone gets sleepy after lunch. You can prevent this afternoon slump by eating protein first during lunch, then carbohydrates. The protein triggers an energy-promoting amino acid in the brain.

Foods that are high in complex carbohydrates, such as whole-grain bread, fruits and vegetables, are good for you, but they contain an abundance of the amino acid *L-tryptophan*, which promotes relaxation and sleepiness. High-protein foods, such as meats and fish, contain *L-tyrosine*, which makes you more alert and less likely to feel tired. Your energy level after lunch will depend on which of these amino acids reaches your brain first.

What to do: Start your meal with a bite or two of protein. This allows the L-tyrosine to reach the brain before the L-tryptophan. But don't just eat protein—carbohydrates are your body's main source of fuel.

GET HAPPY WITH OMEGA-3s

In countries such as Norway and Japan, where people eat the most fish—the best source of omega-3 fatty acids—the incidence of depression and suicide is much lower than in countries where people eat less. Omega-3s can help prevent and treat a variety of disorders, including bipolar disorder and attention deficit hyperactivity disorder (ADHD).

Unfortunately, Americans get excess amounts of another fatty acid group, the omega-6s, found mainly in meats, cooking oils and soybeans. In the last century, the ratio of omega-6s to omega-3s has soared, increasing the risk of mood disorders, including depression.

What to do: Eat three to four fish servings weekly to get more omega-3s. (Avoid fish high in mercury, such as shark, swordfish, tilefish and king mackerel, as well as large tuna, such as albacore, yellowfin, bigeye and bluefin.) Or you can eat nuts if you prefer. Ten to 15 walnut halves or 15 to 20 pecan halves provide the recommended daily amount of omega-3s.

REST—BUT DON'T NAP

The inventor Thomas Edison was famous for getting by on only two to four hours of sleep a night. When he was working on a particularly difficult problem, he would rest for five to 10 minutes. In the brief period between wakefulness and sleep, he often would experience an "A-ha!" moment and find the solution to his problem.

Scientists have found that when the brain goes into an "alpha state"—characterized by brain waves that are slower than the beta waves of wakefulness—people often develop insights, along with more focus and energy.

What to do: Shut your eyes and let your mind relax for five to 10 minutes. Resting in this fashion is not sleeping. People who slip into true sleep are groggy and less alert when they wake up.

PREVENT ALZHEIMER'S WITH "IDEA DENSITY"

The important Nun Study funded by the National Institute of Aging—a 15-year study of 678 members of the School Sisters of Notre Dame, ages 75 to 106—revealed that cloistered nuns with brain changes characteristic of Alzheimer's disease didn't necessarily have cognitive impairments. Why do some people with these brain changes (apparent during autopsies) develop Alzheimer's, while others do not?

When researchers analyzed short biographies that the nuns had written upon taking their vows decades earlier, they found that those with a high "idea density" (many thoughts woven into a small number of words)—a marker of educational level and vocabulary—were less likely to develop Alzheimer's symptoms later in life, even when their brains showed signs of the disease.

The brain continues to form neurons and connections between neurons throughout life. People who are mentally active form the most connections and develop brain reserves that can slow the onset of Alzheimer's symptoms.

What to do: Stay mentally engaged. Take classes at a university or community college. Read challenging books and periodicals. Keep a diary or do crossword puzzles. Learn a new language.

TAKE LEARNING BREAKS

You'll learn most efficiently when you focus on one thing at a time, then take a break before moving on to new material.

Example: Someone learning a new golf swing needs about six hours for the new neural pathways to become established. If he/she tries to learn a second swing within that six-hour window, the new information will crowd out the previous learning.

What to do: If you're in school, studying for a professional exam or just trying to learn a new skill, save the beginning of each day for major new learning. Use the rest of the day for practice and repetition.

Suppose you're learning a new language, such as Spanish. You might spend the morning memorizing verbs with "–ir" endings. Practice this during the day or practice material learned on previous days, but don't introduce verbs with "–er" endings until the next day.

Six Simple Steps to A Sharper Mind

Sandra Cusack, PhD, Guttmann-Gee Research Fellow in Educational Gerontology at the Gerontology Research Centre at Simon Fraser University in Vancouver, Canada. She is coauthor, with Wendy Thompson, of *Mental Fitness for Life*. Bull.

Most people, including many doctors, believe that memory and cognitive abilities inevitably decline at middle age—even though there's virtually no scientific proof to support this belief.

What most people don't realize: Even though some brain cells (neurons) die with age, the brain retains the ability to form new neurons and connections between neurons. In fact, the number of nerve endings (dendrites) in the part of the brain that processes information increases between ages 50 and 80.

Imaging tests allow us to see changes in brain physiology that occur in response to brain exercises and new learning. Age-related diseases, such as dementia—and even some medications —can lead to memory loss and reduced mental function, but such problems are not an inevitable part of aging.*

CREATING A "BRAIN WORKOUT"

People who exercise their minds regularly and develop positive psychological traits, such as optimism and self-confidence, can literally "rewire" their brains (that is, new neurons can be formed, and existing neurons can form new connections). *Here's how...*

Step 1: Set goals. Goals create a sense of purpose and promote feelings of self-worth. Goals that are especially meaningful or that require a good deal of effort and concentration, such as raising money for charity or researching your genealogy, are believed to promote brain health.

Goals are particularly important for older adults who have a tendency to stop challenging themselves mentally in the assumption that their cognitive abilities decline with age. Any goal that improves overall health, such as losing weight or reducing stress, contributes to brain health.

Helpful steps...

•Write down 10 things that you want to do before you die.

Example: Short-term goal—lose 10 pounds in the next three months...long-term goal—become a part-time teacher. Choose goals that stretch your abilities but aren't impossible.

•Write down the advantages of reaching your goals.

Examples: "I'll be healthier and look better if I lose weight," and "It makes me happy to help people learn."

•Make your goals measurable. Suppose your goal is to complete a university degree that was abandoned years ago. Measurable goals might include applying for admission to a local college and enrolling in courses that are challenging.

*Caution: If you have experienced a sudden memory decline, consult a physician. You may need to be evaluated for a memory disorder.

•Set deadlines. Choose a date for each goal, and identify key steps along the way.

Step 2: Be a power thinker. Because many older adults have negative perceptions of their mental abilities, they often say things like, "I can't remember your name because my memory isn't as good as it once was." Such statements indicate a willingness to accept the status quo and often lead to a self-fulfilling prophecy.

Better: Think—and phrase things—positively. Tell yourself, "I don't want to forget names, so I'm going to take the necessary steps to retain my memory."

Step 3: Cultivate creativity. We used to believe that creativity declined with age. But some people reach their prime later in life.

Examples: Goethe finished writing *Faust* at age 83...Grandma Moses began painting in her 70s.

There are many ways to be creative. Humor is a form of creativity. So is keeping a journal, cooking or rearranging furniture in a room. Every activity is creative if you put your personal stamp on it.

Creative people are natural problem-solvers. Studies show that they engage both sides of their brains and reap the rewards of cognitive effort—including better memory and more efficient processing of information.

Step 4: Adopt a positive mental attitude. In the 1960s, Mayo Clinic researchers classified 839 patients as either optimists or pessimists, depending on the number of positive words that appeared in written statements they provided. Thirty years later, many more of the optimists were still alive, having lived an average of six years longer than the pessimists. Optimism, the hallmark of having a positive mental attitude, appears to have powerful effects on mental health, which may help protect cognitive abilities.

Step 5: Perform memory-boosting exercises. Memory is like a muscle—the more you use it, the stronger it gets. Brain stimulation caused by learning new, challenging material triggers an increase in the number of dendrites as well as synapses (connections between dendrites).

Helpful: Create a "brain workout" schedule.

Example: *Sunday*—Read an engaging book...visit a museum. *Monday*—Listen to tapes or CDs to learn a foreign language. *Tuesday*—Do a crossword puzzle...take a meditation class. *Wednesday*—Play bridge...write in your journal. *Thursday*—Take an art class. *Friday*—Volunteer as a tour guide at an art gallery. *Saturday*—Host a dinner party...try out a new recipe.

Also helpful: Learn one new word a day. Write it down and repeat the definition a few times. The next day, write down a new word and review the one from the day before. Review all seven words at the week's end. Doing this daily will increase your vocabulary as well as your ability to retain new information of all kinds. To receive a free word-a-day E-mail, go to *www.wordsmith.org*. Or for free Sudoku puzzles, the popular number-logic game, go to *www.free-sudokus.com*. Nintendo's "Brain Age," which includes math and logic activities, and similar video games also give your mind a good workout.

Step 6: **Speak your mind.** People who assert themselves—by being active in their communities, meeting new people or simply feeling free to say what they're thinking—develop a tremendous amount of self-confidence. Knowing that your thoughts matter will encourage you to think clearly, critically and creatively. It's also a way of engaging the world and keeping your mind active.

Important: Take every opportunity to speak your mind. Join in casual discussions with your family and friends—everyone has something to contribute. Talk to people when you're waiting in line at the post office or grocery store—and, just as important, listen to what they have to say. As we hear different points of view, we develop mental flexibility and open-mindedness. You can practice this skill one-on-one, or in groups, such as book clubs or adult-education classes.

■ **More from Dr. Cusack...**

Are You Mentally Fit?

Rate yourself on a scale of 1 to 10 (10 being the highest rating).

1. Confidence in your mental abilities
2. Setting and achieving goals
3. Willingness to take risks
4. Optimism
5. Creativity
6. Mental flexibility
7. Ability to learn new things
8. Memory
9. Ability to express opinions clearly
10. Overall mental fitness

Add up your score...

Less than 40: Poor. Get started on this program right away!

40–54: Fair. You could significantly improve your brain health with this program.

55–69: Good. You stand to gain from this program.

70–84: Very good. You're well on your way to a rich and fulfilling life, but you could be doing better.

85–100: Excellent. You are an inspiration to others—keep it up!

Surprising Reasons Why People Overeat

Brian Wansink, PhD, professor of marketing and nutritional science, and director of the Food and Brand Lab at Cornell University, Ithaca, NY. He is author of *Mindless Eating: Why We Eat More Than We Think.* Bantam. *www.mindlesseating.org.*

Our minds, not our stomachs, control our eating habits—but our minds don't always do a good job of making food decisions. Most people put on weight because their minds don't accurately keep track of how much they have eaten, not because they lack the willpower to put down their forks.

Surprisingly, when our minds tell us which foods we enjoy, it's often for reasons that have little to do with how they taste.

Example: Approximately one-third of World War II veterans who served in the South Pacific love Chinese food 50 years later. A similar percentage hate it. It turns out that almost all the veterans who love Chinese food did not experience frequent heavy combat when in Asia, but those who hate it did.

Brian Wansink, PhD, a noted food psychologist, has done extensive research on how our minds trick us into unhealthy eating habits. *Here are some of the ways...*

•If it looks like a small meal, it feels like a small meal. Our eyes, not our stomachs, tell us when we're full. In a study conducted by our research team, when we replaced eight-inch dinner plates with 12-inch plates, diners consumed 20% to 35% more because their portions looked smaller on the larger plates. After the meal, they were certain that they hadn't eaten any more than usual.

What to do: Use smaller plates, bowls and spoons if you want to eat less. Drink from tall, thin glasses—not short, fat ones—so you will think you are drinking more. When possible, serve food over a bed of lettuce so that the plate looks full.

•We feel full when there's visual evidence that we have had a lot to eat. In one study, we gave chicken wings to graduate students while they watched the Super Bowl. When we left the bones in front of the students, they ate an average of four wings apiece. When we cleared the bones away frequently—removing the visual evidence of earlier consumption—each student ate an average of six wings. After the game, students in both groups estimated that they had only four wings each.

What to do: When you're eating—particularly when you're snacking—leave out candy wrappers, peanut shells and other evidence of snacking so that your eyes can warn you about how much you have eaten.

•When there's no distance to the food, there's no thinking before eating. Office workers consumed an average of nine Hershey's Kisses per day when we put bowls of the chocolate candies on their desks. Their consumption dropped by more than 50% when these bowls were positioned just six feet away. Six feet is only two steps, but even a short distance forces us to think twice before we eat.

What to do: At home, fill individual plates at the stove, and leave the leftovers on the stove

or a sideboard. The more hassle it is to eat, the less we eat. You will have fewer additional helpings if you must stand up to get them. A bowl of salad or vegetables can be brought to the dinner table because second helpings of these foods won't add many calories.

With snack foods, pour a serving into a bowl rather than eating straight from the bag. Then if you want more, you have to go to the kitchen to get it.

•"Comfort foods" cause overconsumption. Comfort foods improve our moods. These foods pick us up when we're feeling stressed or unhappy and serve as rewards when we're feeling good.

Women's comfort foods tend to be unhealthy dessert or snack items, while men's comfort foods are more likely to be hot meals. Why the difference? Men tend to associate home-cooked meals with someone taking care of them, because men's meals often are prepared by their wives. Women associate home-cooked meals with the chore of cooking, so they prefer prepared snack foods and desserts.

What to do: We get nearly as much emotional benefit from a small serving of a comfort food as from a large one—for example, a single scoop of ice cream instead of a pint.

Also, we get nearly as much emotional benefit from our second- or third-favorite comfort food as from our absolute favorite. If your top comfort food is chocolate ice cream but tomato soup is a close second, keep plenty of microwavable tomato soup in the house so that low-calorie comfort is just seconds away.

•We underestimate beverage calories. When people are asked to gauge the calories in a drink, they typically undershoot by 30% or more. Beverages don't seem to be filling, so we don't assume that they have as many calories as they actually do.

What to do: As a rule of thumb, estimate that you're consuming 10 calories per ounce for "thin" beverages, such as juice, soda and milk...and 20 calories per ounce for "thick" beverages, such as smoothies and meal-replacement shakes. That adds up quickly when you're drinking a 32-ounce soda—to an estimated 320 calories.

Interestingly, if you load that drink with ice, you'll actually burn off a few of those calories. Since your body has to use energy to heat up an iced beverage, you actually burn about one calorie for every ice-cold ounce you drink. If you drink the recommended eight eight-ounce glasses of water a day and if you fill those 64 ounces with ice, you'll burn about 70 extra calories a day, the equivalent of about seven pounds a year.

•Exercise might make you fatter. You have forced yourself to jog three miles every day for months—yet you weigh just as much as when you started. What are you doing wrong?

Most exercisers overestimate the calories their exercise burns and reward themselves with high-calorie foods after their workouts because they think they've earned it. They don't realize that the six Oreo cookies they treat themselves to as a reward have more calories (around 320) than the number of calories they burned while running three miles (around 300).

What to do: If you need a reward, opt for nonfood treats, perhaps a half-hour doing something you enjoy, such as reading a good book or watching a favorite TV show.

•Birth order might affect your eating habits. Oldest children and only children tend to save their favorite foods for last. Give them a chocolate chip cookie, and it might become a special treat for after dinner.

Youngest children and middle children of large families are more likely to polish off favorite foods as soon as they receive them—probably to ensure that older siblings won't snatch the food away. These birth-order eating patterns tend to continue into adulthood.

For adults who are the youngest or middle children, the result can be unnecessary pounds. Favorite foods tend to be unhealthy foods, and people who eat unhealthy foods as soon as they get them may be inclined to eat larger quantities in the long run.

What to do: Don't bring favorite snacks into the house in large quantities, especially if you are a youngest or middle child. You might polish off a box in a single sitting.

Music Helps Lower Your Blood Pressure... Ease Pain and More

Suzanne B. Hanser, EdD, chair of the music therapy department at Berklee College of Music in Boston and past president of the American Music Therapy Association and the World Federation of Music Therapy. She is a research associate at the Dana-Farber Cancer Institute, an affiliate of Harvard Medical School, also in Boston, where she investigates medical applications of music therapy.

Everyone knows the soothing effect of listening to a favorite piece of music. But until recently, there was little scientific evidence to support its effectiveness in helping to combat specific health problems.

Now: A growing body of research has found that music can affect key areas of the brain that help regulate specific physiological functions necessary for good health. The best choice of music and the time spent listening depends on an individual's needs and preferences. *Medical conditions that can be improved by listening to appropriate music...*

HIGH BLOOD PRESSURE

The hypothalamus helps control the autonomic nervous system, which regulates our breathing, heartbeat and other automatic responses in the body. It also is linked to emotional activity.

How music helps: When a person listens to music that stimulates positive memories and/or images, the activity of the hypothalamus helps slow a person's heart and respiration rates as well as blood pressure.

Scientific evidence: In a study published in the *British Journal of Health Psychology,* 75 adults performed a stressful three-minute math problem. Afterward, they were randomly assigned to sit in silence or listen to classical, jazz or popular music. Those who heard classical selections had significantly lower systolic (top number) blood pressure levels. Blood pressure did not significantly improve in people who listened to the other selections.

What to do: Observe how you respond to different types of music. Match your state of mind to the tempo and dynamics.

Example: If you are agitated, listen to something with a strong, fast beat, then gradually switch to slower and softer music. This can reduce stress and lower blood pressure.

INSOMNIA

Although healthy adults typically fall asleep within 30 minutes, adults age 50 and older often have more trouble falling—and staying—asleep.

How music helps: Soft, restful music can act as a sedative by reducing the amount of the stress-related neurotransmitter noradrenaline that circulates in the bloodstream.

Scientific evidence: Sixty people ages 60 to 83 who reported sleep difficulties took part in a study at Tzu-Chi General Hospital in Taiwan. After three weeks, researchers found a 35% improvement in sleep quality, length of sleep, daytime dysfunction and sleep disturbances in subjects who listened to slow, soft music at night. The most effective types of music used in the study were piano versions of popular "oldies," New Age, harp, classical and slow jazz.

What to do: Make sure your bedroom temperature is comfortable, then lie in bed at your usual bedtime, with the lights out (light interferes with the production of the sleep hormone melatonin) and your eyes closed while listening to music. Experiment with different types of music until you discover what's relaxing for you. (Earphones are optional.) If you wake during the night, try listening to music again.

PAIN

Listening to music does not eliminate pain, but it can help distract your brain by creating a secondary stimulus that diverts your attention from the feeling of discomfort.

Scientific evidence: In a 14-day study published in the *Journal of Advanced Nursing,* 66 older adults with osteoarthritis pain sat quietly for 20 minutes daily, while another group listened to music. Those who listened to music reported a significant decrease in pain.

What to do: For pain reduction, it's important to identify music that engages you—that is, it should elicit memories and/or make you want to tap your foot, sway or even dance. Singing, which requires deep breathing, or using a simple percussion instrument (such as chimes or a drum), which does not require playing specific notes, also helps.

Tired? Moody? Adrenal Fatigue May Be to Blame

Dr. Mark Stengler is a licensed naturopathic medical doctor and a leading authority on the practice of alternative and integrated medicine. An associate clinical professor at the National College of Naturopathic Medicine in Portland, OR, Dr. Stengler has served on a medical advisory committee for the Yale University Complementary Medicine Outcomes Research Project and is the author or coauthor of 16 books, including two best sellers—*The Natural Physician's Healing Therapies* and *Prescription for Natural Cures.* Dr. Stengler is the founder and director of the La Jolla Whole Health Clinic in La Jolla, CA. *www.DrStengler.com.*

The epidemic of exhaustion affecting so many Americans today may have at its root a condition that is common and easy to correct—yet that condition often goes unrecognized by medical doctors. The culprit is adrenal fatigue (AF).

Adrenal glands produce stress hormones in response to stressful situations. With AF, the hormone response mechanism is so overwhelmed that it becomes ineffective. AF is usually triggered by long periods of mental, emotional or physical stress, and it is worsened by poor nutrition and unhealthful lifestyle choices.

In my estimation, 20% of Americans suffer from some degree of AF. And I find that this disorder often causes—or contributes to—the development of numerous other illnesses, particularly chronic fatigue syndrome and diabetes. When AF is correctly diagnosed and treated, the other conditions often are relieved as well.

STRESS HORMONE FACTORY

Located on top of each kidney is a crescent-shaped adrenal gland. The hormones these glands secrete affect blood pressure, heart rate, metabolism, liver function, immunity and the body's response to stress. Although the adrenal glands produce many hormones, two in particular become depleted in cases of AF—*dehydroepiandrosterone* (DHEA) and *cortisol.*

•**DHEA.** The body converts DHEA into estrogen and testosterone. Abnormally low DHEA levels may contribute to cardiovascular disease, autoimmune disorders, poor resistance to infection, diabetes, weight gain, osteoporosis, sexual dysfunction, menopausal symptoms and mood disorders. DHEA also plays a role in aging.

•**Cortisol** plays an important role in fighting infection...stabilizing blood sugar...controlling the body's use of proteins, carbohydrates and fats...and regulating the sleep cycle. Cortisol is secreted at higher levels during the fight-or-flight response to stress, providing a burst of energy, heightened alertness and decreased pain sensitivity. But when cortisol levels are elevated for long periods, production by the adrenal glands drops. Insufficient cortisol can make you prone to fatigue, infection, allergies, diabetes and thyroid dysfunction.

Depletion of DHEA and cortisol adversely affects the way your body handles stress, inflammation, blood sugar regulation, energy production, immune response and cognitive function. That's why AF can be a contributing factor in a surprising number of ailments. A weakened immune response plays a part in cancer as well as in recurring infections, particularly of the respiratory tract. And poor regulation of blood sugar can contribute to both diabetes and alcoholism.

MAKING THE DIAGNOSIS

Conventional medical doctors often don't recognize AF—even though the condition was described in medical literature in the early 20th century. It was known then as *hypoadrenia*, which means low- or under-functioning adrenal glands.

If you show signs of AF, your best bet for diagnosis and treatment is to see a holistic doctor. For a referral, consult the American College for Advancement in Medicine (888-439-6891, *www.acam.org*). *In addition to assessing your symptoms, the doctor may perform...*

•**Saliva testing** to measure cortisol levels. This test is more accurate than a blood test. A pattern of low cortisol levels throughout the day indicates AF. I ask patients to collect saliva samples in test tubes upon waking...before lunch...in the late afternoon...and before bed. Cortisol levels are normally highest in the morning and decrease throughout the day. People with severe AF usually have below-normal cortisol readings during at least two of the four time periods. I also use a saliva test that measures the DHEA level in the morning, when it is normally highest.

Saliva testing of cortisol levels is used by many research institutions, particularly to assess the effects of stress. Several commercial labs offer saliva hormone testing—including Quest Diagnostics, the nation's largest conventional medical lab, which is used by medical and naturopathic doctors. To use Quest, you must have a prescription for the test from a doctor. A lab I have used for years that usually doesn't require a doctor's order is ZRT in Beaverton, Oregon (866-600-1636, *www.salivatest.com*). The adrenal function test, including four cortisol samples and a morning DHEA reading, costs $150, which is not covered by insurance. If your state does not allow residents to order lab testing directly (check the list on the ZRT Web site), you can order the kits at the same price through my clinic (call 858-450-7120).

•**Blood pressure measurements,** taken three times—first while you lie on your back, then when you sit upright and again when you stand up. Normally, systolic (top number) and diastolic (bottom number) blood pressure will increase between 5 mm Hg and 10 mm Hg from the first reading to the third. If blood pressure *drops*, it may indicate AF—the adrenal glands may not be producing the stress hormones needed to maintain blood pressure.

•**Pupil testing,** performed in a darkened room. A practitioner shines a flashlight from the side across one eye, and the pupil should continue to get smaller. With AF, the pupil first contracts and then dilates again.

HEALING STRATEGIES

Lifestyle changes and treatment reduce symptoms in most people with AF in four to six weeks. In severe cases, full recovery may take several months. *My advice...*

•**Curb stress.** A hectic lifestyle sets the stage for AF. Are you working too hard? Is your job emotionally draining? Are your relationships unsatisfying? Try to alleviate stress and seek out emotional support.

•**Get enough rest.** Go to bed by 10 p.m., and aim for eight to nine hours of sleep nightly. On weekends, nap for an hour or two.

•**Eat right.** People with AF are prone to blood sugar swings that sap energy, so it is imperative to eat breakfast. I also recommend between-meal snacks, such as whole-grain toast or whey protein drinks. My favorite is Jay Robb's Whey Protein, which is naturally sweetened. It is available at major health-food stores and at *www.jayrobb.com* (877-529-7622). Almonds, walnuts and macadamia nuts are good snack foods, since they provide protein for blood sugar stabilization.

Aim for 2,400 mg of sodium daily. Limit caffeinated beverages, such as coffee, tea and cola, to one cup daily because caffeine stimulates the already overtaxed adrenal glands. Avoid alcohol, which contains simple sugars.

•**Exercise in moderation.** Too little exercise is harmful, since exercise helps balance stress hormones. But overexercising worsens fatigue.

General guideline: If you're exhausted after your workout or feel more worn-out than usual the next day, you're doing too much. Start by walking 15 minutes daily. As your adrenal glands recover, you can gradually increase to 45 minutes of moderately intense exercise daily.

•**Avoid lung irritants.** Cigarette smoke, air pollution and allergens can worsen AF by stimulating cortisol release. If you smoke, please quit. Avoid secondhand smoke, and reduce exposure to allergy triggers with a high-efficiency particulate air (HEPA) filter.

•**Clear up infections.** Acute and chronic respiratory infections as well as other types of infections can exacerbate AF symptoms. To speed recovery, work with a holistic doctor, who can recommend natural immune boosters, such as the herb astragalus.

■ **More from Dr. Stengler...**

Adrenal Fatigue Symptoms

Patients with AF typically experience low energy or exhaustion (even after a good night's sleep), plus one or more of the following...

•**Light-headedness upon standing up**

•**Mood swings, especially irritability**

•**Decreased ability to cope with stress**

•**Low libido**

•**Poor concentration**

•**Impaired memory**

•**Slow recovery from illness**

•**Low back pain**

•**Salt and/or sugar cravings**

•**Inability to lose or gain weight,** despite calorie reduction or increase

---

Hormone Injection May Ease Post-Traumatic Stress

University of Texas Southwestern Medical Center news release.

An injection of a natural stress hormone may help decrease post-traumatic stress, a study in mice suggests.

THE STUDY

In the study, researchers at the University of Texas Southwestern Medical Center at Dallas placed mice in a plastic box and subjected them to a mild electrical shock.

A couple of days later, the mice were returned to the box, and the researchers gauged their fear, based on how long they "froze" in place. After a few minutes, the researchers injected the mice with *corticosterone,* a natural stress hormone produced by the body.

When the mice were returned to the box again a day later, they showed significantly less fear, the researchers reported. The higher the dose of corticosterone the mice had been given, the less fear they showed.

Giving the mice the injection before returning them to the box did not reduce their fear when they were tested again a day later. But when the injections were given over four days, whether before or after their second visit to the box, their fear was reduced one day later.

EXPLANATION

The researchers believe the effect is due to a mechanism called *extinction,* in which the release of corticosterone causes a memory to gradually diminish.

"Corticosterone appears to enhance new memories that compete with the fearful memory, thereby decreasing its negative emotional significance," said study author Craig Powell, a professor of neurology and psychiatry at UT Southwestern.

"The natural release of stress hormones during recall of a fearful memory may be a natural mechanism to decrease the negative emotional aspects of the memory," said study coauthor Jacqueline Blundell, a postdoctoral fellow in neurology at UT Southwestern.

"Conversely, patients with post-traumatic stress disorder have blunted stress hormone responses and thus may not decrease fearful memories normally over time," Blundell said.

MORE RESEARCH WITH HUMANS

Another UT Southwestern study is in progress to see if receiving a stress hormone while reliving memories can reduce fear responses in veterans suffering from post-traumatic stress disorder.

info The American Academy of Family Physicians' Web site has more about post-traumatic stress disorder at *http://familydoctor. org* under "Conditions A to Z."

Layoffs Stress Everyone— Even Those Who Keep Their Jobs

Mika Kivimaki, PhD, department of epidemiology and public health, University College London, England.
Rosemary K. Sokas, MD, MOH, director, division of Environmental and Occupational Health Sciences, University of Illinois at Chicago School of Public Health.
Journal of Epidemiology and Community Health.

Workers are familiar with corporate downsizing and the toll it takes on those laid off, but mental health problems can also rise in those who keep their jobs, a European study shows.

"Employees who remain in work after downsizing may be at increased risk of being prescribed psychotropic drugs," said lead author Mika Kivimaki, from the Department of Epidemiology and Public Health at University College London.

"In other words, enforced redundancies may boost mental health problems among those who keep their jobs," he added.

PAST RESEARCH

Kivimaki's previous research on municipal organizations showed that in downsized groups, cuts resulted in greater levels of job demands and job insecurity, along with declines in perceived job control, in those workers remaining. "Indeed, we have previously also shown organizational downsizing to be a strong predictor of stress-related physical health outcomes, including cardiovascular mortality," he said.

NEW STUDY

Kivimaki's team based its findings on data on the use of psychotropic drugs—including antidepressants, antianxiety drugs and sleeping pills—in a group of almost 27,000 municipal workers in Finland between 1994 and 2000.

Among these workers, about 4,800 worked in units that experienced layoffs but kept their jobs, almost 4,300 lost their jobs, and close to 17,600 did not work in units that were downsized.

RESULTS

Men who lost or left their jobs were most at risk of getting a prescription for a psychotropic drug. Compared with men who worked for units with no layoffs, these men were 64% more likely to be given a prescription for one of these drugs, the researchers found.

However, men who kept their jobs after a layoff were also almost 50% more likely to be given a prescription for one of the drugs, compared with those who worked for units that were not downsized, Kivimaki's group found. Women in downsized units were 12% more likely to be given a prescription.

Sleeping pills were most often prescribed to men, while antianxiety drugs were most often prescribed to women, Kivimaki said.

"Policy makers, employers, and occupational health professionals should recognize that organizational downsizing may pose mental health risks among employees," Kivimaki said.

REACTION

One expert believes the findings confirm that layoffs affect *everyone* in the workplace.

"This is an important study that supports the negative impact downsizing has on survivors who keep their jobs, as well as on those who lose them," said Dr. Rosemary K. Sokas, the director of the division of Environmental and Occupational Health Sciences at the University of Illinois at Chicago School of Public Health.

As pointed out by the authors, job loss has devastating consequences, including increased risk of death, Sokas said. "In the aftermath of the collapse of the former Soviet Union, death rates among men soared in both Russia and in the newly independent states of Eastern Europe. This study, which takes place in Finland, a country with universal health insurance and a relatively intact social net, confirms that work matters," she said.

This study also confirms the harmful effects of organizational downsizing on those who continue in the workplace, Sokas said. "Downsizing is a workplace hazard."

info There's more information on job stress at the American Psychological Association Web site at *http://apa.org*. Search under topics for "Workplace Issues."

Men, Too, Will Shop 'Til They Drop

Lorrin Koran, MD, emeritus professor, psychiatry and behavioral sciences, Stanford University, Stanford, CA.

Helga Dittmar, PhD, senior lecturer, psychology, University of Sussex, England.

American Journal of Psychiatry.

One in 20 American adults said they find themselves unable to stop shopping for items they may not even want or need. And men are just as likely as women to suffer from "compulsive buying," according to the largest survey of its kind ever conducted.

"That's the biggest surprise—that men engage in this behavior almost as commonly as women," said Dr. Lorrin Koran, emeritus professor of psychiatry at Stanford University.

He said the finding runs counter to the conventional view of compulsive buying as a "woman's disease." That impression grew out of the fact that women have typically made up the vast majority of volunteers for studies looking at the disorder.

However, Koran said men who obsessively shop are probably more reluctant than women to come forward and admit they have a problem. "Generally, in psychiatry, men seek care less often than women," he pointed out. "It's not 'manly' to seek help."

The study also found that compulsive shopping usually begins in a person's teens or early 20s, and is associated with lower—not higher —incomes.

SHOPPING ADDICTION

According to Koran, compulsive shopping is more than the occasional splurge, later regretted.

Instead, the urge to shop becomes constant and overwhelming. For most, the act of browsing and buying gradually takes the place of time spent at work, with family or in other pursuits. To qualify as a disorder, "the behavior has to be associated with marked distress and interfere with functioning," Koran said.

The typical compulsive shopper usually feels a sense of euphoria while engaged in shopping, but that "high" later gives way to remorse and distress. "It's afterward, when you realize that you spent money that you didn't have or you argue with your husband about why you have all these clothes in your closet that you never wear," Koran said. "That's when you regret it."

RISK FACTORS

The root causes of shopping addiction remain unclear. But British researcher Dr. Helga Dittmar, a senior lecturer of psychology at the University of Sussex, said two factors—highly materialistic values and poor self-image—appear to be risk factors. In this scenario, buying things is viewed as a path to self-improvement.

"They'll buy those consumer goods that symbolize a part of their ideal self," Dittmar explained.

But just how prevalent is compulsive buying? Previous estimates, based on small samples, had ranged from about 2% to 16% of the population.

NEW STUDY

In this new study, Koran's team conducted a nationwide phone survey of more than 2,500 adults. After gathering data on demographics and income, the researchers used a standard screening instrument called the Compulsive Buying Scale to determine whether a person fit the criteria for the disorder.

They discovered that 5.8% of those interviewed did, in fact, meet the threshold for compulsive buying. Rates differed little between women (6%) and men (5.5%). Compulsive buyers tended to be younger than people unaffected by the disorder and more likely to make less than $50,000 a year, the study found.

Koran said men who compulsively shop tend to purchase different items than women. "Men tend to buy tech items, cameras, CDs, books, tools and gadgets," he said. "Women tend to buy clothes, jewelry, makeup, items for the homes, craft goods."

Whatever their gender, compulsive buyers are usually not made any happier by their ceaseless spending, the experts said. In fact, many find themselves deeply in debt and filled with remorse and shame as they hide their addiction from family and friends. Some studies have even linked the condition to a heightened risk for suicide, Koran said.

GETTING HELP FOR COMPULSIVE BUYING

That's why he and Dittmar are advocating formal inclusion of compulsive buying in the next *Diagnostic and Statistical Manual of Mental Disorders*—the standard guidebook for psychological and psychiatric treatment worldwide.

Based on the new study numbers, "compulsive buying is at least as prevalent as many other clinical disorders," Dittmar noted. "I think, in the end, that I would favor its inclusion in the *DSM,* given that it would acknowledge and help raise public consciousness about the severity of compulsive buying."

She added that, up until now, "there has been a tendency to belittle 'shopping addicts.' It's time that the serious consequences of compulsive buying—psychological, social, financial—are highlighted."

Koran agreed, noting that effective treatments, which include antidepressant drugs and psychotherapy, do exist. But he said those affected must first come forward.

"It's always important to encourage people who have these types of disorders to seek treatment," he said. "There are things we can do to help."

info For more on compulsive buying, visit the Illinois Institute for Addiction Recovery's Web site at *www.addictionrecov.org/spendad dict.htm.*

<big><big><big><big>8</big></big></big></big>

Family Health

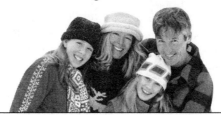

Medical Conditions Doctors Often Misdiagnose

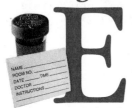

Each year, up to 40% of Americans who are seen in an emergency room or intensive care unit are misdiagnosed. In some cases, a patient's condition is correctly diagnosed, and appropriate treatment is administered later. In other cases, the time that is lost through a misdiagnosis can be life-threatening.

Example: A patient who has painful abdominal cramping may be diagnosed with "gastroenteritis" (inflammation of the gastrointestinal tract) when the real culprit is a potentially fatal bowel obstruction.

Important: Listen to your intuition, but don't try to self-diagnose your problem. Get a complete evaluation from your doctor and a second opinion, if desired.

Here are some conditions that are frequently misdiagnosed…

Wrong diagnosis: Gastroenteritis. Gastroenteritis can be caused by ingesting food or water contaminated with a virus (Norwalk virus, adenovirus)…a bacterium (*Salmonella, Escherichia coli*)…a parasite (*Giardia*)…rare microorganisms (amoebas or parasitic worms)…or a food allergy. Gastroenteritis can result in cramping, vomiting and/or diarrhea.

But these symptoms also can characterize bowel obstruction (commonly caused by scar tissue from previous abdominal or pelvic surgery)… appendicitis…gallbladder disease…or antibiotic-associated colitis.

Self-defense: Do not accept a diagnosis of "gastroenteritis" if your symptoms include…

•**Crampy abdominal pain** that comes and goes. This could indicate a bowel obstruction.

Vicki Rackner, MD, a board-certified surgeon and clinical instructor at the University of Washington School of Medicine in Seattle. She is founder of Medical Bridges, a patient-advocacy consulting firm. Dr. Rackner is the author of *The Biggest Skeleton in Your Doctor's Closet*. Five Star.

•**Pain that begins around the navel** and migrates to the lower right abdomen. This could be appendicitis.

•**Sudden pain in the upper-right abdomen** after eating a high-fat meal. This symptom could be due to a gallbladder attack.

•**Severe diarrhea, abdominal pain and/or fever.** These symptoms could be caused by pseudomembranous colitis, an inflammatory condition of the colon that occurs in some people who have used antibiotics. It's usually caused by overgrowth of the bacterium *Clostridium difficile*.

To diagnose your condition correctly, your doctor should take a thorough medical history and perform a physical exam. Tests may include blood work, X-rays and an ultrasound or computed tomography (CT) scan.

Wrong diagnosis: **Migraine.** More than 45 million people seek medical care each year for headaches. Many have a true migraine, a severe headache often accompanied by nausea, vomiting and/or extreme sensitivity to light and sound. Others have a tension or cluster headache.

In rare cases, a headache can signal a potentially serious condition, such as a stroke…a ruptured brain aneurysm (a weakened blood vessel that has burst)…a contusion (bruising of the brain)…a concussion (a head injury that can cause headache, confusion and amnesia)…a subdural hematoma (bleeding from veins between the outer and middle layers of tissue covering the brain, usually following a head injury)…a brain tumor…meningitis (a bacterial or viral infection of the membrane that surrounds the spinal cord and brain)…or a sinus infection.

Self-defense: Do not accept a diagnosis of "migraine" if your symptoms include…

•**Headache with confusion,** weakness on one side of the body, double vision and/or trouble speaking. This could indicate a stroke.

•**"The worst headache of my life"** or a headache that "hits like a lightning bolt." These are signs of a possible stroke or ruptured brain aneurysm.

•**Headache that gets worse after coughing,** exertion, straining or sudden movement. This can indicate a ruptured brain aneurysm.

•**Headache after a head injury,** especially if the headache gets worse over the next day or two. It could be a brain injury, such as a contusion, concussion or subdural hematoma.

•**New headache pain or changes in headache pattern** (location, intensity or frequency), especially in people age 55 or older. This could signal a brain tumor.

•**Headache with a fever,** stiff neck and/or rash. These are red flags for meningitis.

•**Headache after a recent sore throat,** cold or flu. This could indicate a sinus infection.

Ask your doctor whether you should be seen by a neurologist. Tests may include blood work, a CT or magnetic resonance imaging (MRI) scan, sinus X-rays or a spinal tap, in which a sample of the fluid that surrounds the brain and spinal cord is withdrawn with a needle and sent to a lab for analysis.

Wrong diagnosis: **Muscle strain.** Muscle strain often is diagnosed when a person overexerts himself/herself and then experiences pain and/or swelling.

Among the more serious conditions characterized by these symptoms are an infection…or an aortic dissection (a potentially fatal condition in which the inner layer of the wall of the aorta, the main artery of the body, tears).

Self-defense: Do not accept a diagnosis of "muscle strain" if your symptoms include…

•**Fever and/or a joint that is red and hot.** These are red flags for infectious arthritis (infection of the tissues of a joint).

•**A "ripping" or "tearing" sensation in the upper back.** This commonly occurs in patients who have suffered an aortic dissection.

An evaluation may include X-rays, a CT or MRI scan, blood tests and/or arthrocentesis (removal of joint fluid that is analyzed for bacteria, other microorganisms or gouty crystals).

Wrong diagnosis: **Pleurisy.** Pleurisy is an inflammation of the pleura, the lining of the lung and inner chest wall. This condition is often diagnosed when a sharp chest pain occurs during inhalation.

But chest pain also accompanies heart attack and pulmonary embolism (a blood clot that travels from a leg to the lungs). In addition, pleurisy usually has an underlying cause—such as influenza, pneumonia or fractured ribs—which doctors sometimes fail to identify.

Self-defense: Do not accept a diagnosis of "pleurisy" if your symptoms also include…

•**Shortness of breath,** numbness in your arm and/or sweating. These are all symptoms of a heart attack. In women, heart attack symptoms may include jaw pain, indigestion, back pain and/or fatigue.

•**Rapid heart rate,** shortness of breath and/or sharp chest pain that worsens with deep breathing. These could be red flags for a potentially fatal pulmonary embolism.

Your doctor may order a chest X-ray, electrocardiogram (EKG) or lung scan to look for blood clots.

Wrong diagnosis: **Rash.** Rashes are often harmless immune responses to a substance that a person touches or eats. They usually go away on their own or when treated with over-the-counter cortisone cream.

But rashes also can be due to a bacterial or viral infection.

Self-defense: Do not accept a diagnosis of "rash" if your symptoms also include…

•**Fever, chills, severe headache, aches and pains.** This can indicate an infection, such as Rocky Mountain spotted fever or scarlet fever.

•**Fatigue, muscle and joint stiffness,** and a bull's-eye–shaped rash. These are some signs of Lyme disease.

•**Chills, fever, nausea and/or fluid-filled blisters** in a band on one side of the body. These are signs of shingles.

Your doctor will perform a physical exam and order a blood test and/or other tests, if necessary.

Seeing Your Dentist Can Save Your Life

Alan Winter, DDS, a periodontist in private practice and associate professor of implant dentistry at the New York University College of Dentistry, both in New York City. He has published more than a dozen medical journal articles on gum disease.

If you think that regular dental exams are just for your teeth and gums and aren't very important, you could be putting yourself in danger. Dentists are able to identify signs of a variety of serious diseases that affect other parts of the body.

Recent finding: About 78% of periodontists (dentists who specialize in the diagnosis and treatment of gum disease) have referred patients age 60 or older to be evaluated for diabetes, and 21% have made referrals for osteoporosis, according to a poll conducted by the American Academy of Periodontology. All dentists are trained to identify these diseases and others.

How can an oral exam yield such crucial health information? While you're sitting in the dentist's chair to be treated for tooth or gum problems, your dentist is also checking for signs of cancer and other diseases. By monitoring changes in your gum tissue, your dentist can look for oral manifestations of diseases or other serious health problems.

Adults should get dental exams at least twice a year, or three to four times if they have gum (periodontal) disease. During a thorough exam, a dentist inspects all the soft tissues, including the gums, tongue, palate and throat, and feels (palpates) the patient's neck and under the chin. Signs of possible health problems include ulcerations, thickened tissue, pigmentation changes and abnormal color or consistency of gums and other soft tissues.

No one should consider a dental exam an adequate screening of overall physical health. However, your dentist can serve as a valuable adjunct to your other doctors in helping to spot signs of serious medical conditions.

CANCER

Dentists can spot possible malignancies that form in the gums, palate, cheek or other soft tissues. They also can identify tumors in the jawbone, which either originated there or metastasized (spread) from the breasts, bones, lungs or elsewhere in the body.

Warning signs: A newly formed lesion (open sore) or bump anywhere in the mouth that doesn't go away after seven to 10 days... swelling of the gums...teeth that suddenly become loose...and/or nonspecific oral pain that doesn't seem to be related to a tooth problem. Less commonly, a cancerous lesion in the jawbone may be seen on an X-ray, but many people who have cancer that has spread to the jaw are already being treated by an oncologist or surgeon. On rare occasions, a dentist may be the first to identify such a metastasis.

Self-defense: If you have a bump or lesion that doesn't heal in seven to 10 days without treatment, see your dentist. He/she will decide whether you should see a specialist, such as a periodontist, oral surgeon or ear, nose and throat specialist.

Important: Although some bumps and lesions are cancerous, most are benign and due to canker sores, routine gum problems, root canal problems—or they are the result of trauma, such as hitting your gum with the head of your toothbrush. To reach a proper diagnosis, your dentist will do a thorough examination, get a detailed medical history and may even take a biopsy.

DIABETES

Periodontal disease develops over a period of years. If a dentist sees gum breakdown that is more rapid than expected or there has been extreme bone loss that can't be explained, diabetes should be suspected.

Warning signs: Poor healing after oral surgery, inflammation in the gums and other periodontal problems. These may be signs of diabetes or diabetes that is not well controlled. Such problems can occur because diabetes suppresses the immune system, which impairs the infection-fighting function of white blood cells.

Self-defense: If your dentist suspects diabetes, you should see your primary care doctor or an endocrinologist for a glucose tolerance test.

OSTEOPOROSIS

Most people associate osteoporosis with bone loss in the spine or hips, but it also can occur in the jawbone.

Warning sign: On an X-ray, the jawbone will look less dense than it should.

Self-defense: Follow up with your primary-care doctor. A bone-density test may be needed.

Caution: Bisphosphonate drugs, such as *alendronate* (Fosamax), have been linked to osteonecrosis of the jaw—death of areas of jawbone. Most reports of this side effect are associated with bisphosphonates taken intravenously by cancer patients whose malignancy has spread to their bones, but a handful of cases have involved people who took the oral form of the medication.

A LINK TO HEART DISEASE

Contrary to what many people believe, dentists cannot diagnose heart disease based on the appearance of a person's gums. Much has been written about a possible link between gum disease and heart disease. However, the research that showed a connection was retrospective—that is, it reviewed the characteristics of a particular group.

One such study was conducted by Robert Genco, PhD, of the State University of New York at Buffalo, and colleagues at the University of North Carolina at Chapel Hill. The researchers noted that cumulative evidence supports—but does not prove—an association between periodontal infection and cardiovascular disease. In a recent Finnish study, people with gum disease were found to be 1.6 times more likely to suffer a stroke.

Additional research is needed to determine whether gum disease is, in fact, a risk factor for cardiovascular disease. In the meantime, it makes sense to keep your gums healthy to help minimize the possible risk for heart disease. Studies have shown that people with heart disease are more likely to smoke, not exercise regularly and/or have poor diets.

Dentists often send people with diagnosed heart disease for a cardiovascular evaluation.

Reason: These patients need to get medical clearance for dental surgery. During these evaluations, the cardiologist checks the patient's blood pressure, use of blood thinners and overall risk for heart attack and stroke. A cardiovascular evaluation also helps determine which anesthetic to use—an additive used in some anesthesia can stimulate the heart.

Hate to Floss?
What to Do Instead...

Matthew Messina, DDS, a practicing dentist in Fairview Park, OH. He is a consumer adviser for the American Dental Association.

Daily flossing removes plaque, bacteria and food particles from between teeth where toothbrushes can't reach. It's the best way to protect teeth and gums.

Flossing can even protect your overall health. Research has clearly shown links between periodontal (gum) disease and heart disease and diabetes and, very recently, possible links to Alzheimer's disease and pancreatic cancer. Yet about half of Americans don't floss each day.

Nonflossers often complain that flossing is painful, awkward or time-consuming. *If you can't bring yourself to floss, consider these alternatives...*

FLOSS ALTERNATIVES

•**Water picks.** Water picks use small, high-powered bursts of water to flush debris from between the teeth. This is not as effective as daily flossing, and the sensation takes some getting used to, but it's a lot better than nothing. Water picks are particularly useful for those who have braces or other dental work that makes flossing difficult.

Important: Set your water pick to its medium pressure setting, not the highest. Excessive water pressure can blast bacteria further under your gum line.

•**Mouthwash.** Antibacterial mouthwashes cannot remove plaque from between your teeth, but they can at least kill bacteria. Swish with mouthwash for at least 30 seconds—a full minute is even better. Select a mouthwash with the American Dental Association seal of approval to ensure that it is truly antimicrobial.

You also can fill a water pick with a diluted mouthwash solution (one or two parts water to one part mouthwash). The water pressure will dislodge much of the debris from between your teeth, and the mouthwash will kill most of the bacteria that remain.

•**Interdental cleaners.** These plastic tools are similar to toothpicks, only their blunted ends are less likely to damage the gums. Though not as effective as floss, they can remove much of the debris from between the teeth when used carefully. Ask your dentist to show you how to use one.

BETTER FLOSSING

These floss products can make flossing more pleasant...

•**Floss holders.** Arthritis sufferers and others with limited dexterity often find it difficult or painful to maneuver dental floss around the mouth. A floss holder, available at any drugstore, solves this problem by supplying an easy-to-grip handle.

•**High-quality flosses.** Premium flosses, such as Crest's Glide, are slicker and stronger than economy brands, making flossing easier, especially between tight teeth.

Killer Pneumonia
Is on the Rise

Donald M. Yealy, MD, professor and vice-chair of emergency medicine at the University of Pittsburgh Medical Center/Presbyterian University Hospital. He has written more than 150 articles, reviews and book chapters focusing on pneumonia and pneumonia-related sepsis.

If the current flu season is typical, an estimated 30 million Americans will come down with the illness. That's bad enough—but many of these people will go on to develop secondary pneumonia, a much more serious condition.

Pneumonia, whether it follows another infection or occurs on its own (primary pneumonia), is the sixth leading cause of death in the US. More than 60,000 Americans die from it annually, and many more require hospitalization.

Beware: A rare—but particularly lethal—form of pneumonia is resistant to standard antibiotics. It is caused by the bacterium methicillin-resistant *Staphylococcus aureus* (MRSA), which has appeared in recent years in hospitals and increasingly in the wider community. The death rate from MRSA pneumonia is roughly double that of other pneumonias.

What you need to know...

WHO GETS PNEUMONIA

Pneumonia is an illness of the lungs and respiratory system in which the *alveoli* (tiny sacs in the lungs) become inflamed and flooded with fluid. Pneumonia can be caused by bacteria, viruses or fungi. The viral form is the most common.

People get pneumonia in the same ways that they get the flu—by touching their eyes, nose or mouth after shaking hands, for example, with someone who has the virus on his/her hands—or through airborne droplets from coughs or sneezes.

Bacterial pneumonia is usually the most serious form. It is most commonly acquired by inhaling or aspirating bacteria. Hospital patients have a high risk of contracting bacterial pneumonia—their immune systems tend to be weakened, and germs are prevalent in this setting. Other vulnerable people include those with diabetes, heart or lung disease...adults age 65 and older...young children...and anyone who abuses alcohol or smokes.

Surprising risk factor: People who take acid-suppressing heartburn drugs, such as *cimetidine* (Tagamet), *ranitidine* (Zantac), *omeprazole* (Prilosec) and *esomeprazole* (Nexium), have been found to be 27% more likely to develop pneumonia—especially hospital-acquired pneumonia—than people not taking such medication.

Researchers theorize that these drugs may increase a person's vulnerability to infection by reducing stomach acid, a major defense mechanism against pathogens ingested through the mouth. People should not use over-the-counter acid-reducing drugs for more than a few weeks unless they are prescribed by their doctors.

HOW IT'S DIAGNOSED

It can sometimes be difficult for patients to distinguish the symptoms of pneumonia from those caused by a cold or the flu. Therefore, anyone with a high fever (102° F or higher)...chills...a persistent cough...shortness of breath ...and/or pain when inhaling should see a doctor right away.

What the doctor will look for...

•**Abnormal chest sounds** heard through a stethoscope. The doctor will listen for crackling sounds (rales) or rumblings (rhonchi), caused by air passing through mucus and/or other fluids in the lungs.

•**X-ray showing a cloudy area,** caused by fluid in the lungs.

Caution: An X-ray often will look normal in patients with early-stage pneumonia. A second X-ray is typically taken if symptoms do not improve in two to three days or worsen, especially if the first X-ray looked normal.

A sputum test is also recommended to identify the cause of the pneumonia—and help the doctor choose the best treatment. After an X-ray, it's the best test for diagnosing pneumonia, but only 20% to 25% of patients are able to bring up sputum (by coughing) for analysis.

TREATMENT

An antiviral drug, such as *oseltamivir* (Tamiflu), is sometimes prescribed for viral pneumonia. In viral pneumonia patients who are otherwise healthy, doctors may recommend the same therapy as for the flu—rest, plenty of liquids (up to one gallon daily) and medication to reduce fever and/or pain.

Because bacterial and viral pneumonia can appear quite similar, doctors typically err on the side of caution and assume that it's bacterial in origin when uncertain and prescribe antibiotics.

Studies show that older patients as well as those with underlying health problems do better when they're given antibiotics promptly—preferably within four to eight hours of the initial diagnosis. Most bacterial pneumonias are treated (orally or intravenously) with a penicillin antibiotic, such as Augmentin...a cephalosporin antibiotic, such as *cefaclor* (Ceclor) or *ceftriaxone* (Rocephin)...and/or *azithromycin* (Zithromax).

At-home treatment: Patients with pneumonia are sometimes advised to use an incentive spirometer (a tubelike device that patients breathe into, as hard as they can, at least two to three times a day). It increases pressure in the bronchial tubes and helps maintain open breathing passages.

Preventive: An incentive spirometer also can be used by patients who don't have pneumonia but who have underlying lung disease, such as chronic bronchitis, emphysema or some other obstructive lung disease. It helps keep the airways open and less vulnerable to pneumonia.

AN EMERGING THREAT

MRSA is primarily a skin infection that can enter the body through cuts or scrapes. MRSA was originally found only in healthcare settings. In the 1990s, it began showing up in the general community. This form of infection has the prefix CA, denoting community-acquired.

CA-MRSA pneumonia isn't as dangerous as the hospital-acquired form. It's usually treated with the antibiotics sulfamethoxazole and *trimethoprim* (Bactrim). Hospital patients with MRSA-related pneumonia require a much stronger antibiotic—*vancomycin* (Vancocin), given intravenously.

Self-protection: CA-MRSA is spread by airborne droplets. It also can be present on drinking glasses, toothbrushes, etc. In community settings, such as health clubs, people should never share their personal items.

In the hospital: Patients should wash their hands after touching any object. MRSA can survive on doorknobs, faucet handles, bedrails, remote controls, telephones, food trays, etc. Patients also should wash after using the bathroom and before eating. For convenience, a 62% alcohol hand sanitizer gel can be used. Patients should insist that all medical personnel wash their hands before and after performing any procedure—and even before and after touching any object in the room.

PREVENTION

Not smoking and frequent hand-washing help prevent pneumonia.

Also important…

•**Annual flu vaccine.** People who don't get the flu are far less likely to get pneumonia. The Centers for Disease Control and Prevention (CDC) recommends the flu vaccine for adults age 50 and older…children ages six months to five years old…women who are pregnant during flu season (typically October to as late as May)…and health-care workers or others who have close contact with people in a high-risk group. However, flu vaccine, if available—and there appears to be a good supply this season—can help most people reduce risk.

Important: The FluMist nasal vaccine, which has been approved for healthy people ages five to 49, may be more effective than conventional flu shots. There appears to be a greater immune response in the nose, where the vaccine is administered. This can make it harder for an inhaled flu virus to cause infection.

Caution: FluMist is not recommended for people with asthma or lung disease.

•**Pneumococcal vaccine.** It's recommended for adults age 65 and older as well as for those with pneumonia risk factors, such as cardiovascular or lung disease, cancer or a previous illness with pneumonia. People with certain illnesses, such as kidney or severe lung disease, may need a second dose after five or more years.

Drug Blocks Flu Spread Up to 81%

Fred Hutchinson Cancer Research Center news release.

The antiviral drugs *oseltamivir* (Tamiflu) and *zanamivir* (Relenza) help reduce the spread of seasonal flu within families, a new study suggests. Researchers from Seattle's Fred Hutchinson Cancer Research Center, the University of Michigan and the University of Virginia also suggested that oseltamivir may reduce the infectiousness of flu patients, but further research is needed to confirm this.

THE STUDY

The authors reviewed four studies of 1,475 households where a family member had the flu. The two studies that looked at zanamivir found that the drug's effectiveness in reducing pathogenicity (the ability of the flu virus to cause overt disease) was 52% and 56%. In the two studies on oseltamivir, it was 56% and 79%.

The study also found that use of either drug reduced by 75% to 81% the chance that a person exposed to a flu virus would become ill.

"Preventing the spread of influenza within families is an essential part of influenza management, regardless of the strain. This study shows that there is a clear benefit to be gained by giving antivirals to people who have been exposed to the virus to prevent the onset of symptomatic illness," said lead author Dr. M. Elizabeth Halloran, a Fred Hutchinson Cancer Research Center–based biostatistician.

"While the efficacy of antivirals to protect against influenza is critical, the effect of these drugs on infectiousness also has important public health consequences. Further studies to determine antiviral efficacy for reducing infectiousness would therefore be of great value," said Halloran, who is also a professor of biostatistics at the University of Washington School of Public Health and Community Medicine in Seattle.

info The Centers for Disease Control and Prevention Web site has more about flu prevention at *http://www.cdc.gov/flu/protect/ preventing.htm*.

Germ-Fighting Secrets

Philip M. Tierno, Jr., PhD, director of clinical microbiology and immunology at New York University Medical Center, and associate professor, department of microbiology and pathology at New York University School of Medicine, both in New York City. He is the author of *The Secret Life of Germs*. Atria.

Everyone knows about the disease-causing potential of germs. Yet few people realize that microorganisms are essential for human health.

Of the 65,000 known species of germs, only about 1,400 cause disease. The rest are "good" germs, which establish our immune response, help us digest food and protect our bodies from potential pathogens. However, the germs that do promote disease can be deadly. Infectious diseases, such as pneumonia and septicemia (blood infection), are leading causes of death in the US.

Foodborne germs have made headlines due to the recent outbreaks of *Escherichia coli*–related illnesses. Even so, a surprising number of people are still not aware of the best ways to guard against infection through proper hygiene. Fortunately, most infections—everything from colds and the flu to life-threatening Legionnaires' disease—usually can be prevented. *My germ-fighting secrets…*

•**Wash properly.** The Centers for Disease Control and Prevention (CDC) estimates that proper hand-washing could prevent thousands of deaths annually, but studies show that less than 10% of people wash their hands as long or as thoroughly as they should.

To effectively remove germs: Wash with warm water and soap for about 20 to 30 seconds (roughly the time it takes to sing "Happy Birthday" twice) and rinse. Warm water dissolves soap more readily and makes it easier to remove germs. Rub the soapy water all over your hands—including the wrists, between the fingers and under the fingernails. (Use a fingernail brush, if possible.)

Best: Wash your hands several times a day—always before eating…after using the bathroom …after coughing or sneezing, especially when using your hands or a tissue…after shaking hands…and after handling anything touched by many people, such as door handles and automatic teller machines (ATMs). If soap and water aren't available, use an alcohol gel containing at least 62% alcohol.

•**Use antibacterial products when necessary.** Our hands pick up *millions* of potentially harmful organisms during daily activities—handling raw meats, poultry and/or fish…changing diapers…picking up pet wastes in the yard, etc. Washing with soap and water removes (rather than kills) most germs, but some are left behind —potentially causing illness.

Interesting: Some experts worry that the regular use of antibacterial soaps will promote the emergence of antibiotic-resistant organisms, but there is no evidence that links these products to resistance. More study is needed to determine the long-term effects of antibacterial soaps.

Best: After washing your hands with soap, use an antibacterial cleaner if you've handled materials such as those described above. Some antibacterial products (such as Dial Complete hand wash) contain triclosan, a germicide that kills virtually all harmful bacteria.

Also important: Never allow a pet to lick your mouth, nose, eyes or an open wound. Many people believe that the mouths of dogs and cats are relatively germ-free—however, dogs and cats can carry *Pasteurella*, a bacterium that can cause skin infection in humans. And turtles, frogs and snakes can harbor *Salmonella*, a bacterium that causes gastroenteritis and other illnesses.

•**Limit kissing to close friends and family.** Mouth-to-mouth kissing clearly spreads germs, but even face kissing (kissing anywhere on the face, except the lips) can be dangerous if someone is ill. Flu viruses, for example, can be spread by an infected person during face kissing up to three days before full-blown symptoms develop and five days after they subside, depending on the germ.

Here's how: Before the kiss, the infected person may have touched his/her mouth or nose, then touched his face, contaminating it with infected saliva or mucus.

Best: Instead of kissing someone who may be sick, hug him. That way, you'll avoid face-to-face contact.

•**Air-dry toothbrushes and razors.** Bacteria thrive on toothbrushes and razors that stay damp. Bacteria on a razor could cause a staphylococcal infection of the skin, while a contaminated toothbrush can spread cold or flu viruses. Rinse and let them air-dry after every use—and store them upright so that they dry completely. To sanitize a toothbrush, put it in a cup of antiseptic mouthwash or 3% hydrogen peroxide (enough to cover the brush head), leave for one minute, then rinse and air-dry. Razors should be replaced after two or three uses...toothbrushes should be replaced when the bristles become worn.

•**Clean your showerhead.** The *Legionella* bacterium causes a potentially fatal, pneumonia-like condition called Legionnaires' disease, which is contracted by inhaling infected water droplets. The organism feeds on *cysteine*, a substance produced by a wide variety of waterborne organisms and bacteria found in potable water. Legionella can survive in tap water for many months, and showerheads provide a hospitable environment.

Best: Remove showerheads once a year. Disassemble and clean them thoroughly with a wire brush to remove any organisms that might be present. Use a solution of one ounce of bleach mixed with one quart of water.

Also important: Replace the standing water in humidifiers with fresh water at least once a week. Before adding fresh water, clean the filters/trays according to the manufacturer's directions.

•**Close the toilet lid.** Flushing an older toilet with the lid up can hurl droplets of water that contain fecal matter (and potentially other disease-causing organisms) up to 20 feet. The droplets can then contaminate toothbrushes, combs, faucets, etc. The risk for disease is even higher if the toilet bowl isn't cleaned regularly. Among the diseases that can be transmitted by fecal matter from an infected person are stomach flu and hepatitis A.

Best: In addition to closing the toilet lid, sanitize the bowl weekly with a commercial cleaner or a mixture of one ounce of bleach added to one quart of water.

•**Launder with hot water.** Bath towels can harbor fecal bacteria, including E. coli, along with hepatitis A and other harmful viruses—and these germs aren't necessarily killed by running them through a cold- or warm-water wash.

Warning: Because washing in cold or warm water doesn't kill germs, it's possible to get infected just by removing wet clothes from the washer if you then touch your nose, mouth or eyes.

Best: Use a "hot" washer setting (150° F or hotter) to kill most germs. Another option is to add bleach to the wash, which is effective even in cold or warm water. If you live in a sunny climate, consider line-drying clothes rather than using the dryer. Like the hottest cycle of a clothes dryer, the sun's ultraviolet rays will kill most germs.

Also important: Launder underwear separately in hot water to avoid contaminating other clothes. For added safety, use bleach to ensure that germs are killed when washing underwear.

■ **More from Dr. Tierno...**

What Is a Germ?

A germ is a microorganism, such as a virus, bacterium or protozoan. Some germs help the body produce vitamins, aid in digestion and enable the immune system to work efficiently. Other germs cause disease. Germs, which can live on surfaces for minutes to days, can be transmitted through direct contact, such as sneezes and coughs, or indirect contact, including touching a contaminated doorknob.

What You May Not Know About Diarrhea

Douglas L. Seidner, MD, director of nutrition in the department of gastroenterology and hepatology at the Cleveland Clinic.

D iarrhea—bowel movements that are looser and more frequent than usual—is the second most common medical complaint (after respiratory infections) in the US.

Most people associate a bout of diarrhea with a viral infection or food poisoning.

Now: Researchers are identifying new—and sometimes surprising—triggers, including the use of some medications.

Latest development: *The Journal of the American Medical Association* recently published a study that links the use of acid-lowering heartburn drugs, such as *omeprazole* (Prilosec), *lansoprazole* (Prevacid) and *ranitidine* (Zantac), to increased infection with the bacterium *Clostridium difficile*—a cause of severe and persistent diarrhea (*c. difficile*).

In an unexpected finding, the same researchers identified an association between diarrhea and regular use of nonsteroidal antiinflammatory drugs (NSAIDs). More study is needed to confirm this NSAID-diarrhea link.

HOW DIARRHEA DEVELOPS

What's left of food after most of it has been digested reaches the large intestine as a sort of slurry. There, the body absorbs water from this material, creating a solid mass to be excreted. Normal stool is 60% to 90% water. Diarrhea occurs when stool is more than 90% water.

When stool does not remain in the large intestine long enough, it is excreted in a watery form. This "rapid transit" diarrhea can be caused by stress, overactive thyroid (hyperthyroidism)

and certain drugs, such as antacids and laxatives that contain magnesium, and chemotherapy for cancer.

Other types of diarrhea…

•**Osmotic diarrhea** occurs when too much food remains undigested or unabsorbed. Water is drawn into the colon to dilute unabsorbed chemicals, which makes the stool looser.

Large amounts of certain fruits and beans as well as sugar substitutes (sorbitol and xylitol) that are used in some brands of fruit juice, chewing gum and candy are common causes of osmotic diarrhea. When the diarrhea sufferer stops eating the offending food, the condition stops.

Lactase deficiency—a lack of the enzyme needed to break down milk sugar (lactose)—is another cause of osmotic diarrhea. Most people know if they have this deficiency and avoid milk products.

Osmotic diarrhea also may develop in people taking antibiotics. That's because the drug eliminates beneficial bacteria that live in the intestinal tract, allowing harmful bacteria to proliferate. These microorganisms normally help the body process and absorb the small amount of food that hasn't been digested yet. Diarrhea usually develops within a few days of treatment. If it's bothersome enough, your doctor may prescribe a different antibiotic.

More rarely, diarrhea develops toward the end of antibiotic treatment—or even up to a month later. This may be caused by C. difficile or another bacterium that can flourish and cause inflammation of the large intestine when beneficial bacteria are eliminated.

Helpful: This infection is usually treated with the antibiotics *vancomycin* (Vancocin) or *metronidazole* (Flagyl).

•**Secretory diarrhea** occurs when an excessive amount of water, salt and digestive fluids are secreted into the stool. Viral infections, bacterial toxins that cause some types of food poisoning and rare tumors of the small intestine and pancreas can trigger the secretions that lead to secretory diarrhea.

With food poisoning, excess secretions are stimulated by chemicals produced by bacteria that have contaminated something you ate. This diarrhea usually lasts for 12 to 24 hours and stops without treatment. If it persists, your doctor may order tests, such as stool cultures, to determine whether a virulent bacterium, such as *Salmonella, Shigella* or *Campylobacter,* is involved and will require medication.

•**Travelers' diarrhea** has a similar cause. The culprit is generally a mild strain of a toxin-producing bacterium, such as *Escherichia coli,* that is present in food and/or water. Natives of the region you're visiting have been exposed to the microorganism for years and usually are immune to it. You're not. Traveler's diarrhea typically goes away within one to two days.

•**Exudative diarrhea** occurs when the large intestine's lining becomes inflamed. This triggers the release of blood, mucus, proteins and other fluids. Infection with the bacterium Shigella can cause this type of diarrhea. Crohn's disease (chronic inflammation of the small bowel or colon) and ulcerative colitis (chronic inflammation and ulceration of the colon) can also cause exudative diarrhea.

An antibiotic is sometimes used to treat a bacterial infection. Medication, such as the corticosteroid *prednisone* (Deltasone), and sometimes surgery are used to treat the inflammatory conditions.

BEST RELIEF STRATEGIES

In some cases, diarrhea can be a sign of a serious infection and should be treated by a doctor. *Even though most types of diarrhea run their course within a few days, the following steps can hasten the process and ease your discomfort…*

•**Eat right.** If food poisoning is the problem, you should abstain from all food until symptoms resolve, usually one to two days.

For other acute diarrhea, follow the "BRAT" diet: Bananas, rice, applesauce and toast. Bananas and applesauce contain pectin, a water-soluble substance that helps firm up the stool…the carbohydrates in white rice and white toast are easy to digest. If you eat other foods, stick to small portions and avoid dairy products.

•**Yogurt is an exception.** If it's made from live and active cultures, such as *Lactobacillus bulgaricus* and *Streptococcus thermophilus,* yogurt may replace beneficial bacteria in the colon, helping to relieve antibiotic-related diarrhea.

When the diarrhea subsides, return to your normal diet cautiously. For the first few days, avoid fatty foods (they're harder to digest).

Important: Drink 64 ounces of fluids daily to replace what you're losing. Choose weak tea, water and/or small amounts of clear juice or soda, such as apple juice or ginger ale.

If diarrhea is severe: Drink "replacement fluids," such as CeraLyte, Pedialyte or Enfalyte. These contain salt and simple sugars that help the body retain water. Diarrhea-related dehydration isn't a danger for most adults, but it is a danger for children and many adults over age 65. Young children do not have as large of a reserve of water in the body as healthy adults. Older adults may have heart or kidney disease, which can be exacerbated by dehydration.

•**Medication.** Several over-the-counter preparations can help relieve diarrhea…

•*Loperamide* (Imodium) is a semi-synthetic narcotic that slows food as it passes through the bowel, allowing more time for water to be absorbed. Try loperamide if diarrhea is mild and hasn't been resolved in one to two days. It should not be taken if you have a fever or the stools are bloody.

•*Bismuth subsalicylate* (Pepto-Bismol, Kaopectate) absorbs toxins—it's quite effective for traveler's diarrhea. It should not be taken with aspirin. Do not take it if you have a fever or bloody stools. Children should not take this product.

■ ■ ■ ■

Call the Doctor…

S eek medical attention if any of these danger signs appear…

•**The diarrhea is severe** (six or more stools a day), especially if there are signs of dehydration (parched lips, sunken eyes).

•**The diarrhea is bloody or includes mucus,** rather than just water.

•**It has lasted more than two days**—if mild, two weeks.

•**You have a fever over 101.5° F.**

•**Diarrhea is accompanied by severe abdominal pain** (anything more than moderate cramping).

Fight Kidney Stones With Lemonade!

Glenn M. Preminger, MD, professor of urologic surgery and director of the Comprehensive Kidney Stone Center at Duke University Medical Center in Durham, NC.

When a kidney stone creates a blockage in a ureter (one of the tubes that connect the kidney to the bladder), it can be excruciatingly painful. Each year, more than 250,000 Americans are hospitalized because of this condition. Fortunately, new research is identifying highly effective prevention and treatment options.

Recent findings…

•**Lemonade fights kidney stones.** Researchers recently tracked stone-prone patients for up to four years and found that those who drank two quarts of lemonade daily had fewer new stones…and little or no growth of existing ones.

Why it works: Lemon juice contains high amounts of citrate, a substance that inhibits kidney stones by reducing urine acidity and binding with urinary calcium. Potassium citrate, in pill or liquid form, is routinely prescribed for stone prevention. Lemonade isn't as potent as potassium citrate, but it does appear to be a viable alternative for patients who can't take or tolerate the drug (people with impaired kidney function, for example), or for those who wish to avoid another medication.

MAKE LEOMNADE

To reap the study-proven benefits, you need to drink two quarts of homemade lemonade daily.

The lemonade should be made by mixing two quarts of water with four ounces of reconstituted lemon juice. To reduce or eliminate sugar and/or calories, consider using artificial sweeteners. Since stone formers are advised to drink three quarts of fluid daily as a preventative, you'll benefit even more if two of those quarts are lemonade.

MORE NEWS FOR THOSE WITH KIDNEY STONES

•**Alpha blockers can speed stone passage.** For years, researchers have searched for ways to facilitate spontaneous passage of kidney stones that are stuck in a ureter so that patients would be spared stone removal via a procedure such as an endoscopic technique, using a thin, telescopic tube.

Good news: In multiple trials conducted over the last five years, alpha blockers—prescription drugs traditionally used to treat an enlarged prostate—have proven to be remarkably effective for speeding and easing the elimination of small stones (less than six millimeters in diameter) from a ureter. These drugs increase the likelihood of spontaneous passage of small stones by about 90%.

Alpha blockers work by relaxing smooth muscle cells lining the ureter, improving urine flow and preventing the painful contractions that can slow or block stone movement. It's now become the standard of care to start most ureteral stone patients on a trial of alpha blockers. In a majority of cases, the drugs allow the stones to pass spontaneously. A small percentage of patients who take alpha blockers experience orthostatic hypotension—light-headedness when quickly standing up.

•**Obesity and weight gain elevate kidney stone risk.** Several recent studies confirm that being overweight and/or gaining weight significantly increases kidney stone risk. A recent large-scale, long-term study shows that obese men are 44% more likely, and obese women 90% more likely, to develop stones than are their leaner counterparts. Gaining more than 35 pounds during adulthood also heightens risk (by 39% for men and up to 82% for women), compared with maintaining a stable weight.

What's the connection between kidney stones and weight gain? As recent studies show, many adults who are significantly overweight also have type 2 diabetes (often undiagnosed) or are insulin resistant—that is, their bodies have a reduced ability to respond to insulin, which causes the pancreas to secrete excessive amounts of insulin. Insulin resistance and diabetes raise the acid levels in urine—a primary risk factor for stones. Losing weight is the ideal antidote. But if that's not possible, alkali therapy, in the form of potassium citrate, may be prescribed to reduce the acid load in urine to prevent stones.

■ **More from Dr. Preminger...**

Foods That Prevent Kidney Stones

For prevention, people with a personal or family history of kidney stones should...

•**Drink three quarts of fluid daily,** mostly noncaffeinated. Coffee and tea are fine in moderation.

•**Get enough calcium.** Though stone formers had long been advised to limit calcium intake, recent studies link insufficient calcium to increased risk for stones.

That's because calcium can bind with stone-producing oxalates in the digestive tract, preventing these minerals from concentrating in the urine. Aim for two to three servings daily of low-fat milk, cheese, yogurt or calcium-fortified juice or cereal.

Caution: Calcium supplements may not be the best source. Studies show that they may raise urinary calcium excretion, a risk factor for stones. If you have a personal or family history of kidney stones and wish to take calcium supplements, have your urine tested after three months to check for elevated calcium levels.

•**Limit salt.** Excess sodium steals calcium from your bones and causes it to accumulate in your urine, increasing your risk for kidney stones. Don't add salt to your food...and avoid highly processed, prepackaged foods.

•**Avoid high-oxalate foods,** such as spinach, tea, chocolate, nuts, asparagus and rhubarb. Our bodies also convert some vitamin C into oxalates, and studies suggest that too much can raise urinary oxalate levels. Stone formers should not exceed 2,000 mg (2 g) of vitamin C daily.

•**Cut back on meat.** Animal protein, particularly from red meat, raises acid levels in the urine, increasing kidney stone risk. Aim for three or fewer red meat servings weekly.

■ ■ ■ ■

What Is a Kidney Stone?

A kidney stone is a hard mass that forms when certain minerals—calcium, oxalate and uric acid—fail to dissolve in the urine and then accumulate into solid crystals. Normally, urine contains chemicals, such as citrate, that inhibit stone formation. But some people are prone to stones due to diet, lifestyle and certain medical conditions, such as inflammatory bowel disease. Kidney stones can trigger sudden, searing pain in the back and side, often accompanied by blood in the urine, nausea and/or vomiting.

Orange Juice Best at Stopping Kidney Stones

University of Texas Southwestern Medical Center news release.

An independent study finds that orange juice beats lemonade and other fruit juices in helping to keep kidney stones at bay. Experts have long known that potassium citrate—found in citrus juice—can slow stone formation in people with a history of the condition.

But this study, by a team from the University of Texas Southwestern Medical Center at Dallas, found that other components also affect a juice's ability to prevent stones.

THE STUDY

Thirteen volunteers (some with a history of kidney stones and some without) took part in the multi-phase trial, which was funded by the US National Institutes of Health. For one week, participants drank distilled water, for another week orange juice, and then lemonade for another week. There was a three-week interval between each of these weeks.

During each phase, the participants drank 13 ounces of orange juice, lemonade or distilled water three times a day with meals. They were also put on a low-calcium, low-oxalate diet, which also helps cut stone formation.

RESULTS

The study found that orange juice increased levels of citrate in the urine and reduced the crystallization of uric acid and calcium oxalate, common components of kidney stones. Lemonade did not increase citrate levels.

EXPLANATION

The study's lead author was Dr. Clarita Odvina, assistant professor of internal medicine at the Charles and Jane Pak Center for Mineral Metabolism and Clinical Research at University of Texas Southwestern's General Clinical Research Center where the study took place. Odvina explained that the citrate in orange and grapefruit is accompanied by a potassium ion, while the citrate in lemonade and cranberry juice is accompanied by a hydrogen ion. While hydrogen ions counteract the beneficial effects of high citrate content, potassium ions do not.

info For more information about kidney stones, visit the Web site of the National Institute of Diabetes & Digestive & Kidney Diseases at *www.niddk.nih.gov.*

Study: US Babies Getting Fatter

Matthew Gillman, MD, associate professor, ambulatory care and prevention, Harvard Medical School, Boston.
David L. Katz, MD, MPH, associate professor of public health, director, Prevention Research Center, Yale University School of Medicine, New Haven, CT.
Obesity.

American babies carry more "baby fat" now than ever before, a new study finds. Researchers say infants are 59% more likely to be overweight today than they were two decades ago.

"The obesity epidemic in our country has spared no age group, even our very youngest children," said lead researcher Dr. Matthew Gillman, an associate professor of ambulatory care and prevention at Harvard Medical School. "Overweight rates are going up in young children, and ours is the first study to show that they are going up in infants, in addition to toddlers and preschoolers," he said.

THE STUDY

In the study of 120,680 children under age six, Gillman's team found that children, especially infants, are now more likely to be overweight. Looking at records collected from pediatricians working with a Massachusetts HMO for the years 1980 to 2001, they found that the prevalence of overweight children climbed from 6.3% to 10% during those 22 years. In addition, the proportion of children at risk of becoming overweight grew from 11.1% to 14.4% overall.

Compared with 20 years ago, infants had a 59% increased risk of being overweight, and the number of overweight infants increased by 74%, the researchers found.

RISK FACTORS

The data suggest that obesity prevention may need to start even *before* babies are born, Gillman said. There are a number of factors that appear to be responsible for the trend, he noted.

The first is that women who become pregnant weigh more than they ever have, Gillman said, and "maternal body mass index is a determinate of infant weight at birth and after."

In addition, more mothers are putting on excess weight during pregnancy compared with decades past, Gillman said. "There is also an increase in type 2 diabetes and gestational diabetes among mothers, which are determinants of infant weight at birth and after birth," he added.

How babies are fed may also play a role. "Infants that are breast-fed tend to gain weight more slowly than formula-fed infants," the Harvard expert said.

IMPLICATIONS

Gillman said early weight gain can have dire consequences for long-term health. Studies suggest that gaining excess weight during the first months of life is associated with becoming overweight and developing high blood pressure years later. Other data suggest that infants who gain excess weight are more likely to suffer from wheezing, which can lead to asthma, Gillman noted.

EXPERT CONCERNS ABOUT OBESITY

One expert called the finding just one more facet of the ongoing obesity epidemic.

"This news is disturbing, but not surprising," said Dr. David L. Katz, an associate professor of public health and director of the Prevention Research Center at Yale University School of Medicine. "The progression from lean to overweight to dangerously obese occurs slowly, one pound at a time. The widely publicized increases in childhood obesity indicate that weight gain is beginning at an ever younger age. These data merely confirm the obvious," he said.

The message is troubling for several reasons, Katz said. "As weight gain becomes problematic earlier in life, other chronic disease can be expected to do the same. If overweight becomes commonplace among babies, heart disease may well become commonplace among adolescents, as type 2 diabetes is already," he said.

The nature of weight gain varies with age, Katz said. Infants and adolescents are far more adept at generating new fat cells than adults, he explained, and obesity caused by a high number of fat cells is harder to reverse than obesity caused by enlarging preexisting fat cells.

"As difficult as weight control is for us, it will be that much harder, and more elusive, for our children," he said.

"The findings reported here are from a single HMO in one part of the country, but they contribute to an overwhelming body of evidence that childhood obesity is a crisis throughout the United States," Katz said.

info For more on childhood obesity, go to the Web site of the Obesity Society at *www.obesity.org*. Under "Information" click "Fact Sheets" and then "Childhood Overweight."

Kids and Cold Medicines —A Deadly Mix

Adam Cohen, MD, officer, Epidemic Intelligence Service, Centers for Disease Control and Prevention, Atlanta.

Michael Marcus, MD, director, pediatric pulmonology, allergy and immunology, Maimonides Infants & Children's Hospital, New York City.

Gwen Wurm, MD, director, community pediatrics, University of Miami Miller School of Medicine.

Morbidity and Mortality Weekly Report.

Over-the-counter cough and cold medications can be harmful—even deadly—to very young children, US government research shows. In 2005, three infants under the age of six months died from taking such medications. And, from 2004 to 2005, more than 1,500 children under the age of two were treated in emergency rooms for problems related to taking such medications.

"Cough and cold medicines can be harmful, and even fatal, and should be used with caution in children under two years of age," said study author Dr. Adam Cohen, an officer in the Epidemic Intelligence Service at the Centers for Disease Control and Prevention. "They are drugs, so they have risks as well as benefits."

BACKGROUND

The Food and Drug Administration has only approved the use of over-the-counter cough and cold medicines in children over the age of two. In children younger than two, studies have concluded that such medications are no more effective than a placebo. As a result, appropriate dosing is not known.

"Cold and cough medications, especially medications containing *pseudoephedrine* (a nasal decongestant), have never been shown to have any beneficial effect on children less than two years of age, yet they clearly can have significant harmful effects," said Dr. Michael Marcus, director of pediatric pulmonology, allergy and immunology at the Maimonides Infants & Children's Hospital in New York City.

"There are no studies to support the use of cold medicine in infants," said Dr. Gwen Wurm, director of community pediatrics at the University of Miami Miller School of Medicine. "The thing to keep in mind is that colds go away. Kids might benefit from a humidifier by the bed and saline nose drops, but this kind of loving care is all most kids need."

Various professional groups, including the American Academy of Pediatrics and the American College of Chest Physicians, have issued guidelines recommending caution when using these medications in young children.

NEW DEVELOPMENTS

In June 2006, the FDA took action to stop the manufacture of medications containing *carbinoxamine* (an antihistamine) that were inappropriately labeled for use in infants and young children. Manufacturers were required to stop production by September 2006, but some products might still be in distribution.

The Combat Methamphetamine Epidemic Act of 2006, passed in March 2006, banned over-the-counter (though not behind-the-counter) sales of products containing pseudoephedrine. As a result, many companies have taken this ingredient out of their products.

But products that might be harmful to young children are still available, so officials at the CDC and the National Association of Medical Examiners (NAME) investigated deaths of children under the age of one that were associated with cough and cold medicines.

The three infants who died ranged in age from one to six months. Autopsy and medication investigation records revealed that cough and cold medications were responsible for all three deaths. All three babies had high levels of pseudoephedrine, ranging from nine to 14 times the levels expected from recommended doses for children ages two to 12.

One of the infants had received both a prescription and an over-the-counter cough and cold medicine at the same time, both of which contained pseudoephedrine.

Two of the children had taken prescription medications containing carbinoxamine, although there were no detectable blood levels of the substance. Two of the infants had detectable blood levels of *dextromethorphan* (a cough suppressant) and *acetaminophen* (a fever-reducer and analgesic).

WARNING FOR PARENTS

"Parents should absolutely avoid these medications unless they are being supervised by a physician," Marcus said. "Parents should realize that nonprescription medications may contain similar products to medications that the pediatrician is also prescribing, therefore, they should let the pediatrician know all treatments the child is receiving when discussing a child's treatment."

info For more about colds and cold medications in young children, visit the Web site of the American Academy of Pediatrics at *www. aap.org/patiented/coldsandyoungchild.htm.*

Study Finds Potential Early Warning Sign For Autism

Andy Shih, PhD, chief science officer, Autism Speaks, New York City.
Archives of Pediatrics & Adolescent Medicine.

A new study suggests that some babies who fail to respond to their name by one year of age may be at heightened risk for an autism spectrum disorder. Early identification can mean possible early intervention and better outcomes for affected children, say the authors of two studies aimed at early detection of the disorder.

BACKGROUND

Autism spectrum disorder seems to be becoming more prevalent. According to the US Centers for Disease Control and Prevention (CDC), one in every 150 American eight-year-olds has some form of the disorder. That number is higher than prior estimates.

Autism's causes remain cloaked in mystery, although prior research has pointed to a strong genetic component.

Children and adults with autism experience difficulty with social and language skills and often display repetitive behaviors. However, the disorder is usually not diagnosed until age three or four—even though as many as half of parents with autistic children report problems with development progress before their child's first birthday.

STUDY #1

Researchers at the M.I.N.D. Institute at the University of California, Davis, found that one-year-old infants who don't respond to their names are more likely to be diagnosed with autism or another developmental problem by the time they're two.

This cue could represent an easy way to spot the disorder early on, experts said.

"One of the challenges has been finding an early exam in the general practitioner's or pediatrician's office that can serve as a warning sign or diagnostic indicator," said Dr. Andy Shih, chief science officer for the nation's leading autism advocacy group, New York City–based Autism Speaks. "That's what this paper is getting at. It doesn't mean that (a nonresponsive child) is destined to become autistic, but there seems to be a higher proportion who later go on to develop autism. This, along with many other clues, such as language development, eye contact and even head circumference, are potentially simple diagnostic tools that could be used in the general practitioner setting."

SECOND STUDY ALSO POINTS TO COMMUNICATION SKILLS

A team at Vanderbilt University in Nashville, Tennessee, found that younger siblings of children with autism perform below par on tests of social and communication development compared with younger siblings of normal children. These deficits may represent the early indications of an autism spectrum disorder, the researchers said.

"This is demonstrating that even though siblings may not meet the diagnostic criteria of autism, they seem to also have deficits in language and the social domain. They're not developing as typical, normal children," Shih said. "This highlights the importance of paying attention to siblings of autistic children in terms of development. It also shows the importance of early diagnosis. If these deficits or delays can be identified earlier, it's a great opportunity to provide intervention."

FINANCIAL IMPLICATIONS

A third study, from researchers at Harvard University and ABT Associates Inc., of Lexington, Massachusetts, found that each individual with autism accrues about $3.2 million in costs over a lifetime, with lost productivity and adult day care making up the lion's share.

It was already known that autism costs society more than $35 billion annually in direct and indirect expenses.

info For more information about autism, go to the Web site of Autism Speaks at *www.autismspeaks.org.*

SIDS Linked to Abnormal Brain Biology

David Paterson, PhD, instructor, Children's Hospital Boston.
Debra E. Weese-Mayer, MD, professor of pediatrics, Rush University, and director, pediatric respiratory medicine, Rush University Medical Center, Chicago.
Journal of the American Medical Association.

While there are steps parents can take to help protect their babies from sudden infant death syndrome (SIDS), such as putting babies to sleep on their backs, these measures can't stop all cases of this syndrome, characterized by the sudden and unexplained death of an infant younger than one year old.

That's likely because some children have abnormalities in the serotonin system in their brains that make them more susceptible to SIDS, according to a new study by researchers at Children's Hospital Boston.

"This study confirms that SIDS is a disease process that's biologically based and not this mystery," said one of the study's authors, Dr. David Paterson, an instructor at the Harvard Medical School–affiliated hospital.

As to what might cause these abnormalities, Paterson said, "I think it's going to be a complex combination of factors. I don't think these problems are exclusively genetic or environmental."

THE SEROTONIN SYSTEM

The serotonin system is located in an area of the brain stem called the *medulla oblongata*, and it's believed to regulate many vital body functions, including heart rate, breathing, blood pressure and temperature regulation, according to Paterson.

So, an abnormality in this critical area might stop a baby from having a normal response when not getting enough air. For example, if a baby is sleeping face down, he may be breathing in exhaled air and getting high levels of carbon dioxide. When the brain's serotonin system is working normally, it signals the baby to wake up and move his head to get fresh air. In babies that succumb to SIDS, however, it appears that the serotonin system doesn't send the right signals to the rest of the body, Paterson said.

Paterson said the new study builds on previous research that he and his colleagues have done that found serotonin-receptor defects in two other populations of SIDS babies.

"Now that we've confirmed these abnormalities in a third data set, we're confident there's a problem in the serotonin system," he said.

NEW STUDY

The new research included tissue samples from 31 babies who died of SIDS, and 10 babies who died of other causes. The researchers found that babies who died of SIDS had abnormalities in their serotonin-receptor cells, that they had more serotonin-producing cells, and that they had too few serotonin-transporter cells when compared with the control group of babies.

"Now that we know there's a problem here in the biology of the brain stem, hopefully we can do something about this," Paterson said.

REACTION

"This is a very good study. It takes us one step further in terms of focusing on the role of serotonin and SIDS," said Dr. Debra Weese-Mayer, director of pediatric respiratory medicine at Rush University Medical Center in Chicago.

But, she added, the study does have limitations, such as its small size and the underrepresentation of black infants. Like Paterson, she said she believes that the ultimate cause of SIDS will likely be multifactorial. The serotonin system will likely play a large role, though she said she thought it would probably be serotonin abnormalities along with other factors, such as genetics and environment.

ADVICE

Both experts said there needs to be a renewed focus on getting parents to have babies sleep on their backs. The majority of the infants included in this study were sleeping on their stomachs or sides.

Babies should sleep by themselves on a firm crib mattress with no soft bedding, Paterson said. Also critical is that parents don't smoke around their babies and don't allow anyone else to do so, either. Pregnant women shouldn't smoke or drink any alcohol, Paterson cautioned.

info To learn more about SIDS, visit the Web site of the Nemours Foundation at *www.kidshealth.org/parent/general/sleep/sids.html*.

Sleep Apnea in Children Linked to Lower Learning Ability

Ann Halbower, MD, medical director, Pediatric Sleep Disorders Program, Johns Hopkins University Children's Center, Baltimore.

Ronald D. Chervin, MD, associate professor, neurology, and director, University of Michigan Sleep Disorders Center, Ann Arbor.

Public Library of Science Medicine.

Children with untreated sleep apnea, a condition associated with repeated nighttime awakenings and daytime grogginess, perform significantly worse on IQ tests, according to new research from Johns Hopkins University.

These children also may have some brain impairment that could hinder their ability to learn new tasks.

THE STUDY

Dr. Ann Halbower, medical director of the pediatric sleep disorders program at the Hopkins' Children's Center in Baltimore, and colleagues looked at 31 children between the ages of 6 and 16. Nineteen of them had untreated severe sleep apnea.

Using a special type of magnetic resonance imaging (MRI), the researchers found that the children with sleep apnea had significant changes in two brain regions associated with higher mental function, the hippocampus and the right frontal cortex. They also determined that the children had altered ratios of three brain chemicals—N-aceytl aspartate, creatine and choline—which are indicative of brain damage.

The kids with sleep apnea had lower mean IQ test scores than the healthy children (85 compared with 101) and performed significantly worse on standardized tests that measure executive functions such as verbal working memory and verbal fluency.

"Executive function is the ability to take an old memory and put it to use in a new situation," Halbower explained. "It's what makes smart people smart. The clinical implications are that doctors need to understand that sleep apnea is more of a problem than we thought it was. It's not just a disease of old people."

Because untreated sleep apnea appears to impair brain chemistry, its effects could be permanent, Halbower added.

DETECTING SLEEP APNEA

Because untreated sleep apnea may have even more severe effects in children than in adults, the sooner it's detected, the better, Halbower said.

Parents should be aware that one of the most important symptoms of sleep apnea is frequent pauses in breathing that result in arousal from sleep and stirrings in bed. Other symptoms include snoring, labored or loud breathing, coughing, choking, gasping, excessive nighttime sweating and, sometimes, bedwetting by children older than six.

"If you're looking at an infant or young child, they may sleep in odd positions," said Dr. Ronald D. Chervin, the director of the University of Michigan Sleep Disorders Center. "They may sleep with their rear end up in the air and their head tilted back, which is probably an effort to open their airway."

Daytime signs of sleep apnea include sleepiness, an inability to concentrate and poor performance in school. "But it should be remembered that younger children with sleep apnea aren't just sleepy," Halbower pointed out. "They also show signs of hyperactivity and irritability."

TREATMENT

Halbower's next study will try to determine whether sleep apnea treatment can restore normal brain chemistry and cognitive function.

The standard treatment for sleep apnea in children is surgical removal of enlarged tonsils and adenoids, which can obstruct breathing. Other treatments include removal of excess tissue in the back of the throat or nose and the use of continuous positive airway pressure (CPAP) machines to maintain normal airflow during sleep.

"I would describe [this study] as preliminary news, because it opens up a whole area

that needs further investigation," Chervin said. "It'll be fascinating to see if the neurochemical changes that were present before treatment are still present after treatment."

info For more on sleep apnea, visit the Web site of the National Institute of Neurological Disorders and Stroke at *www.ninds. nih.gov.* Under "Disorder Index" click on "Sleep Apnea."

Taller Moms More Likely to Have Twins

Long Island Jewish Medical Center news release.

Taller women are more likely to have twins, and a protein called *insulin-like growth factor* (IGF) may be the reason why. That's the conclusion of a study by Dr. Gary Steinman of Long Island Jewish Medical Center in New Hyde Park, New York. Steinman is an obstetrician specializing in multiple births.

THE STUDY

In his study, Steinman compared the heights of 129 women who gave birth to twins or triplets with the average height of women in the United States.

He found that the multiple-birth mothers were an average of 65 inches tall, compared with the average female height of 63¾ inches.

EXPLANATION

IGF—released from the liver in response to growth hormone—has a number of effects in the body, including stimulating the growth of cells in the shaft of long bones.

Steinman noted that IGF also increases the sensitivity of ovaries to follicle-stimulating hormone, thereby boosting ovulation. Some previous studies have suggested that IGF may help embryos survive the early stages of development.

Countries with taller women tend to have higher rates of twins than countries with shorter women. Research has also found that shorter people have lower levels of IGF.

Infant Car Seats Might Pose Breathing Risks

Christopher Greeley, MD, medical director, newborn nursery, Vanderbilt Children's Hospital, Nashville.

Linda White, injury prevention coordinator, Cincinnati Children's Hospital Medical Center, OH.

Marjorie Marciano, director, safety education office, New York City Department of Transportation, New York City.

Alistair J. Gunn, MD, associate professor, physiology and pediatrics, University of Auckland.

British Medical Journal

Babies should not be left alone to sleep in car safety seats, especially if they were born prematurely, New Zealand pediatricians report. Their warning is based on a study of nine infants, ages three days to six months, whose alarmed parents described them as "blue," "scrunched up" or "not breathing."

"All but one case occurred when the infants had been left in the car seats indoors, allowing them to fall asleep unrestrained in an upright position," said a report by the group, led by Dr. Alistair J. Gunn, an associate professor of physiology and pediatrics at the University of Auckland.

All the infants survived, but the parents were given advice on better positioning to prevent future problems, and warnings about not leaving the babies in the car seats for excessive periods of time.

CAR SEAT SAFETY

Dr. Christopher Greeley, medical director of the newborn nursery at Vanderbilt Children's Hospital in Nashville, said the paper demonstrates the potential dangers of car seats, which are regarded as essential for protecting children if accidents occur.

"The take-home message is that parents should not leave babies unattended in car seats," Greeley said. "If you leave a very young baby in a car seat, the structure of the head, bigger in the back, can cause the airway, the trachea, to be narrowed."

Vanderbilt follows the recommendation of the American Academy of Pediatrics—that all babies born before 37 weeks of pregnancy get a car seat test before they leave the hospital, he said.

"They get the test for the potentially longest duration of the ride home, so that they don't have this kind of positional occlusion," Greeley said. "The test is done for premature babies or full-term babies who have issues with their airways. If they are born really small, have poor nutrition or have poor neck control, we do the test."

EXPERT RECOMMENDATIONS

When the children do get home, leaving them in car seats for a prolonged period is not a good idea, Greeley said. "The more they are left in, the more predisposed they are to have partial blockage of the airways," he noted. "Sleeping in a car seat is not necessarily a cause of death, but there is a higher likelihood that a baby somewhere will have difficulty with breathing."

"Car seats should only be used for transportation purposes," said Linda White, injury prevention coordinator at the Cincinnati Children's Hospital Medical Center. "Bringing one into the house and leaving a child in it, that is not what they are intended for."

Parents sometimes bring a car seat into the house and leave a baby in it "because they don't want to disturb them," White said. "But you don't want them (the babies) to be at that extended angle for a long period of time. We encourage families, even when they are traveling, to stop often and take the baby out of the car seat. The extended period of time is the key."

Marjorie Marciano, director of the safety education office at the New York City Department of Transportation, offers this advice on car seat installation. "We do know that using a car seat that is installed correctly can reduce the risk of injury significantly, for example by 70% for children under one year old," she said. "Installed correctly means that it should be at an angle of 45 degrees. When working with parents, we always say that it is important that the seat be at the right angle to keep the airway open."

She's Got Her Dad's Smile, Literally!

Gili Peleg, doctoral student, Institute of Evolution, University of Haifa, Israel.

Charles Goodstein, MD, psychoanalyst and clinical professor of psychiatry, New York University Medical Center and New York University School of Medicine and former president, Psychoanalytic Association of New York, New York City.

Proceedings of the National Academy of Sciences.

D id your mother ever tell you to stop making a funny face because it might "freeze" that way? Well, in a way, she was right. New research shows that facial expressions may be "frozen" by your genes.

Comparing the expressions of blind people to other family members, Israeli researchers discovered there's probably a genetic component to facial expressions and that human faces may be programmed from the start to look, and act, the same as those of their parents and siblings.

"There is evidence for a hereditary basis for facial expressions," said the study's lead author, Gili Peleg, a doctoral candidate at the University of Haifa in Israel.

"This study paves the way for discovering genes that influence facial expressions, understanding their evolutionary significance, and elucidating repair mechanisms for syndromes characterized by lack of facial expression, such as autism."

GENETIC FACTOR

"This is an interesting study that raises yet another question about those qualities that we have thought of as having a purely emotional basis," commented Dr. Charles Goodstein, a psychoanalyst and clinical professor of psychiatry at New York University Medical Center. "Many more qualities may be based on physiology and genetics than we've realized."

He said that having families share similar facial expressions might perform some evolutionary function. "If you have the genetically linked capacity to emulate the facial expressions of your parents, in terms of evolution, you'd probably be the most likely to survive," he said.

"There's evolutionary value to having similar facial expressions; you may be more likely to gain the care, love and attention of your parents."

THE STUDY

Peleg, under the supervision of professors Eviatar Nevo and Gadi Katzir at the Institute of Evolution at the University of Haifa, compared the facial expressions of 21 people who were blind from birth to the expressions of 30 of their relatives.

The facial expressions of congenitally blind people could not have been influenced by their environment, the researchers pointed out, since they remain visually unaware of their relatives' faces.

Each study volunteer was interviewed individually and all experienced sadness, anger and joy at some point during the interview. Facial expressions were photographed and indexed.

RESULTS

In most cases, families did exhibit a unique family facial expression "signature," according to the researchers. In fact, in about 80% of cases, family members could be accurately linked to individual participants, based on their range of facial expressions.

"There will always be debate about what traits are nature versus nurture," said Goodstein. "This study eliminates an important consideration, however: What could have been envisioned by the child."

ENVIRONMENT'S ROLE

Environment could still play a role in the development of facial expressions, even in blind children, he added. Goodstein theorized that when a child first smiles, a parent might recognize the expression and be pleased by it.

"What if the parent rewards the baby's smile and pats the baby? That smile is more likely to become a habitual smile," noted Goodstein.

info To read more about facial expressions, visit the American Psychological Association at *www.apa.org/monitor/jan00/sc1.html*.

Air Bags Dangerous for Tall or Small People

Craig Newgard, MD, assistant professor of emergency medicine and public health and preventive medicine, Oregon Health & Science University, Portland.

Toben Nelson, DSc, assistant professor of epidemiology, University of Minnesota School of Public Health, Minneapolis.

Society for Academic Emergency Medicine annual meeting, Chicago.

Short people and tall people can receive serious injuries from air bags, a new study found. "This is the first time that there is proof to substantiate the concern about small-stature occupants, and it is the first time that there has been any implication that tall people are also at risk," said lead researcher Dr. Craig Newgard, an assistant professor of emergency medicine and public health and preventive medicine at Oregon Health & Science University.

While there have been reports that short people are at risk from air bags, that risk has never been conclusively demonstrated, Newgard said. "We found that small-stature and large-stature people, male and female, were at risk for injury from an air bag as opposed to having a protective benefit," he said.

THE STUDY

Newgard said that the study researchers examined more than 11 years of data. That data included results for both older air bags and the newer "smart" air bags, which are designed to compensate for a person's weight. But, it was impossible to determine how many of each type of air bag was reflected in the data, he said.

Newgard and coauthor John McConnell collected data on 67,284 drivers and front-seat passengers involved in car crashes. They found that while air bags were effective for people of medium height—from 5 feet 3 inches tall to 5 feet 11 inches tall—they were actually harmful to people shorter than 4 feet 11 inches tall and those more than 6 feet 3 inches tall. Body weight was not a factor in injury rates.

"If you are of short stature or tall stature you may be putting yourself at risk for injury by riding in the front seat of a vehicle that has an air bag," Newgard said. "Right now, there is no federal safety guideline regarding occupant size for adults and air bags."

MORE STUDY NEEDED

One expert said he wasn't sure that the study findings were conclusive, especially when it comes to tall people.

The study didn't include separate data for new air bags, said Toben Nelson, an assistant professor of epidemiology at the University of Minnesota School of Public Health. "There should be enough data to look at revised air bag design to see if that has made a difference," he said.

Nelson also questioned the findings on air bags and tall people. "Maybe it's an artifact of not having many people of taller stature to see significant findings," he said. "Most of the evidence has been about kids and shorter individuals. There needs to be more evidence on tall people."

info To learn more about air bags, visit the Web site of the US National Safety Council at *www.nsc.org/library/cristext.htm*.

Hot Air Blows Away Head Lice

Dale Clayton, PhD, professor, biology, University of Utah, Salt Lake City.

Craig Burkhart, MD, MPH, dermatologist, Medical University of Ohio, Toledo.

Pediatrics.

A contraption that looks like a cross between a vacuum cleaner and a hair dryer could rescue children from the scourge of head lice, a new study claims. According to one of its creators, the device has a near-perfect success rate at killing off both lice and any of their eggs lurking in kids' hair. And the little critters shouldn't become immune to the so-called "LouseBuster," as they already have to some pesticides.

"It's extremely effective and extremely safe, and we think evolution-proof," said study coauthor Dr. Dale Clayton, a University of Utah biology professor. "It would be very hard for insects to develop resistance to this assault."

TRADITIONAL LICE TREATMENTS

According to Clayton, head lice will infect an estimated one in four American children. The tiny insects—about the size of a sesame seed—can be very difficult to eradicate.

One way to get rid of them is to repeatedly use special lice combs on children's heads, but this approach is so time-consuming that it can overwhelm parents. A variety of antilice shampoos are also available, but some parents don't like the idea of using insecticides—including malathion—on their kids. Also, the Centers for Disease Control and Prevention says some lice have developed immunity to the chemicals used to kill them, although such problems are scattered.

NEW STUDY

Enter hot air, which some specialists think may be better at killing lice and their eggs.

Clayton and his colleagues tested a variety of hair dryers—including handheld and "bonnet" models—on 169 children who were infested with lice.

All the hair dryers killed at least 89% of lice eggs. But only one—the specially designed "LouseBuster"—managed to both kill eggs (98%) and wipe out high numbers of living lice (80%). The remaining living lice appeared unable to breed, perhaps due to stress or sterilization, the team said.

So, according to the study, the heads of children treated with the LouseBuster were free of lice one week after the half-hour treatment.

"We think it has a delayed effect on the lice it doesn't kill," Clayton said. "When you go back a week later, there's nothing there."

The air produced by the LouseBuster is hot—much warmer than a typical hair dryer. Also unlike a hair dryer, it has a special hand piece designed to expose the roots of the hair.

The device apparently works by drying out the lice and their eggs, not by heating them, Clayton said.

The cost of the device is unknown, although Clayton estimated it should be in the hundreds of dollars, not the thousands, making it affordable for school districts. He predicted it could be on the market within a year, and added that the time required for treatment could eventually shrink to 15 minutes.

EXPERT REACTION

Dr. Craig Burkhart, a dermatologist at the Medical University of Ohio who studies lice, doubted that the device would be a success, however.

"The problem with the treatment is that it takes a half an hour at least to destroy the lice, and the contraption is somewhat expensive and very cumbersome," he said.

What to do? "As with all bugs, insecticides remain the treatment of choice," Burkhart said.

info For more information on head lice, visit the Web site of the US Centers for Disease Control and Prevention at *www.cdc.gov*. Type "Head Lice" into the search box.

■ ■ ■ ■

Some Herbal Supplements Dangerous for Kids

Garlic can thin blood and increase bleeding …Saint John's wort can reduce the effectiveness of chemotherapeutic and/or immunosuppressive drugs. Parents should also watch out for supplements that older children might buy themselves, such as weight-loss products, which could cause heart arrhythmias, irritability and poor appetite.

Self-defense: Tell your pediatrician about all medicines and supplements your children take. Studies indicate that between 11% and 15% of parents give their children some sort of herbal medicine.

Cora Collete Breuner, MD, MPH, University of Washington Children's Hospital and Medical Center, Seattle.

■ ■ ■ ■

Acne Prevention

A 13-year-old who's starting to have acne problems today has several natural alternatives to harsh drugstore acne products.

Acne affects more than 85% of adolescents and young adults. Hormonal changes cause glands of the skin to produce more oil, which clogs hair follicles. This sets the stage for the overgrowth of bacteria and yeast on the skin, leading to acne.

Natural treatments are helpful. Facial washes containing tea tree oil, available at health-food stores, can destroy bacteria and fungi associated with acne. Wash the face with a gentle, unscented soap in the morning, and use a tea tree oil facial rinse—such as Desert Essence Thoroughly Clean Face Wash—at night. Taking 500 mg to 750 mg of the herb chasteberry helps balance hormones in the body, which in turn reduces the production of facial oils. Fish oil is also useful, since it reduces skin inflammation. A daily dose of 1,000 mg of combined EPA and DHA is probably right for the teenager. To help heal the skin, he can take 30 mg to 50 mg of zinc and 2 mg of copper daily until the acne is gone.

Encourage him to limit processed foods (including soda, candy, white bread and chips)…to get more fiber from vegetables and fruits…and to drink plenty of water. These dietary habits will moderate his blood sugar levels, reducing inflammation.

Dr. Mark Stengler, ND, director of the La Jolla Whole Health Clinic, La Jolla, CA…associate clinical professor at the National College of Naturopathic Medicine, Portland, OR…author of 16 books, including *The Natural Physician's Healing Therapies*, and coauthor of *Prescription for Natural Cures* (both from Bottom Line Books)…and author of the *Bottom Line/Natural Healing* newsletter.

Checklist May Help Cut Sudden Death in Athletes

American Heart Association.

It's customary for young athletes to need a doctor's exam before being allowed to play on the school team. What should it include?

According to new guidelines by the American Heart Association, a simple 12-step screening process could help reduce sudden cardiac deaths in young athletes. The recommended screening process includes 12 questions about personal and family medical history and a physical examination.

"Although the frequency of these deaths in young athletes appears to be relatively low, it is more common than previously thought and does represent a substantive public health problem," says Dr. Barry J. Maron, chair of the panel that wrote the new screening guidelines.

About one in 200,000 high school athletes die from a heart attack while on the playing field. Most deaths occur among football and basketball players, according to studies.

THE DREAM SCREEN

What should doctors screen in your young athlete? *According to the AHA guidelines, physicians should ask questions about…*

- **Chest pain/**discomfort upon exertion
- **Unexplained fainting** or near-fainting
- **Excessive and unexplained fatigue** associated with exercise
- **Heart murmur**
- **Family history,** asking specifically about one or more relatives who died of heart disease (sudden/unexpected or otherwise) before age 50, and
- **Any close relative under age 50** with disability from heart disease
- **Specific knowledge of certain cardiac conditions** in family members such as hypertrophic or dilated cardiomyopathy, in which the heart cavity or wall becomes enlarged; "long QT syndrome," which affects the heart's electrical rhythm; or Marfan syndrome, in which the walls of the heart's major arteries are weakened.

The physical examination should note…

- **Heart murmur**
- **Blood pressure**
- **Femoral pulses** to exclude narrowing of the aorta
- **Physical appearance of Marfan syndrome**
- **Brachial artery blood pressure** (taken in a sitting position).

If any of the 12 screening elements indicate potential problems, the patient should be referred for further cardiovascular examination before joining a sports team.

info The National Heart, Lung, and Blood Institute has more on sudden cardiac death at *www.nhlbi.nih.gov.* Type "Sudden Cardiac Death" into the search box.

■ ■ ■ ■

Surprising Athletic Predictor

A study of 607 female twins found that the difference in lengths between the second and fourth (ring) fingers indicated athletic ability. Women with ring fingers longer than their index fingers (typical in men) were more likely to excel in running, soccer and tennis.

British Journal of Sports Medicine.

Mother's Beef Consumption May Affect Son's Fertility

Shanna Swan, PhD, associate chairwoman for research and professor of obstetrics and gynecology, University of Rochester School of Medicine and Dentistry, NY.
Human Reproduction.

If you want longevity for your family tree, check what's on your plate. New research finds that pregnant women who eat beef seven days a week or more daily may give birth to sons with low sperm counts.

The exact reason for the association isn't clear. But hormones, pesticides or other chemicals in beef might affect the development of the testes of the still-developing fetus, say researchers.

"We're not saying that people should stop eating beef, and it's particularly important in pregnancy that women get enough protein," says study lead Shanna Swan of the University of Rochester School of Medicine and Dentistry. "Women have to eat protein, although they don't necessarily have to eat meat."

Alternatively, opting for hormone-free or organic beef during pregnancy—or reducing overall meat consumption—may also side-step potential low sperm counts in offspring, Swan adds.

THE STUDY

For this study, the first one to examine beef consumption and semen quality, researchers analyzed semen samples and questionnaires from 387 male partners of pregnant women. The men, born between 1949 and 1983, had reported (with the help of relatives when possible) on their own mothers' diet during pregnancy.

Sperm concentration was inversely related to how much beef the mother had consumed each week. Sons of women who ate more than seven beef meals a week had sperm concentrations 24% lower than those whose moms ate less beef.

Overall, low sperm concentrations were three times higher among sons of women who consumed more than seven meals of beef a week, compared with men whose mothers ate less beef while pregnant. This pattern was only seen in beef—not veal, pork, fish or chicken, say researchers.

None of the men studied were infertile, but about one in five whose mothers ate the most beef had sperm counts classified as "sub-fertile" by national standards.

"They may have taken a longer time to conceive," says Swan. "They were twice as likely to have visited a doctor because they thought there were problems, so it's not to say there's no effect on fertility."

WHAT TO BLAME?

The study authors can't say that anabolic hormones in beef are to blame. Most American cattle were given anabolic hormones to stimulate growth and the hormone residues were present in the beef consumed while these women were pregnant. Beef also contains residues of pesticides and other industrial chemicals.

Currently, six different anabolic hormones are used in cattle in the US and Canada to stimulate growth. Three are natural hormones—estradiol, progesterone and testosterone—and three are synthetic hormones—zeranol (an estrogen), trenbolone acetate (a steroid with androgen effects) and melengestrol acetate (a progestin), say researchers.

The use of these hormones has been banned in Europe since 1988.

info For more on infertility, visit the American Society of Reproductive Medicine at *http://www.asrm.org.*

Couples Often Share Risk For Problem Drinking

Julia D. Grant, research assistant professor of psychiatry, Washington University School of Medicine, St. Louis, MO.
Alcoholism: Clinical & Experimental Research.

People at risk for drinking problems are more likely to marry someone who's also at risk for alcohol dependence, according to a team of American and Australian researchers. "As the say, 'like marries like,'" first author Julia D. Grant, a research assistant professor of psychiatry at Washington University School of Medicine in St. Louis, said in a statement.

Grant and her colleagues studied almost 6,000 twins born in Australia between 1902 and 1964 and interviewed more than 3,800 of the twins' spouses.

"Spouse selection is not a random process, and we call this nonrandom mating. People tend to choose mates who are similar to them, not only from the same neighborhood or socioeconomic background but also alike in personality and other behaviors. We found that people at risk for alcohol dependence tend to marry others who are at risk," Grant said.

But researchers said this doesn't necessarily mean that both spouses will end up with drinking problems. In some cases, one spouse's excess alcohol consumption may actually lower the risk that the other spouse will abuse alcohol.

"We don't really know how this works," Grant said. "It is possible that an individual decreases his or her alcohol consumption in reaction to the other's excessive alcohol use. Maybe one person is responsible for getting the kids up and out for school in the morning, for example."

She noted that alcohol dependence is influenced by both genetic and environmental factors, such as employment, interests, family and friends.

"There's lots of room for different factors to influence the behavior of two people who are married. One spouse could work at a place where the coworkers go out for a drink after work. Or one spouse could be a regular churchgoer, while the other prefers to sleep," Grant said.

9

Heart Disease

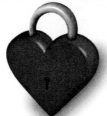

Shake Off the Salt
For a Healthier Heart

Reducing the amount of salt in your diet has been reported to lower your risk of developing heart disease by 25%, and the risk of dying from heart disease by 20%. A recent review of clinical trials has revealed these results.

"Dietary intake of sodium among Americans is excessively high," said lead researcher Nancy Cook, an associate professor of medicine at Harvard Medical School. "Our study suggests that reducing the level of salt in the diet would lead to a reduced risk of cardiovascular disease."

Sodium is known to affect blood pressure levels, particularly among people with high blood pressure. "Among hypertensive individuals, lowering sodium is pretty well established to lower blood pressure," Cook said. "Now it looks like reducing sodium also has an effect on cardiovascular disease."

THE STUDY

Cook's group examined people from two trials completed in the 1990s that analyzed the effect of reduced salt consumption on blood pressure. All the participants in the trials had "high-normal" blood pressure—sometimes called "pre-hypertension"—and were at increased risk of developing heart disease.

The first trial consisted of 744 people; the second trial had 2,382 participants. People in both trials reduced their salt intake by about 25% to 35%. Each trial also included a control group that didn't reduce salt intake.

FINDINGS

The researchers found that those participants who reduced their salt intake were 25% less likely to develop cardiovascular disease 10 to 15 years after the trials ended. There was

Nancy Cook, DSc, associate professor of medicine, Harvard Medical School, Boston.
Christine Gerbstadt, MD, RD, national spokeswoman, American Dietetic Association, Chicago.
David Katz, MD, MPH, director, Prevention Research Center, Yale University School of Medicine, New Haven, CT.
British Medical Journal.

also a 20% lower death rate from cardiovascular disease among those who cut their salt consumption.

IMPLICATIONS

One expert believes this study successfully argues for reducing dietary salt intake.

"Finally, a new affirmation that salt may be more harmful than its casual use or overuse warrants," said Dr. Christine Gerbstadt, a spokeswoman for the American Dietetic Association. "The pendulum may soon shift back to stricter sodium intake guidelines should this study be reproduced in another study of similar rigor in design and results."

HOW TO AVOID EXCESS SALT INTAKE

Dr. Gerbstadt advises consumers to avoid salt in processed foods such as "salted, salt-cured and salt-smoked foods such as lunch meat, hot dogs, ham, olives, pickles and regular salted canned foods and other prepared foods, which often use more salt than homemade equivalents."

EXPERT'S VIEW

Dr. David Katz, director of Yale University School of Medicine's Prevention Research Center, said, "Our food supply makes meaningful reductions in salt intake all but impossibly difficult for most people. The salt we shake on our food contributes far less to most diets than salt processed into foods. Even foods we would never think of as salty, such as breakfast cereals, cookies, and even some soft drinks, often contain copious amounts of sodium.

"This new study hints at the size of the potential benefit from widespread salt reduction," Katz said. "But advice about reducing salt intake can only get us so far. To see the benefits play out at the population level will require modification of the food supply, so that eating less salt requires a lot less work," he said.

info For more information on reducing salt intake, visit the American Heart Association Web site, *www.americanheart.org,* and search "Cutting Down on Salt."

Silent Heart Disease

Prediman K. Shah, MD, director of the division of cardiology and the Atherosclerosis Research Center at Cedars-Sinai Heart Center in Los Angeles. He is a professor of medicine at the David Geffen School of Medicine at the University of California, Los Angeles, and was the leader of the Screening for Heart Attack Prevention and Education (SHAPE) Task Force editorial committee.

Up to 50% of people who have a first heart attack—which often results in sudden death—don't experience prior chest pain, shortness of breath or other red flags for cardiovascular disease. A heart attack is their first and only symptom.

In the past, cardiologists relied solely on the presence of risk factors—a family history of heart disease, smoking, diabetes, etc.—to identify "silent" heart disease.

New approach: An international task force of leading cardiologists has just issued new guidelines that could prevent more than 90,000 deaths from cardiovascular disease each year in the US. Most of these patients have no prior symptoms.

RISK FACTORS AREN'T ENOUGH

Most heart attacks and many strokes are caused by atherosclerosis, buildup of cholesterol and other substances (plaque) within artery walls.

Over time, increasing accumulations of plaque can compromise circulation—or result in blood clots that block circulation to the heart (heart attack) or brain (stroke).

Plaque can accumulate for decades within artery walls without causing the arterial narrowing that results in angina (chest pain) or other symptoms. Even patients with massive amounts of plaque may be unaware that they have heart disease until they suffer a heart attack or sudden death.

RECOMMENDED TESTS

Guidelines created by the Screening for Heart Attack Prevention and Education (SHAPE) Task Force call for noninvasive screening of virtually all asymptomatic men ages 45 to 75 and women ages 55 to 75.* The tests can detect arterial changes that are present in the vast majority

*Screening for adults age 75 or older is not recommended because they are considered at high risk for cardiovascular disease based on their age alone.

of heart attack patients. The SHAPE Task Force identified two tests—a computed tomography (CT) scan of the coronary arteries and an ultrasound of the carotid arteries in the neck—that are more accurate than traditional risk-factor assessments in identifying high-risk patients.

Most patients require only one of these tests. Which test is recommended will depend on insurance coverage and/or other underlying health conditions and risk factors. Although these tests are widely available, health insurers do not always cover the cost, which ranges from about $200 to $400 each.

• **Coronary artery screening.** Calcium within the coronary arteries always indicates that a patient has atherosclerosis (whether or not blockages are present). Calcium is a marker of actual disease, not just the risk of disease.

What's involved: The patient is given a CT scan of the heart and three coronary arteries. Undressing isn't required—the test is noninvasive and takes about five to 10 minutes.

Dozens of images are taken during the test and then analyzed with computer software. If calcium is present, it's given a score based on severity. A score of 0 is ideal...less than 100 indicates moderate atherosclerosis...100 to 400 represents a significant problem...and more than 400 is severe.

In patients with a score of 0 (no calcium is present), the risk of having a heart attack or stroke over the next 10 years is 0.1%. Patients with a score of 400 or higher are 20 to 30 times more likely to have a heart attack or stroke than those with a score of 0.

• **Carotid ultrasound.** This test measures the intima media thickness (the gap between the inside of the blood vessel wall and a layer called the media) of the carotid arteries. It also measures the amount of plaque that may be present.

A thickening of the intima media (the values are adjusted for age and sex) is a predictor of stroke as well as heart attack. The presence of any plaque is a red flag—patients who have plaque in the carotid arteries generally will also show evidence of plaque in the coronary arteries.

What's involved: The patient lies on an examination table while a technician moves a transducer (a device that emits and receives ultrasound signals) over the carotid arteries on both sides of the neck. Like the CT scan, the test is noninvasive. It takes about 45 to 90 minutes to complete.

TREATING SILENT HEART DISEASE

With screening tests, doctors can target high-risk patients more precisely—and recommend appropriate treatment. The aggressiveness of treatment should be proportionate to the risk level.

It's possible that drugs to reduce levels of existing plaque will be on the market within the next five years. *Until then, patients diagnosed with asymptomatic cardiovascular disease (based on one of the above tests) should...*

• **Get a stress test.** Patients who test positive for calcium or plaque in the coronary or carotid arteries should undergo a cardiac stress test. The test, which uses an electrocardiogram, involves walking on a treadmill or riding a bicycle. The test detects impediments in circulation through the coronary arteries and identifies abnormal heart rhythms (arrhythmias) that can occur during exercise in patients with heart disease. Nuclear stress tests (which involve the use of radioactive dye) or echocardiogram (a type of ultrasound) stress tests generally are more reliable than simple electrocardiogram tests.

Patients with significant blockages in the coronary arteries may require invasive procedures, such as angioplasty or bypass surgery, to restore normal circulation to the heart.

• **Control cholesterol and blood pressure.** They're two important risk factors for heart attack and stroke—and both are modifiable with medication and/or lifestyle changes. A patient who tests positive for asymptomatic cardiovascular disease needs to treat these conditions much more aggressively than someone without it. For cardiovascular health, aim for a blood pressure of no more than 110 mmHg to 120 mmHg systolic (top number) and 70 mmHg to 80 mmHg diastolic (bottom number). An ideal LDL "bad" cholesterol level is no more than 70.

Most patients can significantly lower blood pressure and cholesterol with lifestyle changes —exercising for 30 minutes at least three to four times a week...losing weight, if necessary...eating less saturated fat and/or trans fat...and increasing consumption of fruits, vegetables, whole grains and fish.

Other risk factors to control: Smoking, obesity, diabetes, as well as emotional stress/anger, which may lead to a heart attack or angina. It's important to control all of these risk factors because they can amplify each other—for example, a sedentary lifestyle promotes obesity, which can lead to diabetes—or have a cumulative effect that's much more dangerous than an individual risk factor.

info For more on silent heart disease, consult the Society for Heart Attack Prevention and Eradication, a nonprofit group that promotes heart disease education and research, 877-742-7311, *www.shapesociety.org.*

Hidden Heart Failure

Margaret Redfield, MD, professor of medicine at the Mayo Clinic College of Medicine and director of the Mayo Clinic's Heart Failure Clinic, both in Rochester, MN. She was senior author of a recent *New England Journal of Medicine* study on the increased prevalence of diastolic heart failure.

Until recently, most cases of congestive heart failure were believed to occur when the heart weakens and becomes unable to pump effectively—a condition known more specifically as systolic heart failure (SHF).

Now: A review of nearly 4,600 heart failure cases treated at the Mayo Clinic shows that a long-overlooked form of congestive heart failure, called diastolic heart failure (DHF), is even more common than SHF and is just as deadly. In 15 years, the proportion of heart failure cases caused by diastolic dysfunction jumped from 38% to 54%.

THE AGING HEART

Normally, the heart muscle contracts and relaxes with every beat. The contraction phase, when blood is pumped out to the body, is called systole...the relaxation phase, when the heart refills with blood, is called diastole.* With age or disease, such as high blood pressure, diabetes

*Blood pressure—a measurement of the pressure of blood against the walls of the main arteries—is expressed in terms of systolic pressure (the top number) and diastolic pressure (the bottom number).

or atherosclerosis (plaque buildup in the arteries), the heart muscle may become weak and unable to pump effectively, resulting in SHF...or rigid and unable to relax and fill properly, leading to DHF.

Both SHF and DHF are chronic, progressive and often fatal. They produce identical symptoms—shortness of breath...inability to exercise...and fatigue. They can lead to lung congestion (fluid backup in the lungs) or swelling in the abdomen, lower legs or feet, caused by fluid and water retention (edema).

Important: It's impossible to distinguish SHF and DHF with a physical exam, X-ray or electrocardiogram (a recording of the electrical activity of the heart). To get a definitive diagnosis, you need an echocardiogram (an ultrasound of the heart, which shows pictures of the valves and chambers). If you have been diagnosed with heart failure, ask your doctor about receiving an echocardiogram.

There's evidence showing that the incidence of DHF is rising—perhaps because our aging population is living longer with hypertension, atherosclerosis, diabetes and other diseases that can compromise diastolic functioning (as well as systolic functioning). Most cases of DHF are diagnosed in people over age 70, and, for unknown reasons, a disproportionate number of them are women.

BEST TREATMENT OPTIONS

Although researchers are now beginning to recognize the prevalence of DHF, the treatment approach is less well defined than that for SHF. The goal is to help manage symptoms related to fluid retention, such as edema and shortness of breath, and treat underlying conditions, such as hypertension, atherosclerosis, atrial fibrillation (irregular heartbeat), diabetes or high cholesterol, with medication and/or lifestyle changes.

Treatments for DHF...

•**Diuretics** to reduce excess bodily fluid and prevent pulmonary congestion or edema.

•**Angiotensin-converting enzyme (ACE) inhibitors** or other vasodilators to relax and widen blood vessels and lower blood pressure.

•**Beta-blockers** to slow heart rate, giving the heart more time to fill with each beat. Although the use of beta-blockers is standard in SHF, they're not always appropriate for DHF. That's because beta-blockers not only slow heart rate, but also reduce the heart's ability to relax.

However, in the first major beta-blocker study to include some older DHF patients, participants taking the new beta-blocker *nebivolol* had a 4.2% lower risk for heart failure–related hospitalizations and a 2.3% lower risk for death than the placebo group. Still, more research is needed, and the decision to use beta-blockers for DHF must be made on an individual basis, weighing the potential risks and benefits for the particular patient.

DIET AND EXERCISE

DHF patients—as well as people with SHF—should eat a heart-healthy diet rich in whole grains as well as vegetables and fruits...reduce their intake of sodium (especially if they have hypertension) to 2 g daily...and limit saturated fats and avoid trans fats.

Exercise is difficult for heart failure patients because they may experience shortness of breath, but if they can manage 30 minutes daily of a low-intensity activity, such as walking, cycling or water aerobics, it can help maintain and perhaps improve heart functioning.

Also helpful: Yoga or tai chi. In an Italian study published in *The Lancet*, heart failure patients who practiced yoga-like breathing for one month had higher resting blood oxygen levels, slower normal breathing rates and more endurance for exercise—all signs of improved cardiopulmonary functioning. (To find a yoga teacher, contact the American Yoga Association at 941-927-4977 or *www.americanyogaassociation.org*.)

Meanwhile, in a recent Harvard Medical School study, heart failure patients who participated in a twice-weekly, hour-long tai chi class for three months (in addition to taking medication) were able to walk longer distances without getting winded and reported feeling better overall. (To find a tai chi class near you, visit the Tai Chi and Health Information Center Web site, *www.americantaichi.net*.)

ON THE HORIZON

As DHF becomes more widely recognized, scientists are increasingly making it a focus of their research. *Promising therapies...*

•**Angiotensin receptor blockers (ARBs).** Studies have shown that these blood-pressure–lowering medications are useful for treating SHF. Now researchers at Georgetown University Hospital in Washington, DC, are investigating whether theses drugs also may benefit DHF patients.

•**Alagebrium.** This new drug reduces arterial stiffness. In a recent trial at Wake Forest University in Winston-Salem, North Carolina, it was shown to significantly improve diastolic function in patients with DHF. Study participants taking alagebrium reported having more physical energy for daily activities and improved mental functioning. Larger studies are under way to confirm the effectiveness of alagebrium.

•**Aldosterone receptor antagonists.** These drugs, which act as potassium-sparing diuretics (causing the kidneys to excrete excess fluid while retaining potassium), are typically prescribed for hypertension or edema and have been shown to help SHF patients. In August, the National Institutes of Health launched the first large-scale clinical trial to determine whether an aldosterone antagonist called *spironolactone* (Aldactone) helps DHF patients.

•**Sildenafil** (Viagra). Brazilian researchers recently reported that this impotence drug may safely lower blood pressure as well as resting heart rate and improve exercise tolerance in men who have both erectile dysfunction (ED) and congestive heart failure.

Sildenafil is not FDA-approved for heart failure treatment, but that may change if current studies yield positive results.

•**Cardiac resynchronization therapy (CRT).** In about one-third of heart failure patients, the heart's ventricles fail to beat simultaneously, which reduces pumping efficiency. With CRT, a specialized pacemaker is implanted, which re-coordinates the action of the heart's right and left ventricles.

In a recent study, CRT combined with drug therapy reduced the risk for hospitalizations and fatalities among SHF patients by as much as 20%. Researchers are planning trials to determine whether it may offer similar benefits to DHF patients.

■ ■ ■ ■

15-Second Test

Multidetector computed tomography (MDCT) lets doctors see plaque in arteries with a 15-second scan in the emergency room. Chest pain from heart attacks and angina rarely occurs without plaque buildup. A few hospitals can do MDCT now, and more are expected to in the future.

Udo Hoffman, MD, director of cardiac CT research, department of radiology, Massachusetts General Hospital… assistant professor of radiology, Harvard Medical School, both in Boston…and leader of a study of 103 people with acute chest pain, published in *Circulation*.

New Test Could Mean Early Warning

Ruth McPherson, director, University of Ottawa Heart Institute lipid clinic and lipid research laboratory.
Kari Stefansson, MD, chief executive officer, deCODE Genetics, Iceland.
Science Express.

Two research teams have identified genetic material strongly associated with a significantly increased risk of heart disease.

About one in every four Caucasians are thought to carry the genetic variants located on chromosome 9, and a test to identify those who are at high risk of heart attack could be available by the end of this year.

The discoveries are even more interesting because the same cluster has recently been strongly implicated in raising diabetes risk.

IMPLICATIONS

"This is an important finding, because it was replicated in different populations around the world," added Canadian scientist Dr. Ruth McPherson, director of the Ottawa Heart Institute's lipid clinic and lipid research laboratory, who led one research effort.

The two separate reports do not pinpoint specific genes. Instead, they cite what are called *single nucleotide polymorphisms* (SNPs)—slight variations in the sequence of units that make up the molecule of DNA that carries genetic information.

One report, led by scientists at an Icelandic biotechnology company, and one report from McPherson's group in Canada, cites two different genes. All are clustered together in a region of chromosome 9.

Regardless of where the study participants originated—Canada, Iceland or the United States—the SNPs bumped up heart risk. For example, people carrying the SNP cited in the Icelandic study had about a 60% raised risk for heart attack compared with noncarriers, while people carrying the two SNPs in the Canadian study had a 30% to 40% increased risk of heart disease.

"The discovery that these SNPs can impact heart risk remains puzzling, because they do not involve specific genes," McPherson said. "However, they do lie near two tumor-suppressor genes known to be associated with cell proliferation, aging and death. There might be other explanations for the association.

"They may be in a region that regulates the activity of genes," McPherson added. "It is possible that the region regulates genes that are a bit further away. But the finding so far does not tell us anything about their mechanism of action."

Still, there is "a kind of excitement about such unexpected findings that could lead to genes with entirely different pathways," McPherson said.

Part of the excitement is that the genetic factors identified by the studies do not seem to be linked to known risk factors. That opens the possibility of new preventive measures aimed at whatever in the SNPs influences heart risk.

Another bonus found by a team led by Dr. Francis Collins, director of the US National Human Genome Research Institute, recently reported that the same genetic material is also highly linked to a boost in diabetes risk.

THE NEXT STEP

"The most important story here is that not only does this variant impose the risk of heart attack, but it imposes greater risk on younger people," said Dr. Kari Stefansson, a neurologist, formerly with Harvard Medical School. "For men under the age of 50 and women under the age of 60, it doubles the risk of heart attack."

A test based on the finding will be available probably before the end of this year, Stefansson said. "We plan to launch it ourselves." Regulatory approval is not required.

"The test would be aimed at two groups of people—those with known risk factors such as high cholesterol, high blood pressure and diabetes, and those whose physicians wanted to screen them for risk. When someone is found to carry two risk-associated SNPs, those are the people you want to follow meticulously," with close attention to risk factors, Stefansson said.

"Ultimately, such a test could be added to the whole package that we use to assess risk," McPherson said.

info For more information on SNPs and their role in genetics at the Human Genome Project, visit the Web site at *www.ornl.gov/sci/techresources/.index.shtml*.

Latest Lifesaving Treatments for Heart Patients

Keith A. A. Fox, MB, ChB, British Heart Foundation professor of cardiology, the University of Edinburgh, Scotland.
Louis Teichholz, MD, medical director, cardiac services, and division director, cardiology, Hackensack University Medical Center, NJ.
Journal of the American Medical Association.

The rates of heart failure and death are dropping, as more doctors and medical centers start implementing new heart disease treatment guidelines.

New guidelines call for more aggressive use of medications, such as oral anti-clotting drugs like aspirin, beta-blockers, *angiotensin-converting enzyme (ACE) inhibitors, angiotensin II receptor blockers* (ARBs), and statins. Guidelines also recommend that when appropriate, angioplasty be performed quickly.

Numerous randomized clinical trials have been conducted, and more and more evidence is available to doctors regarding treatment of heart disease.

As a result of all these trials, many organizations, such as the American Heart Association, the American College of Cardiology and the European Society of Cardiology, have issued new treatment guidelines, according to Dr. Keith A. A. Fox, the British Heart Foundation professor of cardiology at the University of Edinburgh in Scotland.

BACKGROUND

Every year, almost eight million Americans will have a heart attack and another five million will have heart failure, according to the American Heart Association. A heart attack occurs when blood flow to the heart is blocked, usually by a blood clot. Heart failure occurs when the heart becomes so damaged that it can no longer pump blood efficiently.

THE STUDY

To assess the impact these new guidelines have had on patient care, Fox and his colleagues gathered data on almost 45,000 people treated at 113 hospitals in 14 different countries. The researchers assessed in-hospital and six months post-discharge outcomes.

Fox said that due to implementation of new guidelines, "survival was markedly improved, and, for the first time in any study, we have shown a marked reduction in the development of new heart failure."

Overall, he said, "deaths in heart attack declined from 8.4% to 4.6%, new heart failure from 19.5% to 11%, and new heart attacks from 4.8% to 2%."

CONCLUSIONS

"The changes must be due to improved treatment of patients after presentation to hospital," said Fox. "The improvement is due to the combined effect of better use of anti-clotting and other heart attack drugs, and greater use of angioplasty."

Dr. Louis Teichholz, medical director of cardiac services and division director of cardiology at Hackensack University Medical Center, agrees that the use of medications and increased use of angioplasty are the biggest contributors to the decline in heart failure and deaths.

"One of the most important changes is the more aggressive use of medications," said Teichholz, who added that the use of angioplasty was also a big factor in the improved mortality and heart failure statistics. "When you take patients to the catheterization lab and open up the artery, it markedly improves mortality and saves heart muscle."

Teichholz pointed out that recent studies have questioned the use of angioplasty and stenting in chronic heart conditions, but in acute situations, such as a heart attack, he said, "Opening up the artery can be lifesaving."

Teichholz said that the six-month, follow-up statistics weren't as impressive. Most of the gains made in the acute-care setting had leveled off, he noted.

"For most people," he said, "what's really important to know is the clock starts ticking as soon as you get chest pains. Don't wait hours before going to the hospital."

info To learn more about acute coronary syndrome, visit the American Heart Association, *www.americanheart.org.*

Breakthrough Stent Relieves Heart Pain

Shmuel Banai, chief medical officer, Neovasc Medical Inc., Tel Aviv, Israel.

Deepak Bhatt, MD, assistant director, Cleveland Clinic cardiovascular coordinating center.

Gregory Barsness, MD, assistant professor of cardiology, Mayo Clinic, Rochester, MN.

Journal of the American College of Cardiology.

A new, different kind of stent brought relief by diverting blood to oxygen-starved heart muscle to people suffering from refractory angina, a kind of heart-related chest pain for which there currently is no effective treatment.

ACTION PLAN

"An effective treatment for refractory angina is definitely needed," said Dr. Deepak Bhatt, associate director of the Cleveland Clinic cardiovascular coordinating center, "because it now affects at least 500,000 Americans, and the number is growing.

"A very substantial portion of these folks I see have no option," Bhatt said. "We've tried everything there is to be tried, and they continue to have chest pain. There is an unmet need for better therapies for this unstable angina."

NEW FINDINGS

A conventional stent is a flexible tube implanted in an artery to keep it open. The new stent is designed to partially block a coronary blood vessel so that blood is diverted to areas of the heart muscle that are in pain because of inadequate blood supply.

"The new stent is an hourglass-shaped, stainless steel, balloon-expandable stent delivered on a proprietary catheter," said Dr. Shmuel Banai, an interventional cardiologist at Tel Aviv Medical Center. The stent partially restricts the flow of blood draining from the heart by narrowing the coronary sinus, a vein that collects blood from the heart, to a diameter of three millimeters.

Researchers studied the results of implantation of the stent in 15 patients with refractory angina in Germany and India. The angina score measuring pain improved in 12 patients with echocardiograph and computed tomography showing a reduction in the ischemic area of the heart.

"There were no total occlusions, clotting or other complications noted at the end of the trial, and that is still the case two years out," Banai said.

FURTHER STUDY NEEDED

The new report is "intriguing" and "provocative," Bhatt said, but the number of patients in the study was small, and there was no control group. "A placebo effect can occur," he said, so that just the thought of having an effective treatment can bring improvement. "These folks have no hope, so if you offer some hope, they can respond positively," Bhatt said.

Still, the concept "definitely is worthy of further study," Bhatt said.

Dr. Gregory Barsness, assistant professor of cardiology at the Mayo Clinic in Rochester, Minnesota, said that while the trial study has not had complete follow-up, it is a "novel strategy that at least has been shown to be safe in a small group of patients.

"Having refractory angina does not necessarily increase the risk of death," Barsness said, "but these people certainly are suffering greatly. This population of patients with refractory angina is growing and will continue to grow as the population ages. Any strategy that improves the quality of life without morbidity and mortality would certainly be welcome."

For more information on angina, go to *www.medicinenet.com/angina/article.htm.*

Beware! Nearly 20% of Defibrillators Fail

Thomas Kleeman, clinical electrophysiologist, Herzzentrum Ludwigshafen, Germany.

Kenneth A. Ellenbogen, MD, director, department of electrophysiology, Virginia Commonwealth University, Richmond.

Circulation.

A German cardiovascular research center reports that the wires through which implanted defibrillators deliver electric jolts that keep hearts beating normally aren't as reliable as many originally thought. This is a potential problem for many Americans who are walking around with defibrillators inside of them—some 68,000 people in 2004—the most recent year for which statistics are available.

BACKGROUND

Even though the wire's composition was changed to improve reliability, both the newer and older versions of these defibrillators show an annual rate of defect of almost 20%, a decade after implantation. Given that these devices are used to treat arrhythmias, dangerously irregular heartbeats that can lead to cardiac arrest, the researchers note that such a significant failure rate poses a public health threat.

"It's a very serious problem because if the leads [wires] have defects, they have to be changed or the device cannot terminate fibrillation," said study author Dr. Thomas Kleeman, a clinical electrophysiologist at Herzzentrum Ludwigshafen. "Surgery to change them is not so easy," he added.

THE STUDY

Kleeman and colleagues looked at the reliability of defibrillators implanted in 990 people by the Ludwigshafen center between 1992 and May 2005. They found an average 15% defect rate in the wires, with a median time of failure of 4.7 years. Other German institutions were facing the same problem.

It's generally a simple issue of wear-and-tear, he said. "If the defibrillator is in for many years, the chance of failure increases," Kleeman said, with the likelihood of failure increasing with the number of leads per defibrillator. "But," he added, "failure appears to be more common in women, younger people and those whose left ventricle was healthier when the device was implanted."

Causes of failure include: insulation problems (56%); fractured wires (12%); loss of ability to detect the abnormal electrical pulse in the heart chamber (11%); abnormal impedance, a problem in the electrical circuit (10%); or a sensing failure (10%).

While 11% of those who got defibrillators during the study died, none of the deaths were attributed to lead failure. Of that group, 55% died of congestive heart failure, 13% died from noncardiac causes, 9% from other cardiovascular problems, and 2% from sudden death. In 21% of the cases, the cause of death remains unknown.

Newer wires are made from different polymers, and Dr. Kleeman suggests that they might be an improvement.

IMPLICATIONS

"But the study is a reminder that eternal vigilance is needed in medicine, especially for devices on which life depends," said Dr. Kenneth A. Ellenbogen, director of the department of electrophysiology at Virginia Commonwealth University, and a spokesman for the American Heart Association.

ICDs (implantable cardioverter defibrillator) should be checked frequently, as often as once a month in some cases, Ellenbogen added. "Certainly with patients living longer and longer and newer technology being developed to make the devices last longer, there can be a significant risk of failure," he said.

The latest technology makes it possible to run what amounts to a continual check on ICDs, with bedside monitors that transmit data to manufacturers, Ellenbogen said. And the news about the latest ICDs is not all that bad, he noted. "That certainly has been my clinical experience, that they are getting better," he said.

info For more information on the implantable defibrillator, visit the Web site for the medical journal *Circulation, circ.ahajournals.org/.*

Fish Oil–Exercise Combo May Boost Cardio Health

American Journal of Clinical Nutrition.

A combination of fish-oil supplements and exercise may help improve cardiovascular health in overweight people, an Australian study suggests.

THE STUDY

The study included 75 overweight men and women, ages 25 to 65, who had at least one of the following cardiovascular risk factors—mild hypertension, elevated total cholesterol and elevated plasma triacylglycerols.

The volunteers were divided into groups that received either six grams fish oil (including 260 milligrams *docosahexaenoic acid* [DHA] and 60 milligrams *eicosapentaenoic acid* [EPA]); six grams fish oil per day and an exercise regimen of 45 minutes of running or walking three times weekly; six grams sunflower oil (placebo)/day; or six grams sunflower oil/day and the exercise regimen.

FINDINGS

The study found that the use of fish oil resulted in a larger decrease in plasma triglycerides, a larger increase in plasma HDL ("good") cholesterol and greater improvement in opening of the blood vessels) than the sunflower oil. Exercise improved small artery flexibility, and the combination of both exercise and fish oil reduced fat mass.

The study confirms the findings of previous research: exercise and fish oil benefit cardiovascular health. The study authors suggested that fish oil could be a useful adjunct to exercise programs designed to improve body composition.

info The US Food and Drug Administration offers advice on their Web site on how to keep your heart healthy at *www.fda.gov.*

Restless Legs Syndrome Linked to Heart Risks

American Academy of Neurology.
Neurology.

R estless legs syndrome may be associated with an increased risk of developing cardiovascular disease, especially in elderly people, a Canadian study suggests.

Restless legs syndrome (RLS) is a neurological disorder in which people have a strong urge to move their legs. Periodic leg movements associated with the disorder are typically most severe at night, and can occur every 20 to 40 seconds.

THE STUDY

University of Montreal researchers monitored the blood pressure and leg movements of 10 patients with untreated restless legs syndrome who spent a night in a sleep laboratory. Patients' blood pressure rates during periodic leg movements increased by an average of 20 points for the systolic reading (top or first number) and by an average of 11 points for the diastolic reading (bottom or second number).

IMPLICATIONS

"This repetitive rise in blood pressure during periodic leg movements could be harmful to the cardiovascular system, especially in severe cases of RLS, the elderly, and those with a long history of the disease," study lead author Dr. Paola Lanfranchi said.

"Past studies have shown that significant blood pressure changes, as shown in our study, are associated with the development of vascular and heart damage. Furthermore, drastic blood pressure surges at night have been associated with a higher rate of stroke in the elderly," Lanfranchi added.

"Further studies are needed to clarify and quantify the damaging effects of such changes on the heart and blood vessels and also to determine how medications for RLS may impact this damaging effect," study coauthor Dr. Jacques Montplaisir said in a prepared statement.

Just 10 Minutes of Daily Exercise Boosts Heart Health

Timothy Church, MD, MPH, PhD, director, Laboratory of Preventive Research, Pennington Biomedical Research Center, Louisiana State University, Baton Rouge.

I-Min Lee, MBBS, ScD, associate professor of medicine, Brigham and Women's Hospital and Harvard Medical School, and associate professor of epidemiology, Harvard School of Public Health, Boston.

Journal of the American Medical Association.

A new study has good news for people who've been avoiding exercise because they don't think they have enough time —even 10 minutes a day can improve cardiovascular fitness.

NEW FINDINGS

The research found that when overweight or obese, sedentary women started to exercise an average of 72 minutes a week, they increased their peak oxygen consumption—a measure of cardiovascular fitness—by 4.2%.

"It was surprising to us, the idea that as little as 10 to 15 minutes of exercise a day could provide benefit in terms of fitness," said the study's lead author, Dr. Timothy Church, director of the Laboratory of Preventive Medicine Research at the Pennington Biomedical Research Center at Louisiana State University.

Church noted that the intensity of exercise the women in the study engaged in was very low, probably equivalent to walking at a speed of about two to three miles an hour. "For people who've been really sedentary, you're getting a benefit almost immediately. Just get off the couch," he added.

The researchers also found that while a little bit of exercise was beneficial, more exercise boosted cardiorespiratory fitness even higher.

"Physical activity is clearly beneficial for your health. This study shows that any activity is good, and more is better," said Dr. I-Min Lee, an associate professor of medicine at Brigham and Women's Hospital and Harvard Medical School, both in Boston.

THE STUDY

Church and colleagues undertook the research, because there have been few studies that have looked at the dose-response effect of exercise—that is, how much exercise do you need to see a benefit and will more exercise continue to produce additional benefits?

To answer those questions, the researchers recruited 464 overweight or obese postmenopausal women. All of the women had some degree of high blood pressure, and none exercised at all.

The women were randomly assigned to one of four groups: The control group that remained sedentary; a light exercise group that averaged 72 minutes a week of exercise; a moderate exercise group that averaged about 136 minutes a week; and a high exercise group that completed nearly 192 minutes of exercise each week.

The researchers measured the women's peak oxygen consumption at the start of the study, and then again after six months of exercise. They found that the women in the light exercise group increased their peak oxygen consumption levels by 4.2%. The moderate exercise group saw a 6% rise, while the heavy exercise group upped their cardiorespiratory fitness by 8.2%.

IMPLICATIONS

"This is great news for couch potatoes and for the aging," said Church. People who can't do the recommended amount of exercise each week can still benefit from a smaller amount.

Current recommendations call for 30 minutes of exercise most days of the week. Church said the three exercise groups roughly translate to 50%, 100% and 150% of the exercise guideline.

"Even with a little bit of physical activity, there was a significant improvement in physical fitness. And, this study showed that you can start seeing health benefits, with a very doable dose of physical activity," he said.

info To learn more about the benefits of exercise, visit the American Academy of Family Physicians Web site, *www.aafp.org*.

Lifesaving Drug Lowers Heart Risks

Deepak Bhatt, MD, associate director, Cleveland Clinic cardiovascular coordinating center.

Stephen A. Siegel, MD, assistant clinical professor, medicine, New York University.

Journal of the American College of Cardiology.

Carvedilol, a newer member of the beta-blocker family of heart drugs, has saved more lives than an older drug, and has also cut the incidence of heart attacks and strokes, according to European researchers.

THE STUDY

The five-year study of more than 3,000 people with heart failure, where the heart progressively loses its ability to pump blood, found a 21% lower incidence of heart attacks and a 25% lower incidence of fatal strokes among those who took carvedilol (brand name *Coreg*) compared with those taking an older medication, *metoprolol* (Lopressor).

"This is quite a different message from what they said before," Dr. Deepak Bhatt, associate director of the Cleveland Clinic's cardiovascular coordinating center, said.

"Earlier, they described reductions in deaths from heart failure," said Bhatt. "Now, they say [Coreg] is good not only for the heart muscle but also for the arteries."

NEW FINDINGS

The new finding is the latest chapter in the history of beta-blockers, which have been in and out of favor for treatment of high blood pressure and heart failure, said Dr. Stephen A. Siegel, assistant clinical professor of medicine at New York University.

"This helps clearly bring into line that beta-blockers can be important tools in the right patient population, especially those with congestive heart failure," Siegel said.

But the results also indicate that all beta-blockers might not be created equal, he said.

"The study results indicate that carvedilol might be different from other beta-blockers," Siegel said. "With the congestive heart failure data, carvedilol had better results than most of the other beta-blockers. Some particular differences in terms of beta-blocking effect might be part of why it is particularly beneficial in treatment of congestive heart failure."

But the results of the European trial are still somewhat controversial, and the choice of a beta-blocker for individual patients might not be clear-cut, Bhatt said. The controversy arises from the dosages used in the European study.

Cost is another element in the decision, Bhatt said. Coreg is much more expensive than metoprolol, which is now available in generic form.

"I don't think the data are strong enough to switch all patients to carvedilol," Bhatt said. "But there surely is no harm in the switch."

info You can learn more about beta-blockers from the Texas Heart Institute Web site, *www.texasheart.org.*

Secondhand Smoke Poses Heart Disease Risk

Andrea Venn, PhD, associate professor, Division of Epidemiology and Public Health, University of Nottingham, United Kingdom.

Byron Lee, MD, associate professor, cardiology, University of California, San Francisco.

Circulation.

Breathing secondhand smoke appears to increase levels of two markers for heart disease, the protein *fibrinogen* and *homocysteine* (an amino acid), British researchers report.

The lead researcher is Andrea Venn, an associate professor at the University of Nottingham's Division of Epidemiology and Public Health.

THE STUDY

For the study, Venn and coauthor Dr. John Britton collected data on 7,599 adults in the third National Health and Nutrition Examination Survey. None of these people had ever smoked.

Study participants had their blood levels of cotinine, an indicator of nicotine, measured. They also had their levels of fibrinogen, homocysteine and C-reactive protein measured, all factors linked to heart disease.

The researchers found that only 18% of the participants had no detectable levels of cotinine. The other participants had either low or high levels of the substance. Eighteen percent of those with low levels of cotinine and 56% of those with high levels said they lived with a smoker or were exposed to tobacco smoke at work.

The researchers also found that the low- and high-cotinine groups had significantly higher levels of fibrinogen and homocysteine, compared with those who had no detectable levels of cotinine. The increased fibrinogen and homocysteine levels were equivalent to about 30% to 45% of levels seen in active smokers. Fibrinogen and homocysteine are markers for heart disease.

"Furthermore, our study showed that these effects were not restricted to people exposed to high levels of secondhand smoke but were also evident in our low-exposure group, the majority of whom reported not living with a smoker and not being exposed at work," Venn said.

LOW LEVELS OF SECONDHAND SMOKE STILL DANGEROUS

The findings suggest that secondhand smoke has a significant effect on susceptibility to cardiovascular disease, even at relatively low levels of exposure, Venn said. "Secondhand smoke is likely to be an important avoidable cause of cardiovascular disease in the population, and it is therefore important that measures are implemented to minimize the public's exposure to secondhand smoke," she said.

"Contrary to what the tobacco companies will tell you, there is overwhelming evidence that even secondhand smoke is harmful," said Dr. Byron Lee, an associate professor of cardiology at the University of California, San Francisco.

info To learn more about secondhand smoke, visit the Web site of the Centers for Disease Control and Prevention at *www.cdc.gov/tobacco/secondhand_smoke*.

Napping Slashes Heart Disease Risk by 30%

Dimitrios Trichopoulos, MD, PhD, professor of cancer prevention and epidemiology, Harvard School of Public Health, Boston.
Gregg C. Fonarow, MD, professor, cardiology, University of California, Los Angeles.
Archives of Internal Medicine.

A large study of Greek men and women suggests that taking a daily midday nap has a stress-reducing effect that may lower your risk of dying from heart disease by more than 30%.

BACKGROUND

Siestas are common in Mediterranean countries and several Latin American nations, where the rate of death from heart disease is comparatively low. Earlier studies had looked at the association between midday naps and heart disease, but the results were inconsistent. The new study is the first large, prospective study of people who were healthy at the start of the study. It's also the first one to take into account risk factors, such as diet and exercise.

"If you have a siesta, it conveys a benefit against coronary mortality, which is considerable," said senior author Dr. Dimitrios Trichopoulos, a professor of cancer prevention and epidemiology at the Harvard School of Public Health. "For those of you accustomed to having a siesta—keep doing it. For the rest, wait to see additional studies, and if they confirm these findings, then you may really have to consider changing your lifestyle."

THE STUDY

For the study, Trichopoulos's team collected data on 23,681 people in Greece. At the beginning of the study, none had a history of heart disease, stroke or cancer. The researchers followed these people for an average of 6.3 years.

They found that people who regularly took a midday nap at least three times a week for an average of at least 30 minutes had a 37% lower risk of dying from heart disease, compared with people who didn't nap.

People who napped occasionally had a nonsignificant 12% reduction in their risk of dying from heart disease.

The apparent protective effect of siestas was particularly strong among men who worked, and was weaker among men who didn't, mainly retirees. The data in this study couldn't determine whether women had the same benefit from a nap.

Trichopoulos believes that naps are a way to relieve stress. "We know there are all sorts of physiological phenomena associated with sleep," he said. "But because sleep is such an important factor for cardiac mortality, it might have a simple stress-relieving impact."

FURTHER RESEARCH NEEDED

Dr. Gregg C. Fonarow, a professor of cardiology at the University of California, Los Angeles, comments that factors other than the siesta may be the reason for the lower rates of death from heart disease.

"Before siestas could be recommended as a means of lowering cardiovascular risk, these findings would need to be confirmed in a large-scale, randomized, controlled trial," Fonarow said. "Individuals wanting to lower their cardiovascular risk should stick to what has been proven to be effective: Don't smoke, get regular exercise, and maintain healthy blood pressure, weight, and cholesterol levels."

info For more on how to alleviate causes of heart disease such as stress, visit the Web site of the American Psychological Association, *www.apa.org.*

Read This Before Saying 'Yes' to Bypass Surgery, Angioplasty or Stents

Michael D. Ozner, MD, a clinical assistant professor of medicine at University of Miami School of Medicine, medical director of the Cardiovascular Prevention Institute of South Florida and medical director of Wellness and Prevention at Baptist Health South Florida, all in Miami-Dade County. He is chairman of the American Heart Association of Miami and author of *The Miami Mediterranean Diet: Lose Weight and Lower Your Risk of Heart Disease.* Cambridge House. *www.cardiacoz.com.*

About 1.6 million Americans undergo heart bypass surgery, angioplasty or stent procedures annually—even though there's no evidence that these procedures prolong life or prevent future heart attacks in the majority of patients.

The three-year survival rate for most patients who have had bypass surgery is almost exactly the same as it is for patients with heart disease who don't have surgery.

Good news: With medications and lifestyle changes, the vast majority of patients with heart disease can reduce the risk of a future heart attack by up to 80%—without undergoing expensive and risky procedures.

FLAWED APPROACH

More than half a million Americans die each year from heart disease. The majority suffer from coronary artery disease (CAD). This is caused by atherosclerosis, a condition in which a buildup of fatty deposits (called plaque) in the coronary arteries causes blockages that restrict blood flow to the heart. The plaque may rupture and result in a blood clot in the artery, which can shut off the blood supply and lead to a sudden heart attack.

Many doctors view CAD primarily as a plumbing problem. When imaging tests reveal blockages in the arteries, their first instinct is to clear out the "gunk," whether or not a patient is experiencing troublesome symptoms.

This approach is often flawed. Most bypass and stent procedures are the equivalent of cosmetic cardiology. They make blood vessels appear healthy but do little to reduce heart attack risk. In fact, most heart attacks are caused by tiny blockages that can be hard to detect—and these blockages often are not in the blood vessels that triggered all the concern in the first place.

Surgical procedures are risky. The mortality rate from bypass surgery ranges from 3% to 5%. More than 50% of patients may experience cognitive difficulties after surgery, and patients who have bypass surgery are nearly four times more likely to suffer a subsequent stroke. Those are poor odds for procedures that don't necessarily prolong life or make patients healthier.

MEDICAL BYPASS

Some patients—those with unstable CAD—do require intervention, such as bypass surgery or a stent procedure.

Example: A person with critical blockages in multiple coronary arteries and a weak heart muscle.

Most patients with CAD, however, are stable and unlikely to benefit from a bypass or stent. They are the best candidates for what might be called a *medical bypass.* With medications and lifestyle changes, most of these patients can eliminate symptoms (if any) and reduce heart attack risk. Only in rare cases, if symptoms get worse, would one of these patients need to consider medical intervention.

One key factor in cardiovascular health is to have an ongoing relationship with your doctor —he/she can advise you on the best steps to take to prevent and treat heart disease. *He may recommend that you…*

•**Follow a Mediterranean-style diet.** Eat lots of fruits, vegetables, whole grains and legumes…olive oil instead of butter or margarine …several servings of fish weekly…and no more than a few weekly servings of lean meats.

The landmark Lyon Diet Heart Study, which followed more than 600 participants for almost four years, showed that people who ate a Mediterranean diet instead of a typical American diet had a 50% to 70% reduction in recurrent cardiovascular disease.

•**Relax with yoga,** meditation, exercise, etc. Doctors don't always ask patients about stress—which is why it is sometimes called the "forgotten" risk factor for heart disease. People who successfully manage stress can significantly lower blood pressure and the risk of heart disease. Stress management also lowers the risk for arrhythmias (heart rate irregularities).

•**Exercise daily for 30 to 45 minutes.** It is one of the best ways to maintain a healthy weight and prevent or control diabetes and high blood pressure. Regular exercise raises levels of HDL "good" cholesterol. It also can contribute to weight control—which can reduce inflammation in the blood vessels, a risk factor for CAD.

All forms of exercise are beneficial. Aerobic exercise, such as brisk walking, is the best choice for most people because it doesn't require a high level of fitness to do it.

•**Get your cholesterol checked**—and take cholesterol-lowering medication if necessary. Everyone should have a blood test for cholesterol annually. Research indicates that aggressive lowering of LDL cholesterol helps reduce risk of heart disease and death from CAD.

Bonus: Cholesterol-lowering statin drugs also reduce inflammation in the blood vessels.

•**Take a baby aspirin daily.** It helps prevent platelets from clumping together and forming clots that can block blood flow to the heart. The anti-inflammatory effects of aspirin are also beneficial. Since aspirin may cause gastrointestinal upset and/or bleeding, talk with your doctor before initiating aspirin therapy for CAD prevention.

•**See your dentist twice a year.** Studies have shown that patients with periodontal disease —gum inflammation that can result in tooth loss—have a higher risk of heart attack and stroke than those without it.

•**Get more omega-3s.** Most Americans are deficient in omega-3 fatty acids. Omega-3s lower inflammation and triglycerides, a fat that can put you at risk for heart disease. Omega-3s reduce the risk of arrhythmias and heart attack. Sources of omega-3s include cold-water fish, such as salmon, and plant sources, such as walnuts and flaxseed. Or ask your doctor about taking a fish oil supplement.

Double Dose of Clot-Buster Cuts Heart Problems in Half!

Gregory Dehmer, MD, professor of medicine, Texas A&M College of Medicine, Temple.

Marc S. Sabatine, associate professor, Brigham and Women's Hospital, cardiovascular division, Boston.

Society for Cardiovascular Angiography and Interventions.

Cardiologists should give more than the recommended dosage of the clot-preventing drug *Plavix* before performing angioplasty.

THE STUDY

The analysis of 10 previous studies found that giving angioplasty patients double the current recommended dose of Plavix—600 milligrams rather than 300—cuts the combined risk of heart attack and cardiac death by half, according to Dr. Anthony Abbate, an assistant professor of medicine at Virginia Commonwealth University.

The 10 studies analyzed by Abbate and Dr. Giuseppe G. Biondi-Zoccai, assistant professor of cardiology at the University of Turin in Italy, included 1,500 patients who had angioplasty. Most had either 300 milligrams or 600 milligrams of Plavix before the procedure.

The incidence of cardiac death or nonfatal heart attack was 50% lower in the following 30 days in those getting the higher dose of Plavix. Only 3.1% of those getting the 600-milligram dose had in-hospital heart attacks, compared with 6.4% of those getting the 300-milligram dose. The overall 30-day incidence of death or heart attack was 3.8% for the higher dose and 7.3% for the lower dose.

IMPLICATIONS

"The evidence shown by this meta-analysis is very strong," said Dr. Gregory Dehmer, past president of the Society for Cardiovascular Angiography and Interventions and a professor of medicine at Texas A&M College of Medicine. "Although Plavix is powerful stuff, the meta-analysis did not find an excessive amount of bleeding. So we have a lower risk of myocardial infarction [heart attack] with no significant increase in adverse side effects."

"This research has important clinical and cost implications," Biondi-Zoccai added.

AHA GUIDELINES

Current guidelines by the American Heart Association, the American College of Cardiology and the Society for Cardiovascular Angiography and Interventions say that physicians should strongly consider giving 300 milligrams of Plavix before angioplasty, a medical procedure to open narrowed or blocked blood vessels of the heart.

"Those guidelines are in the process of being updated," Dehmer said, adding that new guidelines are expected in the next few months.

"In practical terms, many practitioners are concerned about the current recommendations," Dehmer said. "One concern is that should the patient require elective bypass surgery, does a higher dose of *clopidogrel* [the generic name of Plavix] increase the risk of excessive bleeding?

"This bleeding risk is addressed in this meta-analysis, which shows very minimal potential downside," he added.

FUTURE PLANS

But the final word is not in yet, according to Dr. Marc S. Sabatine, associate professor in the cardiovascular division of Brigham and Women's Hospital in Boston. That will come from a major international study, to include up to 14,000 angioplasty patients, which is still enrolling participants.

Timing also plays a role in treatment, he noted. Plavix must be activated in the liver, which takes about six hours, so giving it earlier makes it more effective.

"But even with those side considerations, many laboratories are considering switching to 600 milligrams," Sabatine said.

Drink Tea or Milk— Just Not Together!

Verena Stangl, MD, professor of cardiology, Charite Hospital, Universitatsmedizin-Berlin, Campus Mitte, Germany. *European Heart Journal.*

Plenty of studies have suggested that tea is a boon for cardiovascular health, but new research has found that adding milk to your favorite brew negates those benefits.

BACKGROUND

"There are a lot of studies that show that tea is protective against cardiac diseases," said lead researcher Dr. Verena Stangl, professor of cardiology at the Charite Hospital, Universitatsmedizin-Berlin, in Germany. "If you look at the studies, you see that in Asia there are less cardiac diseases, but in England that's not the case. So the question is, is the addition of milk a reason for this difference between Asia and England, where tea is often taken with milk?" she said.

THE STUDY

Sixteen healthy postmenopausal women drank either half a liter of freshly brewed black tea, black tea with skimmed milk or boiled water on three different occasions under similar conditions. The researchers then measured the

189

function of the cells lining the brachial artery in the forearm, using high-resolution ultrasound before—and two hours after—tea consumption.

Stangl's team found that black tea significantly improved the ability of the arteries to relax and expand. "But when we added milk, we found the biological effect of tea was completely abolished," she said.

Additional experiments on rat aortas and rat endothelial cells—which line blood vessels—also found that tea relaxed the vessels. But adding milk blunted the effect.

The culprit in milk is a group of proteins called caseins, which interact with tea, decreasing its concentration of catechins. Catechins are flavonoids that are responsible for tea's protective effects against heart disease, according to the study authors.

ADVICE

"If you want to drink tea for its health effects, don't drink it with milk," Stangl said. Stangl noted that milk also destroys the antioxidant effects of tea and perhaps its cancer-protective effects as well.

info For more medical news on heart and health, visit *www.news-medical.net*.

■ ■ ■ ■

Not Enough Sleep Increases Hypertension Risk

People who slept an average of five or fewer hours per night were more than twice as likely to be diagnosed with hypertension over a 10-year follow-up period as people who averaged more than five hours a night. Blood pressure drops an average of 10% to 20% during sleep, so less sleep exposes the cardiovascular system to additional stress, which over time can raise blood pressure and lead to hypertension.

Best: Try to get seven to nine hours of sleep per night by allowing adequate time in bed…maintaining bedtimes…having a comfortable sleep environment…avoiding alcohol and caffeine before sleep…and exercising regularly but not too close to bedtime.

James Gangwisch, PhD, assistant professor, department of psychiatry, Columbia University, New York City, and lead author of a study of 4,810 people, published in *Hypertension*.

Surprising Heart Health Facts That Could Save Your Life!

Barry L. Zaret, MD, Robert W. Berliner Professor of Medicine and professor of radiology at Yale University School of Medicine in New Haven, CT. He served as chief of the section of cardiology at Yale from 1978 to 2004. He is coauthor of *Heart Care for Life*. Yale University Press.

One out of every five Americans has some form of heart disease. Literally millions of cases could be prevented if people had better information about the best prevention and treatment strategies.

Despite the abundance of health information reported in the media, many people are endangering their health because they are still ill-informed about key aspects of heart disease. Barry L. Zaret, MD, one of the country's leading specialists in cardiovascular health, clears up five misconceptions.

Misconception 1: High cholesterol is the main risk factor for heart attack.

Fact: While high cholesterol does increase risk, recent studies show that elevated levels (3 mg per liter or higher) of *C-reactive protein* (CRP), a protein that circulates in the bloodstream, may have an even stronger link than high cholesterol to heart attack and stroke.

Everyone has at least a small amount of CRP in the bloodstream. At higher levels, it indicates the presence of inflammation—possibly caused by an underlying bacterial or viral infection that may damage the linings of blood vessels and promote the development of atherosclerosis.

Every patient with a high risk for cardiovascular disease—smokers and/or those with a family history of heart disease, for example—should have a high-sensitivity CRP blood test. This test, unlike the standard CRP test, distinguishes between inflammation due to cardiovascular disease and other inflammatory conditions, such as arthritis. The high-sensitivity CRP test is particularly important for patients who have had a previous heart attack or who have unstable angina (chest pain caused by lack of blood to the heart). An elevated CRP level in these patients indicates a very high risk for heart attack—even if cholesterol levels are normal.

Misconception 2: All adults should take a daily aspirin.

Fact: Daily aspirin therapy is often recommended for patients who have an elevated heart disease risk due to family history, smoking, obesity, diabetes and atherosclerosis. Studies show that it can curb heart attack risk in *men* by more than 40%.

For women, the evidence is less clear. New research indicates that women who take aspirin are more likely to experience gastrointestinal upset or bleeding problems than men. Although research shows that in women age 46 or older aspirin protects against stroke, it does not reduce heart attack risk in all of these women. Aspirin has been shown to lower heart attack risk only in women age 65 or older, whether or not they have risk factors for the disease. Women of any age who smoke or have a family history of heart disease or other risk factors may benefit from aspirin therapy. The standard recommendation for women is 81 mg daily.

There's no evidence to suggest that aspirin helps prevent a heart attack in healthy women who are under age 65. For these women, not smoking, controlling body weight, getting regular exercise and maintaining a healthful diet are the best ways to guard against the development of heart disease.

This also is true for men age 64 and younger who are healthy and have no risk factors for heart disease. However, men age 65 or older, even if healthy, should take 81 mg of aspirin daily to protect against heart disease.

Misconception 3: The greatest danger of smoking is lung cancer.

Fact: Lung cancer is obviously a concern for smokers, but the risk for cardiovascular disease is actually higher. Of the approximately 440,000 premature deaths caused annually by smoking, the majority are due to cardiovascular disease, according to the Centers for Disease Control and Prevention.

Smoking increases levels of carbon monoxide in the blood, which damages artery linings and promotes atherosclerosis. It appears to lower HDL "good" cholesterol and increase blood levels of *fibrinogen*, a substance in the blood that promotes clotting.

Good news: One year after quitting, the risk for heart disease drops to one-half that of current smokers—and within 15 years becomes about the same as for someone who never smoked.

Misconception 4: Exercise is dangerous if you've already had a heart attack.

Fact: Heart attack patients especially benefit from regular exercise. An analysis of 22 different studies that followed more than 4,000 patients for three years found that the death rate among patients who participated in a cardiac rehabilitation program that included exercise was 20% to 25% lower than among those who didn't exercise.

Heart patients who exercise have increased endurance, fewer chest or leg pains and improved heart function. Regular exercise also lowers blood pressure, raises HDL cholesterol and lowers resting heart rate.

Patients who have heart disease or have had a heart attack, or those who have been sedentary, should get a thorough checkup before starting an exercise program. This should include a treadmill stress test, which evaluates blood flow to the heart. Once your doctor determines that it's safe to exercise, aim for 30 minutes at least three to five days a week. Aerobic exercise—fast walking, swimming, etc.—provides the most benefits for heart patients. If you've had a heart attack or other cardiac event, start your exercise routine at a rehabilitation center, if possible. Ask your cardiologist to recommend one near you.

Misconception 5: Reports saying that chocolate is good for the heart are mostly hype.

Fact: The cocoa beans used to make chocolate are extremely rich in flavonoids, plant compounds that appear to relax small blood vessels and lower blood pressure. Some of the flavonoids in cocoa also appear to inhibit the ability of platelets to form clots in the arteries.

Harvard researchers recently studied residents of Kuna (an island off Panama), who drink an average of three to four cups of cocoa a day. (They consume even more cocoa in other foods.) Hypertension among these people is almost nonexistent—until they leave the island

and forgo their cocoa-rich diet. At that point, their rates of hypertension and heart disease rise.

Of course, there is a downside. The high levels of fat and sugar in chocolate can lead to obesity and elevated blood sugar. But one to two small squares daily of dark chocolate that's at least 70% cocoa and low in added sugar does appear to be good for the heart.

Baby Boomer Time Bomb Strikes Without Warning

David Tilson, MD, the Ailsa Mellon Bruce Professor of Surgery at Columbia University and director emeritus of the department of surgery at St. Luke's Roosevelt Hospital Center, both in New York City. He was chairman of a recent international conference on abdominal aortic aneurysm in New York City. He maintains an aneurysm information Web site, *www.columbia.edu/~mdt1.*

Until recently, hypertension, diabetes and other chronic conditions have been identified as America's biggest health threats.

Now: As the baby boomer population ages, abdominal aortic aneurysm (AAA), a potentially far more serious condition, appears to be on the rise.

An aneurysm is a bulge in a blood vessel wall. Some aneurysms affect blood vessels in the brain. Others occur in the aorta, the main artery of the body. About the diameter of a garden hose, the aorta travels from the heart through the chest and abdomen, then forms separate branches that enter the legs. Aortic aneurysms usually form in the abdominal cavity—the artery walls may be weaker in this area.

Surgeons can repair AAAs before they rupture —if they are identified. An AAA can be discovered during tests, such as X-rays or computed tomography (CT) scans, for other conditions. But what makes an AAA so deadly is that it usually is not identified and typically causes no symptoms prior to rupturing.

Caution: If you have symptoms of an AAA— abdominal or back pain, along with a pulsating mass in the abdomen—seek immediate medical attention.

A SILENT THREAT

Most AAAs grow slowly—about 3 millimeters (mm) to 4 mm (about one-eighth inch) per year. A person can have an AAA for decades before it becomes large enough to rupture—if it ever does. Even when doctors detect an AAA, they're unlikely to recommend surgery if the aneurysm is smaller than 5 centimeters (cm)—about two inches—in diameter.

Warning: AAA patients must be closely monitored with imaging tests for the rest of their lives because the risk of dying from a rupture is so high. An AAA that's 5 cm or larger—or that's growing more than 1 cm a year—has a significant risk of rupturing and needs to be surgically repaired.

CAUSES OF AAA

AAAs have some of the same risk factors as those for atherosclerosis, the accumulation of fatty deposits (plaque) that weaken artery walls. The same measures that doctors recommend to prevent heart attacks—not smoking, controlling hypertension and cholesterol, for example— also can help prevent AAAs.

Some patients, particularly those with Marfan's syndrome (a genetic condition that's characterized by extreme height), are born with a weakness in the aorta wall. In rare cases, infection or inflammation (vasculitis) in a blood vessel can predispose patients to AAA.

For small or slow-growing AAAs, "watchful waiting" is usually best. Patients are advised to have ultrasound screenings every six months to determine whether the AAA is getting large enough or expanding fast enough to rupture.

Caution: Patients with high-risk AAAs should avoid heavy lifting and intense aerobic exercises. These activities can cause surges in blood pressure that can increase the risk for a rupture.

Researchers have investigated the use of medications—for example, beta-blockers, such as *propranolol* (Inderal), and tetracycline antibiotics—to slow the growth of AAAs. The results have been disappointing. New drugs are being investigated, but surgery is currently the best option.

NEW TREATMENT STRATEGIES

Surgery to repair an AAA involves opening the abdomen, removing the damaged section of artery and replacing it with a synthetic graft.

Newer approach: A procedure known as endovascular surgery involves the insertion of a catheter into an artery in the leg. The surgeon threads the catheter upward into the damaged section of artery. Once the catheter is in place, it's used to insert and fasten a metal-covered mesh tube (stent) that reinforces the blood vessel.

The initial success rate of both procedures—open surgery and endovascular repair—has been determined to be about 96% to 98%, respectively. However, patients who undergo an endovascular procedure spend less time in the hospital and recover more quickly.

Recent finding: A study of 28,000 Medicare patients, published in the *Journal of Vascular Surgery*, found that the risk for death with endovascular procedures was 1.9%, compared with 5.2% for conventional surgery. It's still not known, however, whether the stent-grafts used in endovascular repair are as durable as the repairs performed in conventional surgery.

Guidelines…

• **Relatively young, healthy AAA patients** are generally advised to have conventional surgery. These patients are typically better able to withstand the operation, and the hand-sewn repair might last longer than an endovascular graft.

• **Older patients** who may not be healthy enough to withstand conventional surgery—and who have a shorter life expectancy—will probably benefit more from an endovascular procedure.

REGULAR SCREENING

Because an AAA rarely causes symptoms but is so deadly, anyone with risk factors—men who are current or former smokers or are age 65 or older…and men and women who are age 65 or older and have a first-degree relative (parent, sibling or child) with an AAA—should undergo an ultrasound test to detect changes in the artery wall. If you have a family history of AAA in one or more relatives who was diagnosed with an AAA under the age of 65, then you should be screened at a younger age.

An initial ultrasound at age 65 for people with any of the above risk factors is recommended. Cardiovascular risk factors, such as elevated blood pressure and/or cholesterol, also may be considered. Patients with no signs of disease at this age don't require additional tests.

Exception: Patients with a family history of AAAs should be retested every five years. Their risk is at least three times higher than that of someone without a family history.

Medicare and most other health insurers will pay for ultrasound screening in patients age 65 and older who have AAA risk factors.

■ ■ ■ ■

Simple Blood Test Can Predict Heart Attack Risk

The test measures blood levels of the protein *NT-proBNP*—a marker of BNP, a hormone that goes up during cardiac stress. The higher the level of this protein, the greater a person's risk of complications. The test is used in hospitals to diagnose heart failure among patients with difficulty breathing. This test should not be part of routine checkups, but it can be helpful to cardiologists trying to determine which patients with known cardiac disease need aggressive treatment.

Kirsten Bibbins-Domingo, MD, is assistant professor in residence of medicine, epidemiology and biostatistics, University of California, San Francisco, and coauthor of a study of 987 heart disease patients, published in *The Journal of the American Medical Association.*

Do You Have a Faulty Heart Valve?

Robert O. Bonow, MD, the Goldberg Distinguished Professor of Cardiology at Northwestern University Feinberg School of Medicine and chief of the division of cardiology at Northwestern Memorial Hospital, both in Chicago. Dr. Bonow is the lead author of the *American College of Cardiology/American Heart Association 2006 Guidelines for the Management of Patients with Valvular Heart Disease.*

About 20 million Americans have at least one dysfunctional heart valve, caused by either a congenital defect or other factors, such as age, high blood pressure (hypertension), coronary artery disease or a previous heart attack.

Until recently, treatment for a person with valvular heart disease depended largely on his/her cardiologist's personal preferences. This lack of standardized care increased a patient's odds of undergoing an operation either earlier or later than necessary or even suffering a preventable death.

Now: Consistent clinical evidence and a consensus among medical experts regarding valvular heart disease have resulted in new treatment guidelines from the American College of Cardiology (ACC) and the American Heart Association (AHA).

WHAT IS VALVULAR HEART DISEASE?

Blood flow through the heart is regulated by four heart valves (mitral, aortic, tricuspid and pulmonic). Mitral valve prolapse (MVP), in which the two leaflets (flaps) of the mitral valve don't close properly, affects about 2% to 5% of adults. MVP typically requires no treatment, except for the use of antibiotics to prevent a potentially fatal valve infection (endocarditis) before certain dental procedures and surgeries.

Many Americans are affected by a complication of valvular disease, known as regurgitation, in which the valves fail to close completely, allowing blood to leak backward through the valve.

In many other people with valvular heart disease, one of the valves stiffens and narrows, compromising blood flow. This condition is called stenosis and has several possible causes. Among people age 60 or older, a common cause is the accumulation of calcium deposits in the aortic valve.

To diagnose valvular heart disease, a doctor will perform a physical exam and review the patient's medical history. He may order one or more tests, such as an ultrasound of the heart, also known as an echocardiogram...a chest X-ray...or an electrocardiogram (ECG), which records the electrical activity of the heart.

Both valvular regurgitation and stenosis force the heart to work harder to pump blood. Medication can't correct valve function. If a valve is severely diseased or damaged, surgery to repair or replace it may be necessary.

Key recommendations from the new ACC/AHA guidelines...

• **Make sure that you receive an echocardiogram.** Doctors typically use a stethoscope to detect valvular heart disease—the abnormal blood flow causes a murmur. However, it's often difficult to distinguish between benign and disease-related murmurs with a stethoscope alone. Without an echocardiogram, it's impossible to gauge the severity of any valve dysfunction.

•**Get a precise diagnosis.** An echocardiogram and other quantifiable data, such as a chest X-ray or ECG, should be used in the diagnosis of valvular heart disease to identify its severity. The diagnosis should characterize the valve problem as mild, moderate or severe.

•**Consider surgery.** Valve disease can be fairly advanced before a patient notices any symptoms...and with today's minimally invasive repair/replacement techniques, surgery is often less risky than waiting for heart damage or heart failure to develop.

Important: Unless you're facing emergency surgery (which rarely occurs in patients with valvular disease), always get a second opinion before undergoing valve repair or replacement.

•**Ask your doctor whether mitral valve repair rather than valve replacement is an option.** Evidence shows that repair leads to better heart function and a greater chance of survival.

Important: Before consenting to mitral valve replacement, consult a cardiologist who specializes in valve repair. Ask your doctor to refer you to a hospital or surgical center where doctors are known to have a successful record of performing the procedure.

It's well established that people who undergo valve repair instead of replacement have a much lower risk of dying within 30 days of the surgery, have a much better quality of life and don't have to worry about the long-term risks of an artificial valve.

•**Talk to your doctor about mechanical and biological replacement valves.** Most mitral valves can be repaired, but diseased aortic valves typically need to be replaced. Patients have two options—a biological valve (from a human cadaver or pig or cow tissue) or a mechanical valve.

Mechanical valves can last a lifetime, but they also heighten the risk for blood clots. That's why anyone who receives a mechanical valve must take an anticoagulant, such as *warfarin* (Coumadin), for the rest of his life.

Biological valves don't pose a clot risk, but they do degrade over time and may eventually need replacing. For this reason, patients younger than age 65 requiring an aortic valve or younger than age 70 requiring a mitral valve were automatically given a mechanical replacement in the past to avoid a second surgery.

Now clinical evidence has shown that the newer biological valves can last much longer than the previous generation of biological valves. If a biological valve is inserted into a 55-year-old, there's a 75% chance that the valve will still be functioning well in 20 years.

In addition, improved surgical techniques have made the possibility of a second operation in 20 years less risky, in many cases, than daily anticoagulant therapy, which poses the constant danger of bleeding. Therefore, a biological valve may be the better choice, especially if you're age 55 or older.

■ ■ ■ ■

Symptoms of Heart-Valve Disease

Many patients with valve disease experience no outward symptoms, but some notice…

- **Shortness of breath** during physical activity and/or while lying flat.
- **Weakness or dizziness.**
- **A feeling of weight or pressure in the chest** during activity or when breathing cold air.
- **Heart palpitations** (racing or fluttering).
- **Swelling in the ankles,** feet or abdomen.

The High Cost of Cholesterol-Lowering Drugs

University of Michigan.
Circulation.

Higher doses of cholesterol-lowering statins can benefit patients who have had a recent heart attack or hospital stay for chest pain, also known as acute coronary syndrome, but may not be particularly cost-effective for all heart patients.

THE STUDY

A team from the University of Michigan Cardiovascular Center and the VA Ann Arbor Healthcare System performed a computer analysis of data from thousands of heart patients. They found that some patients with a recent history of acute coronary syndrome got more than four additional quality-adjusted months of life from receiving higher and more expensive doses of statins.

But this may not be the case for other patients with stable coronary artery disease who have narrowed arteries but haven't recently been hospitalized for heart attack or chest pain. For these patients, the usual statin dose may provide adequate heart protection. Higher doses for more stable heart patients may offer only marginal benefit—only about five weeks of quality-adjusted life.

info For more information, visit the Web site of the American Heart Association, *www. americanheart.org/cholesterol.*

New Drug Fails to Improve Odds for Heart Failure Patients

Robert Hobbs, MD, cardiologist, Cleveland Clinic.
Journal of the American Medical Association.

A new drug is no more effective at improving the survival rates of people with heart failure than an older, widely used medication, says a recent international study.

THE STUDY

There were hopes that the new drug, *levosimendan*, would improve survival because it uses a special mechanism that makes heart muscle cells more sensitive to the calcium that causes them to contract.

However, the study of 1,347 people with acute decompensated heart failure, done at 75 centers in nine countries, found essentially the same death rate for participants who got levosimendan as those who received an established medication, *dobutamine*.

"The trial leaves cardiologists without a totally satisfactory treatment for decompensated heart failure," said Dr. Robert Hobbs, a Cleveland cardiologist specializing in treatment of the condition. Some five million Americans have one form or another of heart failure, and about one million of them are hospitalized for it each year.

Decompensated heart failure is one form of the general condition in which the heart progressively loses the ability to pump blood. It is characterized by a set of symptoms including shortness of breath and intolerance to exercise.

BACKGROUND

"The original therapy, which is still basic, is diuretics," Hobbs explained. "They make the body lose water, so people feel better. In the 1980s, ACE inhibitors came along to make people feel better and live longer, and they were added for long-term benefit. The third group of drugs to be used were beta-blockers."

Dobutamine is a beta-blocker that has been found to improve symptoms, but it has also been associated with an increased risk of death and cardiovascular problems. In the latest trial, participants with decompensated heart failure received levosimendan or dobutamine intravenously.

"The common practice has been to give dobutamine in the belief that the heart is like a battery that has lost its charge," Hobbs said. "By giving dobutamine, you would recharge it. That didn't actually happen [in previous studies]. It appeared to be associated with complications, longer hospital stays and more mortality."

In another study, careful analysis indicated that levosimendan was associated with a lower risk of death than dobutamine. "It did have the different mechanism of action, and it was felt that might translate into improved safety," Hobbs said. "But it proved to be no better in the new trial."

In the 180 days after drug infusion, the death rate was 26% among patients who got levosimendan and 28% in those getting dobutamine. There was no important difference in reported breathing difficulties and in time spent out of the hospital.

Participants who got levosimendan were less likely to experience cardiac failure but they were more likely to experience the abnormal heartbeat called atrial fibrillation, low blood levels of potassium and headache.

"The bottom line on all of this is that it is hard to show benefit for what we do for acute decompensated heart failure," Hobbs said.

Patch That Saves Heart Patients from Dangerous Surgery

Matthew W. Martinez, MD, cardiology fellow, Mayo Clinic, Rochester, MN.

Robert Beekman III, MD, codirector, heart center, Cincinnati Children's Hospital Medical Center.

Society for Cardiovascular Angiography and Interventions.

Emergency use of a patching device can help patients avoid high-risk surgery when a heart attack results in a hole between the ventricles, which are the major blood-pumping chambers of the heart, researchers report.

"These patients are often too ill to go to surgery," explained Dr. Matthew W. Martinez, a cardiology fellow at the Mayo Clinic in Rochester, Minnesota. "What we are doing is bridging these people so that they become stable enough to survive surgery."

These types of dangerous cardiac tears, called a "ventricular septal defect," are fortunately rare and occur in less than 1% of heart attacks, according to Martinez. However, drug treatment leaves patients with a 90% risk of death, while surgery carries a 50% death rate, so any alternative is welcome.

THE STUDY

Martinez studied 10 patients whose ventricular septal defects were treated at the Mayo Clinic with the patching device between 1995 and 2005. The device effectively closed the holes completely in 8 of the 10 cases.

The device is threaded in collapsed form into the heart by a catheter and is opened at the site of the rupture in the ventricle walls. It is made of flexible nitinol metal and covered with a polyester fabric. New heart tissue can grow on this fabric, repairing the hole permanently.

Unless something is done to close the hole, blood shoots backward from the left to the right ventricle—rather than into the body—with each heartbeat causing severe heart failure. The procedures done for the adult heart attack patients at the Mayo Clinic were all successful, Martinez said, although one patient died five days later of an illness unrelated to the ventricular septal defect patch.

FUTURE PLANS

According to Dr. Robert Beekman III, co-director of the heart center at Cincinnati Children's Hospital Medical Center, a version of this device is now the standard of care for a related heart problem called "atrial septal defects"—holes between the two upper chambers of the heart that can appear at birth. Beekman has implanted such devices in hundreds of children with congenital heart defects.

"However, ventricular septal defects are very different heart problems," Beekman said. "There is a lot more morbidity and complications [with the ventricular problem] than with atrial septal defect closure, so it is taking a lot more time for the Food and Drug Administration to approve it.

info For more information about septal defects and their treatment, visit the Nemours Foundation Web site at *www.kidshealth.org.*

Elderly Patients Missing Lifesaving Care

David J. Cohen, MD, director, cardiovascular research, Saint Luke's Mid-America Heart Institute, Kansas City, MO.

American College of Cardiology.

Patients aged 90 and older suffering from angina or heart attack are less likely than younger patients to receive recommended medical treatments in hospital emergency rooms—even though older patients are more likely to survive if they do receive the treatments.

"Having an acute coronary syndrome, even over the age of 90, is not as dire as it once was. With optimal medical therapy and invasive care, the outcomes were nearly as good as in a somewhat younger group of patients," said study author Dr. David J. Cohen, director of cardiovascular research at Saint Luke's Mid-America Heart Institute in Kansas City, Missouri.

BACKGROUND

Acute coronary syndrome is often caused by a blood clot that temporarily or partially blocks the coronary artery.

Recommended therapies include aspirin to prevent clotting; a blood thinner called *heparin* that also prevents clotting; and beta-blocker drugs that slow the heart rate, reduce the force of the heart's contraction, and prevent rhythm abnormalities. The guidelines also recommend that high-risk patients receive cardiac catheterization within 48 hours, along with drugs called *glycoprotein IIb/IIIa inhibitors* to prevent clotting during or after cardiac catheterization.

THE STUDY

Researchers analyzed data from a national study on almost 52,000 patients age 75 and older, with acute coronary syndrome. More than 5,500 were at least 90 years old, and 112 were at least 100 years old.

Age was a major factor in the use of recommended therapies. For example, cardiac catheterization was considered inadvisable in almost 60% of patients age 90 and older, compared with 27% of patients age 75 to 89.

IMPLICATIONS

Cohen noted that the national study found the risk of major bleeding increases with the more therapies that are used to treat acute coronary syndrome—from a 3.5% risk with one treatment to a 17.3% risk with five treatments.

"We shouldn't simply, on the basis of age, say a person is too high risk (for treatment). We should discuss these therapies with patients and their families," Cohen said.

However, patients who receive more therapies—particularly aspirin, beta-blockers and cardiac catheterization—have a better chance of survival.

Women: Know the Signs of 'Broken Heart Syndrome'

Society for Cardiovascular Angiography and Interventions.

Takotsubo cardiomyopathy, or broken heart syndrome, is a rare, life-threatening condition. It's called broken heart syndrome because some form of emotional or physical distress often precedes it. The actual cause of the condition, which almost always strikes women, is unknown. The condition was originally diagnosed in Japan and has been seen in the US only in recent years.

Patients are usually critically ill during the first 48 hours, and it often appears that they're having a heart attack. However, there is no sign of coronary artery blockage.

A BETTER WAY

"These patients can be difficult to manage. They may be in cardiac arrest, cardiogenic shock, or severe heart failure. They may require advanced life support with airway management and mediations to support blood pressure," said Brown University cardiology fellow Dr. Richard Regnante.

A registry developed by Regnante and colleagues at Brown University in Providence, Rhode Island, currently includes 40 patients diagnosed with Takotsubo cardiomyopathy at two major Rhode Island hospitals over a span of 2½ years. Of those patients, 95% were women, and 60% experienced a stressful event—ranging from armed robbery to a major argument, tooth extraction, or preparation for colonoscopy—before they went to a hospital emergency room for treatment of broken heart syndrome.

SYMPTOMS

The most common symptom among the patients was chest pain (70%), followed by shortness of breath (33%). All patients showed electrocardiographic (ECG) changes suggestive of an acute coronary syndrome, a term that encompasses both heart attack and unstable angina.

The registry data also show that a blood test for heart damage was positive in 95% of the patients. Cardiac catheterization detected heart motion abnormalities in all the patients. One patient died of acute heart failure.

Most patients who survived the first 48 hours experienced steady recovery, and heart function was found to be normal in 29 of the 30 patients who had follow-up echocardiography within a few weeks.

"We don't know why some women develop this syndrome after what appears to be minimal stress, while other women experience severely stressful events but don't develop Takotsubo cardiomyopathy," Regnante said.

It's likely that a surge of stress hormones is a factor. It's also possible that a blood clot temporarily blocks a major artery but then dissolves before doctors can detect it.

REGISTRY HELPFUL

Whatever the causes, researchers say this national registry will help doctors more easily recognize and treat this rare, life-threatening condition.

info Contact Johns Hopkins Medicine to learn more about broken heart syndrome, *www.hopkinsmedicine.org.*

Implanted Pumps May Help End-Stage Heart Failure Cases

American Heart Association.
Foundation for the Advancement of Cardiac Therapy.

Implantable heart pumps can improve heart function in some end-stage heart failure patients awaiting transplant, and enable them to be discharged from the hospital without undergoing a transplant of a new heart, a new study suggests.

In end-stage heart failure, the heart weakens, grows larger, and shows other signs of deterioration. Implantable left ventricular assist devices

(LVADs) pump blood through the body and allow the heart's main pumping chamber to rest.

This multicenter study included 67 end-stage heart failure patients who had four different types of LVADs. The patients were evaluated every 30 days for several months after they received their LVADs.

FINDINGS

Nine percent of the patients had their LVADs removed without needing a heart transplant, but another 9% died before the end of the data collection period.

"There are two contrasting, important findings in our study," lead researcher Dr. Simon Maybaum, medical director of the Center for Advanced Cardiac Therapy at the Albert Einstein College of Medicine's Montefiore Medical Center stated. "One, the ability to remove an LVAD from a patient with end-stage heart failure was low. Two, there was a high degree of improvement in heart function during the use of the assist device."

The study also found that after 30 days with an LVAD, about one-third of the patients had a left ventricular ejection fraction (percentage of blood pumped out of the left ventricle with one beat) greater than 40%, measured when the pump flow was decreased. Healthy hearts typically have an ejection fraction of 55% to 60%.

However, the percentage of patients with a 40% ejection fraction decreased as the study progressed. There were 27% at 60 days; 19% at 90 days; and 6% at 120 days.

The researchers also measured the patients' exercise capacity after LVAD implantation and found that between 30 days and 120 days, the patients showed improvements in peak oxygen consumption and exercise endurance.

USEFUL FOR FUTURE RESEARCH

"We now have a much more reliable description of the natural history of the changes in heart function during LVAD support. That makes us optimistic that other strategies (such as drug or stem cell therapy) may allow us to further improve cardiac function," Maybaum said.

Depression Linked to Early Heart Disease

Jesse C. Stewart, PhD, psychology department, Indiana University-Purdue University Indianapolis.

Nieca Goldberg, MD, chief, women's cardiac care, Lenox Hill Hospital, New York City, author, *The Women's Healthy Heart Program*, Random House Publishing Group, and spokeswoman, American Heart Association. *Archives of General Psychiatry.*

Depression, especially its physical signs, such as fatigue and loss of appetite, may contribute to thickening arteries, an early sign of cardiovascular disease.

BACKGROUND

Previous research has suggested that negative emotions like anxiety and anger can increase the risk for heart disease. But in the new study, depression—and its physical symptoms—was the emotional linchpin to early signs of heart disease.

"In other studies, anxiety, depression, anger and hostility have all separately been linked to future risk of heart disease," said lead researcher Jesse C. Stewart, a member of the psychology department at Indiana University-Purdue University Indianapolis. But the problem with those studies was that they didn't look at these negative emotions together. And since their symptoms can overlap, it has been hard to tell which emotion plays the most important role in heart disease.

THE STUDY

Stewart's team looked for emotional links to heart disease among 324 men and women with an average age of 60.6 years old. To determine early signs of heart disease, the scientists examined *carotid artery intima-media* thickness, which is a measure of the inner layers of the arteries and is related to early-stage heart disease. Measurements were taken at the start of the study and again three years later.

"We found that mild to moderate depressive symptoms were associated with greater progression of subclinical atherosclerosis (hardening of the arteries)—greater increase of the artery wall," Stewart said. "In contrast, anxiety symptoms, hostility and anger were not at all related to a change in the blood vessel thickness."

What's more, analysis showed that only the physical symptoms of depression predicted the progression of atherosclerosis. And it appears that the symptoms of depression exist before the signs of atherosclerosis.

Stewart isn't sure why depression has this effect. "Depression has been associated with some physiological changes, including in the immune system. These physiological changes probably explain this association," he said.

The study also found that the 5% of study participants taking antidepressants fared better than those with depression who weren't taking the drugs. "They had significantly reduced progression of atherosclerosis," Stewart said.

But, because the sample was so small, it isn't possible to make a definitive statement about the value of *selective serotonin reuptake inhibitors* (SSRIs) in reducing atherosclerosis. "There is intriguing evidence that SSRIs may be associated with reduced progression of atherosclerosis," Stewart said.

IMPLICATIONS

"Identifying the harmful aspects of emotion could lead to the identification of people who are at risk for heart disease due to their tendency to experience negative emotions and who may benefit from psychological and pharmacological intervention," he said. "Identifying these harmful aspects could also lead to the development of more focused and potent interventions."

Dr. Nieca Goldberg, chief of women's cardiac care at Lenox Hill Hospital in New York City, noted that depressed people are less likely to take care of themselves and have more risk factors for heart disease.

"People who are depressed don't adopt a healthy lifestyle," said Goldberg, a spokeswoman for the American Heart Association and author of *The Women's Healthy Heart Program*. "They overeat, smoke more, and may drink more. In addition, people who have depression have platelets that are more likely to clot."

Goldberg thinks doctors should pay closer attention to depression and other psychological factors that can affect patient health. "For too long, the medical system has amputated the head from the rest of the body," she said. "It is important for us to consider the psychological aspects of our patients' lives, because that is an important factor in our care of a patient."

info For more detailed information on the link between depression and heart disease, visit the Web site of the US National Institute of Mental Health, *www.nimh.nih.gov.*

Low-Dose Aspirin Therapy Effective After Heart Surgery

Shamir R. Mehta, MD, associate professor of medicine, McMaster University, Hamilton, Ontario, Canada. American College of Cardiology.

If you've had angioplasty, stenting or other types of heart procedures, low-dose aspirin may be just as effective as higher doses at preventing post-surgery blood clots.

Lower doses, which can be less expensive, may also be the safest and better than other doses at reducing the risk of bleeding in heart patients, say Canadian researchers.

THE STUDY

Researchers at McMaster University in Ontario compared the safety and efficacy of varying doses of aspirin—low (less than 100 milligrams; intermediate (101 to 199 mg); and high (more than 200 mg)—in 2,658 heart patients.

All study participants had what doctors call "acute coronary syndromes" (ACS)—a group of symptoms linked to chest pain caused by arterial damage that puts them at high risk for heart attack. All had also undergone procedures such as angioplasty; some with and some without the placement of artery-opening stents.

The patients were randomly assigned an aspirin dose following their procedure and tracked for eight months. Researchers found no difference in the rates of death, heart attack or stroke between the difference doses.

And while rates of major bleeding were similar among all groups after 30 days of aspirin therapy, it had improved most significantly after eight months in those taking the "children's" aspirin dose (81 milligrams or one quarter of a normal aspirin).

THE SIGNIFICANCE

"These data are intriguing, since low-dose aspirin is most commonly prescribed in Europe, but, in the United States, higher doses are most commonly used," notes study author Dr. Shamir R. Mehta. "Our data suggest that lower doses may be safer, but this finding needs confirmation in a dedicated randomized trial."

Studies Prove Drug-Eluting Stents Risky Without Blood Thinner

David F. Kong, MD, assistant professor of medicine, Duke University Medical Center, Durham, NC.

Robert O. Bonow, MD, director of cardiology, Northwestern University, Chicago.

John Kao, MD, assistant professor of medicine, University of Illinois, Chicago.

Journal of the American College of Cardiology.
Journal of the American Medical Association.

Heart patients who receive newer drug-eluting stents implanted to keep their arteries open have a higher risk of sudden death if they stop taking the blood-thinning drug *Plavix* than those with older bare-metal stents.

This was the conclusion of two new reports done to evaluate the safety of drug-eluting stents, specifically designed to reduce the high rate of artery reclosure following angioplasty.

There has been growing concern about the long-term safety of drug-eluting stents, which are used 80% of the time when a stent is implanted. Plavix (clopidogrel) is routinely prescribed following stent implantation.

THE STUDIES

In one study by Swiss researchers, 746 people who had 1,113 stents implanted did show that the drug-eluting stents did a better job of keeping arteries open.

But the incidence of death or heart attack for those patients was 4.9%, compared with 1.9% in patients with bare-metal stents.

Reason: Drug-eluting stents cause a higher rate of thrombosis, which is sudden blockage of an artery by a blood clot.

In another study, 4,600 patients were observed by Duke University researchers. Patients who received drug-eluting stents who stopped taking Plavix had more than twice the risk of death or heart attack than those who continued to take the drug.

"The overall risk over the ensuing 18 months was 7.2% versus 3.1%," notes Dr. David F. Kong, a member of the research team. "We also looked at bare-metal stents. The risk of death or heart attack was about 6% for those not taking Plavix, 5.5% for those taking Plavix."

Good news: There was a marked reduction in the need for repeat angioplasties among patients getting drug-eluting stents—one in 12, compared with one in five for those getting bare-metal stents.

LONG-TERM QUESTIONS

Drug-eluting stents now dominate the market —and that should continue, says Dr. Robert O. Bonow, director of cardiology at Northwestern University and a spokesman for the American Heart Association. "They are very effective at preventing restenosis," says Bonow. Restenosis is the closure of the artery, which frequently occurs following angioplasty.

But drug-eluting stents may also prevent the regrowth of the normal tissue that lines the artery, increasing the risk of thrombosis, Bonow adds.

Plavix can counter that risk. But it must be taken on a long-term basis.

"Until we know more, any cardiologist would recommend continued use of clopidogrel," Bonow says. "The uncertainty is how long we keep people on Plavix, indefinitely or for the first two years."

That can get expensive: Plavix therapy costs at least $120 a month. "At least in my practice," says Dr. John Kao, a Chicago cardiologist, "when I evaluate someone who needs intervention, if the patient is on a fixed income and cannot afford to take Plavix for six to 12 months, I put in a bare-metal stent."

info Learn more about heart treatments from the Food and Drug Administration at *www.fda.gov/hearthealth*.

Drugs Work as Well as Angioplasty for Stable Heart Disease

William E. Boden, MD, professor of medicine and public health, University at Buffalo School of Medicine and Biomedical Sciences, NY.

Judith S. Hochman, MD, professor of cardiology, New York University School of Medicine, New York City.

American College of Cardiology.

New England Journal of Medicine.

D rug therapy alone seems as effective as angioplasty for long-term relief of the chest pain and other symptoms caused by angina and other forms of "stable" heart disease, reveals a startling new study.

In the first long-term comparison, patients with significant but stable heart disease (that not requiring emergency care) who took aspirin, cholesterol-lowering statins and other heart drugs had nearly identical levels of symptom relief after five years as those who underwent angioplasty and follow-up treatment with the same drugs.

Angioplasty is a procedure that uses a balloon to open narrowed or clogged blood vessels near the heart. Usually, during the procedure a stent—a wire mesh tube—is placed in the vessel to keep it open. Nearly 1 million Americans a year undergo angioplasty, which can cost upwards of $30,000.

"This is really good news for patients," notes study lead author Dr. William E. Boden, professor of medicine and public health at the University at Buffalo School of Medicine and Biomedical Sciences. "We have more treatment options for patients than we thought we did."

THE STUDY

For the study, called COURAGE, Boden's research team randomly assigned nearly 2,300 patients. At any of 50 treatment centers across the US or Canada, they either received drug therapy alone, or drug therapy plus angioplasty. Among the latter group, 94% received at least one stent.

These patients were representative of the type of heart disease that affects 70% of heart patients in the US—that which requires treatment to lower risk of an eventual heart attack, but typically not emergency care.

During an average five-year follow-up, researchers tracked the rates of heart attack or death. They found that 19% of the angioplasty group had died or had a heart attack, compared with 18.5% in the group that only received drug treatment.

There were also no significant differences between patients who had angioplasty and those who had drug therapy alone in rates of death, heart attack, stroke or hospitalization for any heart-related problems.

The only benefit of angioplasty, says Boden, was that "it offered an immediate reduction in chest pain, a benefit that disappeared as the study progressed."

THE SIGNIFICANCE

Based on these findings, Boden believes that drug therapy for patients with stable heart disease should be tried as first-line treatment. "As an initial strategy, medical therapy is a defendable approach," he notes. "We should no longer consider it to be putting patients in harm's way, or thinking of it as an inferior treatment strategy."

Prior to Boden's study—which generated front-page headlines around the world—the common belief was that patients with chronic stable heart disease needed either an angioplasty or heart bypass surgery. This study suggests that for many, the initial treatment should be drug therapy.

THE REACTION

Dr. Judith S. Hochman, a professor of cardiology at New York University School of Medicine, agrees. "A trial of intensive (drug) therapy without angioplasty, to see how the symptoms respond, is what's indicated."

Angioplasty should be reserved for patients who have continuing symptoms, she adds. "If you have too much angina to do the activities you want to do, despite a trial of intensive medical therapy, then angioplasty is a good option."

However, angioplasty should be the first-line defense in anyone having a heart attack. "If you are having a high-risk unstable syndrome, angioplasty is very effective at reducing the chance of dying."

Don't Ignore Little-Known Signs of Heart Attacks

Susan Bennett, MD, cardiologist and director, Women's Heart Center, George Washington University Hospital, Washington, DC.
Rita Redberg, MD, MSc, professor of medicine, University of California, San Francisco, and scientific advisor, Choose to Move Program, American Heart Association.
European Heart Journal.

It might seem difficult to not recognize a heart attack, yet as many as four in 10 attacks may go undetected…in part because of those having a heart attack do not recognize the symptoms.

Crushing chest pain is the tell-tale sign, but women may not experience that classic symptom as often as men. That may explain, according to studies, while most undetected attacks affect women.

DENIAL CAN BE DEADLY

Both genders need to know the warning signs of a heart attack and to seek immediate help if they suspect one.

"People often ignore the warning signs of a heart attack," says Dr. Rita Redberg, a professor of medicine at the University of California, San Francisco. Sometimes, it's a case of denial.

Other times, people wrongly write it off as indigestion or stress. But it can be deadly if you ignore a possible attack or are sent home from the emergency room with false reassurance that you are fine.

WARNING SIGNS

According to the American Heart Association, the warning signs of a heart attack typically include…

• **Chest discomfort in the center of the chest that lasts more than a few minutes,** or that goes away and then returns. It can feel like uncomfortable pressure, squeezing, fullness or pain.

• **Discomfort in other areas of the upper body,** such as pain or discomfort in one or both arms, the back, neck, jaw or stomach.

• **Shortness of breath,** with or without chest discomfort.

• **A cold sweat,** nausea or light-headedness.

THE GENDER GAP

Women are more likely than men to experience such symptoms as shortness of breath, nausea and vomiting, and back or jaw pain.

After analyzing electrocardiographs (ECGs) of more than 4,000 men and women over age 55, Dutch researchers find that 43% of heart attacks go unrecognized—primarily among women.

Dr. Susan Bennett, director of George Washington University Hospital's Women's Heart program, says that even a doctor may not recognize a heart attack, especially in women. "Physicians typically underevaluate and undertreat women," she notes.

Bennett adds that the decision to evaluate a patient for a possible heart attack depends on the "index of suspicion." Often, that suspicion is not high enough for women, she says, and when doctors see a woman who is white and thin "they get that reflex that this is a lower-risk person."

Of course, even better than recognizing a heart attack early on is focusing on preventing one. "Know your numbers," Bennett advises. That means knowing your blood pressure as well as your cholesterol levels. Focus, too, on a healthful diet and a healthful weight. Aim for a body mass index (BMI—a ratio of weight to height) below 25, which is equal to less than 150 pounds for a person 5-feet, 5-inches tall, and less than 175 pounds for a person 5-feet, 10-inches tall.

info Browse through more articles about heart attack warning signs at *www.news-medical.net.*

10

Natural Remedies

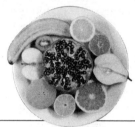

Common Foods with Uncommon Healing Powers

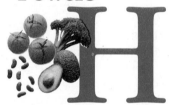

Herbal extracts that are derived from foods may yield medicinal benefits, according to new research reported by the American Chemical Society. Several extracts have been researched.

CHIVES

Chives seem to help protect against salmonella and other foodborne illnesses, says Salam A. Ibrahim, from the department of food science and nutrition at North Carolina A&T State University, in Greensboro, North Carolina.

In his research, Ibrahim finds that among many plant, herb and mushroom extracts tested, the antimicrobial properties of chives proved to have the most potent effect against 38 strains of salmonella—the most common bacterial foodborne illness. But when heated above 121 degrees Celsius—about 250 degrees Fahrenheit—for more than 15 minutes, the antibacterial effect was completely lost.

GRAPE SEEDS

Grape seeds may help lower blood pressure, reports another research team who studied 24 patients diagnosed with "metabolic syndrome," a condition characterized by heart-hurting risk factors such as high blood pressure and obesity. Half were given either 150 or 300 milligrams of grape seed extract each day; the others received a placebo.

After one month, those getting grape seeds experienced a significant drop in both systolic

G. Tissa Kappagoda, MD, PhD, department of internal medicine (cardiovascular medicine), University of California, Davis.

Salam A. Ibrahim, PhD, department of food science and nutrition, North Carolina A&T State University, Greensboro.

Jennifer L. Causey, PhD, nutrition manager, Lipid Nutrition, Channahon, IL.

Ken Fujioka, MD, director, department of nutrition and metabolism, Scripps Clinic, San Diego.

American Chemical Society.

and diastolic blood pressure. Those getting a placebo had no improvement.

"I think this is not going to be a standard treatment for high blood pressure," says researcher Dr. G. Tissa Kappagoda of the department of internal medicine at the University of California at Davis. "But it may be a potential tool for people who are prehypertensive, as part of a lifestyle management routine that includes weight management and exercise."

PINE NUTS

Pine nuts, a main ingredient in pesto, may help with weight loss, according to another study. That's because pine nuts contain high amounts of an oil called pinolenic acid, which has been shown in laboratories to stimulate the release of two appetite-suppressing hormones, CCK and GLP1.

In a study by Jennifer L. Causey, of Lipid Nutrition Co., 18 overweight women consumed three grams of pinolenic acid in gel capsule form. Four hours later, levels of these hormones had risen, and their appetites fell by approximately one third, she says.

These fatty acids induce a feeling of fullness, suggesting that pine nut oil may be useful as part of a weight-loss program that includes diet and exercise.

THE REACTION

Although each study is preliminary and involves a small number of study participants, they deserve notice, says one expert.

"All [these foods] certainly have the possibility to do what the researchers saw," says Dr. Ken Fujioka, director of the department of nutrition and metabolism within the department of endocrinology at the Scripps Clinic in San Diego. "The pine nut, in particular, has been noted before as an appetite-controller, so [this] finding makes sense …The chives finding is not surprising either… and could be a great idea to help cope with a meal that maybe we shouldn't have eaten. And many blood pressure medications—particularly the earlier ones—started off from natural plant sources. So, all of these findings seem reasonable."

info For more on food and health, visit the American Dietetic Association Web site at *www.eatright.org.*

Green Tea—Now Proven To Pump Up Heart Health

Shinichi Kuriyama, MD, PhD, researcher, Tohoku University Graduate School of Medicine, Sendai, Japan.
Kuang-Yuh Chyu, MD, PhD, assistant professor of medicine, University of California, Los Angeles, and staff cardiologist, Cedars-Sinai Medical Center, Los Angeles.
Robert Vogel, MD, professor of medicine, University of Maryland Medical School, Baltimore.
Journal of the American Medical Association.

Green tea has shown to protect against illness in laboratory and animal studies, but until now, its health-boosting effects on people have been scant, with only a handful of studies.

But in the largest study of its kind—on more than 40,000 people living in Japan—researchers have some encouraging news, that is, the more you drink, the better.

THE STUDY

Researchers found that adults who drank at least five cups of the brew daily had a lower risk of death from cardiovascular disease, as well as other causes with the exception of cancer, than those who drank less than one cup a day.

This finding comes after tracking study participants, ages 40 to 79, for 11 years. At the study's start, none had a history of heart disease, stroke or cancer.

Over the course of the study, more than 4,000 participants died—including 892 from cardiovascular disease and 1,134 from cancer.

In comparing death rates and green tea consumption, the researchers led by Dr. Shinichi Kuriyama of Tohoku University Graduate School of Medicine found that those who had consumed five or more cups per day had a risk of death from all causes that was 16% lower than people drinking less than one cup per day.

Meanwhile, deaths from cardiovascular disease were 26% lower for tea drinkers versus those who avoided the beverage. Among women, those who drank five or more cups of green tea daily had a 31% lower risk of death from heart disease and stroke death compared with women who drank less than a cup a day.

"I think our study would provide strong evidence regarding the benefits of drinking green tea in humans on cardiovascular disease," notes Kuriyama, who recommends drinking at least one cup of green tea a day.

THE THEORY

Experts believe green tea may be protective because it contains natural compounds called polyphenols—and one substance in particular, epigallocatechin-3-gallate. These substances have strong antioxidant properties that might help prevent heart disease.

Still, others say that while the study is interesting, more research is needed. "Tea is not harmful, that we know," says Dr. Kuang-Yuh Chyu, a cardiologist at Cedar-Sinai Medical Center in Los Angeles, who was not involved in the study. If you're a tea drinker, continue. But if not, Chyu adds that any real health benefit probably results from long-term consumption.

Another expert, Dr. Robert Vogel, professor of medicine at the University of Maryland Medical School, says that he also has doubts of any direct "cause-and-effect" protection, but acknowledges that green tea consumption is certainly preferable to drinking beverages such as nondiet sodas, which are loaded with sugar.

If you want to regularly drink tea and see if it is effective protection, be aware it should not be consumed steaming hot. "Drinking green tea at high temperature may be associated with increased risk of esophageal cancer and mortality," says Kuriyama.

info To learn more about how antioxidants work, visit the How Stuff Works Web Site at *health.howstuffworks.com/antioxidant1.htm.*

■ ■ ■ ■

Green Tea Boosts Brain Power

In a recent Japanese study of cognitive function in people age 70 or older, participants who drank two or more cups of green tea daily had a 54% lower prevalence of cognitive decline —measured via memory, attention and language-use tests—than those who drank three cups or less weekly.

Theory: Antioxidants in green tea may reduce the buildup of a type of plaque in the brain that is responsible for memory loss in Alzheimer's disease.

Self-defense: Drink two or more cups of green tea daily to help promote brain health.

Shinichi Kuriyama, MD, PhD, associate professor of epidemiology, Tohoku University Graduate School of Medicine, Sendai, Japan.

Miso Soup Ingredient May Fight Fat

Kazuo Miyashita, PhD, professor, Graduate School of Fisheries Sciences, Hokkaido University, Japan.
Connie Diekman, RD, director of nutrition, Washington University, St. Louis.
Hoyoku Nishino, MD, PhD, researcher, Kyoto Prefectural University of Medicine, Kyoto, Japan.
Liangli Lucy Yu, PhD, associate professor, University of Maryland, College Park.
American Chemical Society annual meeting.

Miso soup may please more than your palate—it may help you lose weight, say researchers.

A team led by Kazuo Miyashita, a chemistry professor at the Hokkaido University Graduate School of Fisheries Sciences in Japan, finds that a substance in brown seaweed—an ingredient of miso soup—may be a powerful fat burner.

In animal studies, his team finds that rodents fed the brown pigment in the seaweed—fucoxanthin—experienced a 5% to 10% weight loss through a shrinkage of abdominal fat. The compound is also in a type of kelp called wakame that is widely consumed in Japan.

THE STUDY

Researchers say fucoxanthin appears to stimulate a protein that causes fat oxidation and conversion of energy to heat. This protein is found in belly fat, suggesting that the compound might be particularly effective at shrinking oversized guts, the researchers hypothesized.

In their study, fucoxanthin also stimulated the animals' livers to produce DHA, a beneficial omega-3 fatty acid that reduces "bad" LDL cholesterol. It's also rich in phytochemcials believed to protect against cancer and other diseases.

THE REACTION

"The exciting finding is that fucoxanthin may increase metabolism and weight control," says

Connie Diekman, director of nutrition at Washington University in St. Louis. "But the downside is that this is an animal study, and we can't automatically translate from animals to humans."

Until there's better documentation that eating seaweed can shrink your waistline, Diekman's recommendation is "don't give up on what we know will work—correct food choices, right portions and regular physical activity."

Still, the Japanese researchers hope that further study could eventually lead to a fat-burning pill containing fucoxanthin.

■ ■ ■ ■

Miso Soup with Bean Curd and Wakame Seaweed

Bean curd and seaweed may sound unappealing to eat, but it's very tasty in this recipe.

Ingredients:

4 cups vegetable stock

½ cup dried wakame (a type of seaweed)

½ pound soft, medium or firm bean curd, cut into ¾-inch cubes

2 scallions, cut into very fine rings (use both white and green portions)

2½ to 4 tablespoons miso

Pinch of cayenne

Instructions:

It is first necessary to prepare the seaweed. Place the wakame in warm water, covering it by 1 inch. Let it stand for approximately 15 minutes, or until it is fully reconstituted. Drain in a sieve.

Put the stock into a medium pot and bring to a simmer. Add the bean curd and scallions. Simmer for 30 seconds. Gently stir in the reconstituted wakame. Reduce heat to low.

Put the miso in a small sieve and lower it into the soup (you may have to move the bean curd pieces aside). Push the miso through with a spoon.

Turn off the heat, stir once, sprinkle with cayenne and serve.

Makes 2 to 4 servings.

Spice Up Your Health

University of Michigan Health System.

Hungry for an easy way to improve your recipes…and your health? Look no further than your spice cabinet.

"By replacing traditional seasonings like sugar, salt and fat with herbs and spices, you can improve your overall health—along with the flavor of your food," says Suzanna Zick, a naturopathic physician and researcher at the University of Michigan Health System. "Adding herbs and spices can help you maintain a healthy weight. Plus, they can help prevent certain cancers, and even lower blood pressure, control blood sugar and improve cardiovascular health."

Herb such as oregano, thyme, rosemary, parsley and garlic are excellent replacements for salt, and can bring out the natural flavors in a meal. *These and other spices are a preventative health measure for your diet…*

- **Garlic.** To help lower cholesterol and blood pressure, you need to eat about three medium cloves of fresh garlic per day. Dry garlic, or garlic left out too long, loses its health punch.

- **Rosemary.** It's an antioxidant believed to improve memory and possibly help prevent cancer and help overcome colds.

- **Thyme.** It has long been used to treat coughs, even whooping cough, says Zick.

- **Basil and oregano.** The essential oils in these herbs are also thought to fight against colds.

- **Turmeric.** Researchers find that curcumin found in turmeric has anti-inflammatory properties and can shrink precancerous colon polyps. Turmeric can be consumed alone or as part of curry mixes.

- **Ginger.** It's a popular nausea reliever; credit goes to substances called gingerols that relieve queasiness.

- **"Warming spices"** including nutmeg, cinnamon, allspice, pepper, cayenne pepper and ginger are thought to better disperse blood throughout the body. This may bring better blood flow to skin and extremities, says Zick, and possibly improve blood pressure.

■ ■ ■ ■

Amazing! Spice That Zaps Cancer Cells

A powdered form of ginger kills ovarian cancer cells, according to a new laboratory study. Ginger may be unique because it causes cells to die in two distinctly different ways. This could aid in the development of therapies for treatment-resistant cancers.

University of Michigan Health System.

Curry—The Right Spice For a Better Memory

Milan Fiala, MD, researcher, University of California, Los Angeles, David Geffen School of Medicine and VA Greater Los Angeles Health Care System.

Sam Gandy, MD, PhD, chair, Medical and Scientific Advisory Council, Alzheimer's Association, and director, Farber Institute for Neurosciences, Thomas Jefferson University, Philadelphia.

Journal of Alzheimer's Disease.

P revious research has linked curry consumption with a lower risk of Alzheimer's disease. Now, researchers may be closer to understanding why.

Curcumin, a component in curry and turmeric, is known for its anti-inflammatory and antioxidant properties. The spice, a staple in Indian diets, may help immune system cells called macrophages rid the body of amyloid beta, the protein that builds up to form damaging plaques in the brains of Alzheimer's patients.

"We know that macrophages aren't working properly in Alzheimer's patients, since they seem to be defective in cleaning amyloid-beta from the brain," explains researcher Dr. Milan Fiala, a researcher with the David Geffen School of Medicine at UCLA and the VA Greater Los Angeles Health Care System. "We found that curcumin can help some macrophages to function properly in a test tube."

Next step: To determine if the popular spice works similarly in the human brain.

THE STUDY

Earlier research by another UCLA team found that curcumin-fed mice with amyloid-beta plaques experienced a decrease in inflammation and reduced plaque formation.

In Fiala's study, blood samples were collected from six Alzheimer's patients and three healthy controls. Researchers then isolated macrophages and treated them with a curcumin solution for 24 hours, then added amyloid beta.

In three Alzheimer's patients, macrophages started ingesting the plaque-forming proteins after the curry was added.

This study is the latest by Fiala's team, which has examined the immune function of more 100 Alzheimer's patients. "Our research has helped to identify why the brain isn't being cleared of amyloid beta in Alzheimer's disease patients," he says. "The immune system can attack and remove amyloid-beta from the brain, but the job is not done properly in Alzheimer's patients."

Fiala says macrophages may be as important for Alzheimer's disease as insulin is for diabetes. "If we can improve the immune system, we can help the body's natural ability to clear damaging plaques."

IMPLICATIONS

"In terms of treatment implications, it's very interesting that curcumin seems to help the brain clear away beta amyloid," notes Dr. Sam Gandy, chair of the medical and scientific advisory council at the Alzheimer's Association.

Fiala believes his team's research into the role of macrophages in Alzheimer's disease patients may one day point to new approaches for diagnosing and treating the illness.

Testing immune-cell response may also offer other researchers a novel way to assess the effectiveness of drugs in clearing amyloid beta from the brain. It might also help doctors individualize treatment, Fiala says.

Curcumin appears to have few side effects. "We can only say what we see in test tubes, but we don't see any toxic effects with curcumin, even administered in high doses," notes Fiala.

Curcumin's health benefits may extend beyond Alzheimer's disease. One recent six-month study, completed by researchers at Johns Hopkins University, finds that daily doses of the spice were associated with a nearly 60% lower risk for colon polyps, a known precursor to colon cancer.

info Curry is a name given to many different Indian spice mixes. To learn more about cooking with curry, visit the Penzeys Spices Web site at *www.penzeys.com.*

Fish Oil Boosts Kids' Hand-Eye Coordination

David L. Katz, MD, MPH, director, Prevention Research Center, Yale University School of Medicine, New Haven, CT.

Archives of Disease in Childhood.

Here's another reported benefit of fish oil —toddlers whose mothers took the heart-healthy supplements during pregnancy tend to have better hand-eye coordination than children whose mothers didn't take the supplements, according to a study.

The explanation: Omega-3 fatty acids— predominant in fish oil—are "taken up avidly by the developing eyes and brain of a fetus, and are thought to be important contributors to healthy development in early childhood," explains Dr. David L. Katz, director of the Prevention Research Center at Yale University School of Medicine, who was not involved in the study. "Along with essential omega-6 fats, these compounds influence everything from hormonal balance to immune function."

THE STUDY

In the study, researchers at the University of Western Australia's School of Paediatrics and Child Health tracked 98 pregnant women. They were randomly selected to take daily supplements, containing either four grams of fish oil or four grams of olive oil starting at 20 weeks of pregnancy until their babies were born.

When the children were 2½ years, their growth and development was tested. The tests included tests for language, behavior, practical reasoning and hand-eye coordination.

Researchers found that children whose mothers had taken fish oil supplements consistently scored significantly higher in hand-eye coordination tests. This held true even after the researchers accounted for the mothers' age and length of time they breast-fed.

In addition, in studying umbilical cords, researchers note that high levels of omega-3 fatty acids in the babies' umbilical cord blood was linked to better hand-eye coordination years later.

Among the 72 children tested, there were no significant differences in language skills and growth between children whose mothers had taken the fish oil supplements and those given olive oil capsules.

"These preliminary data indicate that supplementation with a relatively high-dose fish oil during the last 20 weeks of pregnancy is not only safe but also seems to have potential beneficial effects that need to be explored further," write the authors.

THE REACTION

"This study confirms that supplements of fish oil taken by pregnant women can influence the hand-eye coordination of their offspring," says Dr. Katz. "Whether that translates into long-term benefits in vision, coordination, or cognition remains to be seen. But the findings certainly hint at the importance of omega-3s to the health of young children."

His advice: "We know enough already to conclude that fish oil from supplements is generally a good idea, during pregnancy especially. I routinely advise one gram, twice daily, of fish oil to my pregnant patients—and my nonpregnant patients, too."

info For more on fish oil supplements, visit the US National Library of Medicine at *http://medlineplus.gov.*

■ ■ ■ ■

The Right Supplement

When choosing a product, consider the following guidelines…

•**It contains both EPA and DHA** (most provide both at a 1.5-to-1 ratio favoring EPA).

•**It is "molecularly distilled,"** a process used to separate the oils from any metals or other pollutants.

•**It is encapsulated under nitrogen** rather than oxygen—oxygen can turn the oils rancid, giving them a "fishy" taste and smell.

•**It is highly concentrated** to minimize the number of pills you'll need daily. Over-the-counter omega-3 supplements may contain from 30% to 90% fish oil.

•**It is approved by the US Pharmacopeia (USP).**

Laurence S. Sperling, MD, professor of medicine and director of the section of preventive cardiology at Emory University School of Medicine in Atlanta.

The Healing Power Of Mushrooms

Robert B. Beelman, PhD, professor of food science and chair of the Plant and Mushroom Products Impact Group at Pennsylvania State University in University Park. His current research focuses on the nutritional and medicinal values of mushrooms.

For centuries, Asian physicians have used mushrooms for medicinal purposes, but only recently have they become a focus of research in the US.

Latest findings: In addition to being highly nutritious, mushrooms contain chemical compounds that appear to lower the risk for elevated cholesterol, cancer and other serious conditions.

Studies on the medicinal properties of mushrooms—in whole food as well as supplement and extract form—are under way at the National Cancer Institute and other medical organizations.

It's not yet known whether mushroom extracts and supplements are more beneficial than the whole food. Some medicinal mushrooms, such as reishi, have a tough, woody texture and can be taken only as an extract. But most—shiitake, maitake, etc.—are edible and available at supermarkets and specialty stores.

Caution: It's best to avoid wild mushrooms and to eat only those that have been proven safe—that is, store-bought mushrooms.

Aim to eat three to six ounces daily of a variety of mushrooms. Raw and cooked mushrooms contain equal levels of nutrients.

Important health benefits…

CHOLESTEROL CONTROL

High cholesterol is among the main risk factors for cardiovascular disease. Studies have shown conclusively that patients who lower LDL "bad" cholesterol with statin drugs can reduce their risk for heart attacks by 25% to 50%.

New finding: The oyster mushroom contains significant amounts of statin-like compounds, which suppress the activity of HMG-CoA reductase, an enzyme used to make cholesterol in the body.

Bonus: It's possible that oyster mushrooms can lower LDL without suppressing HDL "good" cholesterol.

All mushrooms contain chitin, a structural material that strengthens the cell walls in people who eat them. Chitin, which accounts for 25% to 30% of a mushroom's dry weight, binds to cholesterol molecules in the intestine and prevents them from passing through the intestinal wall into the bloodstream.

ANTIOXIDANT ACTIVITY

The white button mushrooms that dominate the produce bins at American supermarkets were once thought to be insignificant sources of disease-fighting antioxidants—but new research shows that they're high in L-ergothioneine, an antioxidant that's produced only by fungi.

THE BEST CHOICES

Crimini and portobello mushrooms contain even more L-ergo-thioneine than white button mushrooms, and have the highest overall antioxidant content. What's more, all three of these mushrooms contain about 15% more L-ergothioneine than wheat germ or chicken liver, which previously were thought to be the richest sources.

The body has a chemical transport system dedicated solely to L-ergothioneine, which indicates that it's critical for normal metabolism.

In addition to L-ergothioneine, most mushrooms are also rich in selenium. Depending on the variety, one serving of mushrooms (about three ounces) provides about 10% to 20% of the recommended daily intake of this mineral—55 micrograms (mcg) for women and 70 mcg for men. Selenium is a very powerful antioxidant that inhibits blood-fat oxidation and the accumulation of arterial plaques.

Important: Most "specialty" mushrooms, such as oyster, shiitake and maitake, contain only trace amounts of selenium because they are grown on hardwood or sawdust, rather than selenium-rich soil. White button and crimini mushrooms are good sources of selenium.

ANTICANCER ACTIVITY

As far back as the 1950s, studies showed that laboratory animals with cancer that were given mushroom extracts had higher survival rates.

Increasing evidence now suggests that mushrooms contain chemical compounds and nutrients with anticancer properties.

Those anticancer chemicals…

•**Lentinan,** a substance in shiitake mushrooms, has been found in animal studies to increase levels of immune cells (such as T- and B-lymphocytes) that suppress tumor development.

•**Aromatase inhibitors** suppress the enzyme aromatase, which converts androgens (the so-called "male" hormones) into estrogens (the so-called "female" hormones). Lower estrogen levels may reduce the risk for prostate cancer and some kinds of breast cancer. White button, crimini and portobello mushrooms have the highest levels of aromatase inhibitors.

•**5-alpha-reductase,** an enzyme found in white button mushrooms, suppresses the conversion of testosterone to dihydrotestosterone (DHT), a hormone that promotes the development of prostate cancer.

WEIGHT CONTROL

An average serving of mushrooms has only about 28 calories and 0.4 g of fat—nearly ideal for a weight-loss diet. The high water (more than 90%) and fiber (up to 1.8 g in shiitake mushrooms) contents make mushrooms more filling than many other low-calorie foods. The chitin in mushrooms is also beneficial for weight loss because it reduces the absorption of fats.

Delicious Teas That Ease Everyday Ailments

Brigitte Mars, an adjunct professor of herbal medicine at Naropa University in Boulder, CO. She is the author of 12 books, including *Healing Herbal Teas* (Basic Health), and a professional member of the American Herbalist Guild (AHG).

Herbal teas, which are generally rich in vitamins, minerals and other healthful compounds, have been used as healing agents for thousands of years.

However, because of the prevalence of over-the-counter and prescription medications, most Americans don't think of drinking tea to treat common ailments. That's a mistake.

Dozens of scientific studies have supported the use of herbals for a wide variety of health problems.* Herbal teas have the same active ingredients as herbs sold in capsules, powders and extracts. Herbal teas also have fewer side effects than medication and can be much less expensive.

Loose tea herbs, which are available at health-food stores, tend to be more potent than tea bags. To prepare tea with loose herbs, use one heaping tablespoon of dried herb or three tablespoons of fresh herb in eight ounces of boiling water. Steep for 10 minutes.

For best results, drink four eight-ounce cups of herbal tea per day until the problem subsides. If you are age 65 or older, do not exceed three cups daily…or two cups daily if you are age 70 or older.

Best teas for treating common health conditions…

COLDS AND FLU

Echinacea, which has an aromatic, earthy flavor, promotes white blood cell production… acts as an anti-infection agent…and stimulates the immune system.

How to use: Echinacea should be used for no more than 10 consecutive days, because it loses its effectiveness when taken continually. Drink echinacea tea at the onset of cold or flu

*Check with your health-care practitioner before drinking herbal tea, especially if you are a pregnant woman, nursing mother or have a chronic medical condition. Some herbal teas should not be combined with certain drugs.

symptoms, such as sore throat, sneezing and/or nasal congestion.

Caution: Echinacea stimulates the immune system, so people with autoimmune diseases, such as lupus, should consult a doctor before using this herb. People who are allergic to plants in the daisy family, such as ragweed, are more likely to have an allergic reaction to echinacea.

Other teas that fight colds and flu: Elderflower and elderberry.

DIGESTIVE DISORDERS

Peppermint, which has a zesty, fresh taste, calms muscle spasms…eases intestinal cramping …contains antibacterial compounds…soothes ulcers…and freshens breath after a meal.

Caution: Do not drink peppermint tea if you are suffering from an acute episode of a digestive disorder, such as a gallstone attack. Seek immediate medical attention.

Other teas that fight digestive disorders: Cardamom, ginger and cinnamon.

HEADACHE

Lemon balm, which has a gentle lemon flavor and aroma, acts as an anti-inflammatory and antispasmodic…and contains magnesium, which acts as a muscle relaxant.

Caution: This herb may inhibit thyroid function. If you have low thyroid function (hypothyroidism), avoid lemon balm tea.

Other teas that fight headache: Feverfew and rosemary.

INSOMNIA

Linden flower, which has a sweet flavor and jasminelike aroma, is rich in vitamin C…calms nerves…and promotes rest. In Europe, linden flower tea often is given to patients before surgery to help them relax.

Other teas that fight insomnia: Chamomile and passionflower.

LOW LIBIDO

Oat seed, which has a slightly sweet, milky flavor, relaxes the nerves…and is often used as an aphrodisiac.

Caution: Oat seed contains gluten, so this herb should be avoided by people with gluten intolerance.

Other teas that fight low libido: Cinnamon and raspberry leaf.

▪ ▪ ▪ ▪

Top Tummy-Soothing Teas

Herbal teas are great for digestive symptoms, but which tea is best for which symptoms?

Abdominal cramps and ulcers: Chamomile tea. Its essential oils are anti-inflammatory and antispasmodic. Chamomile calms the nervous system, so it is good for digestive symptoms linked to stress.

Gas (flatulence): Fennel tea. Use when gas occurs after meals. Interestingly, fennel was once used in the US as a drug for the treatment of indigestion.

Bloating: Gingerroot tea. It also can help with gas, diarrhea, nausea, vomiting and morning sickness.

Irritable bowel syndrome (characterized by alternating constipation and diarrhea): Peppermint tea. It also can help with cramps, gas and bloating. Peppermint can aggravate heartburn (acid reflux) in some people, so go easy at first.

If you frequently have digestive upset: Try one-half to one cup of tea just before each meal or with meals. For occasional upset, drink a cup as needed to reduce the symptoms. Tea bags work as well as loose tea—use organic, if possible.

Dr. Mark Stengler is a licensed naturopathic medical doctor and a leading authority on the practice of alternative and integrated medicine. An associate clinical professor at the National College of Naturopathic Medicine in Portland, OR, Dr. Stengler has served on a medical advisory committee for the Yale University Complementary Medicine Outcomes Research Project and is the author or coauthor of 16 books, including two best sellers—*The Natural Physician's Healing Therapies* and *Prescription for Natural Cures.* (Both from Bottom Line Books). Dr. Stengler is the founder and director of the La Jolla Whole Health Clinic in La Jolla, CA. *www.DrStengler.com.*

▪ ▪ ▪ ▪

Try Super-Healthy White Tea

White tea is the most healthful tea according to a recent study. Derived from the same plant as green and black teas, white tea (called yinzhen) undergoes less processing than other varieties, so it retains more beneficial flavonoids, antioxidant plant compounds that help reduce the risk for heart disease and cancer. White tea has a sweet, delicate taste. It is available in specialty tea shops and some grocery stores.

Helpful: Drink three mug-sized cups of white tea daily.

Gayle A. Orner, PhD, assistant professor, Linus Pauling Institute of Oregon State University, Corvallis.

'Super Tomato' Could Slice Birth Defects

Andrew D. Hanson, PhD, professor of plant biochemistry, University of Florida Institute of Food and Agricultural Sciences, Gainesville.
Jesse F. Gregory III, PhD, professor of food science and human nutrition, University of Florida Institute of Food and Agricultural Sciences, Gainesville.
Proceedings of the National Academy of Sciences.

Scientists have created a folic acid-enriched "super tomato" that they say could cut the rate of birth defects, anemia and other folate deficiency-linked problems.

"We used the tomato, because it is a very good model to work with," says study coauthor Andrew D. Hanson, professor of plant biochemistry at the University of Florida. "Now we want to move the strategy we have developed into cereal and tuber crops such as sweet potatoes."

MANIPULATING MOLECULES

This discovery could be a boon for nations where nutritional deficiencies are common. Inadequate folate is linked with birth defects such as spina bifida, heart disease and some cancers. In the US, grain products are now fortified with folic acid, and pregnant women are advised to take folate supplements if necessary.

Hanson and colleague Jesse F. Gregory III targeted two molecular pathways by which tomatoes, as well as other plants, make folate. One produces a molecule called pteridine, the other producing another molecule, p-aminobenzoate

(PABA). Those two molecules eventually become linked in the process that creates folate.

"Humans don't have the ability to produce parts of those pathways, which is why we require [folate] as a vitamin," Gregory explains.

BITING BENEFIT

Their genetically engineered tomatoes, when ripened accordingly, contain 25 times more folate than normal, they report.

"We have produced a few experimental plants," Hanson says. Now the goal is to show that the same increase in folate production in their tomatoes can be achieved in others plants that are dietary staples in underdeveloped countries.

info The National Institutes of Health Web site has more on folate at *http://dietarysupplements.info.nih.gov/.*

Coffee May Reduce Cirrhosis Risk

Arthur L. Klatsky, MD, senior consultant in cardiology, Kaiser Permanente Medical Center, Oakland, CA.
Constance E. Ruhl, MD, Social and Scientific Systems Inc., Bethesda, MD.
Archives of Internal Medicine.

Drinking coffee seems to protect alcohol drinkers from developing cirrhosis or liver disease, according to new epidemiological research. Cirrhosis is an often-fatal condition that destroys liver tissue and is usually caused by excessive drinking.

A single daily cup of coffee reduced the incidence of cirrhosis by 22% in a study at Kaiser Permanente Medical Care Program, in Oakland.

But this finding, says study lead Dr. Arthur L. Klatsky, "should not be interpreted as giving a license to drink without worry, because of all the other problems connected with drinking."

Three drinks per day should be the upper limit for most people, he says—at least with most males anyway.

THE FINDINGS

Klatsky's team analyzed data from more than 125,000 people between 1978 and 1985. All were free of liver disease when they had examinations. At those times, they were surveyed on their alcohol, tea and coffee consumption.

By the end of 2001, there were 330 cases of cirrhosis among study participants, 199 attributed to alcohol consumption. After extracting for other factors, researchers determined that regular coffee consumption was linked to a lower risk—and that a daily cup made study participants 22% less likely to develop cirrhosis caused by alcohol.

THE REACTION

These findings come as no surprise to Dr. Constance E. Ruhl, coauthor of an earlier study, published in the medical journal *Gastroenterology*. Her research, pooled from federal data, showed that people at high risk of liver disease were 22% less likely of being hospitalized for cirrhosis if they were coffee drinkers.

"It's encouraging to me that they found something similar," Ruhl says. "It's additional evidence that there might be a relationship there."

Theory: Some researchers believe that caffeine induces the release of adenosine, a molecule that prevents the inflammation that leads to kidney damage. High levels of antioxidants and polyphenols are found in coffee, another reason to enjoy your "joe."

info Get more information about cirrhosis from the National Institute of Diabetes and Digestive and Kidney Disease at *http://digestive.ni ddk.nih.gov/*.

■ ■ ■ ■

Coffee Is a Primary Source Of Antioxidants

Antioxidants, such as vitamins A, C and E (found most abundantly in fruits and vegetables), help prevent cell damage. However, most Americans get the majority of their antioxidants from drinking caffeinated and decaffeinated coffee.

Helpful: Add healthful foods with the highest concentrations of antioxidants per serving (dates, cranberries and red grapes) to your diet.

Joe Vinson, PhD, professor of chemistry, University of Scranton, PA.

Cheers! Red Wine Helps Your Heart

Dr. Mark Stengler is a licensed naturopathic medical doctor and a leading authority on the practice of alternative and integrated medicine. An associate clinical professor at the National College of Naturopathic Medicine in Portland, OR, Dr. Stengler has served on a medical advisory committee for the Yale University Complementary Medicine Outcomes Research Project and is the author or coauthor of 16 books, including two best sellers—*The Natural Physician's Healing Therapies* and *Prescription for Natural Cures*. (Both from Bottom Line Books). Dr. Stengler is the founder and director of the La Jolla Whole Health Clinic in La Jolla, CA. *www.DrStengler.com.*

You might have read the headlines in recent years—moderate consumption of alcohol, especially red wine, decreases the risk of cardiovascular disease. Before you assume that's reason enough to consume alcohol on a regular basis, let's look at this issue more closely.

It is true that alcohol consumption provides some cardiovascular protection. For example, when researchers combined data from 51 epidemiological studies, they found that the risk of heart disease decreased by about 20% when one to two alcoholic drinks were consumed per day. (One drink of alcohol is equivalent to 1.5 ounces of liquor, 5 ounces of wine or 12 ounces of beer.) The people who seemed to benefit most from light drinking (about 1.2 drinks a day) to moderate drinking (2.2 drinks daily) were middle-aged men and women.

Red wine has additional benefits over other alcoholic beverages, studies suggest. That's because several chemicals in red wine may protect the heart, including *resveratrol*, a polyphenol (plant pigment) with antioxidant effects. (White wine has smaller amounts of resveratrol.)

The natural compounds in red wine seem to prevent buildup of plaque in the arteries by reducing inflammation and promoting good tone in blood vessel walls. The compounds also play a role in preventing blood clots, which can obstruct blood flow and cause a heart attack or stroke. Alcoholic beverages of any type increase HDL "good" cholesterol, which removes LDL "bad" cholesterol from circulation, thereby minimizing plaque formation.

Despite these positive effects, I don't recommend that people rely on wine or any alcoholic beverages for heart disease prevention. If you do not drink alcohol on a regular basis, don't start. One of the obvious risks of regular alcohol consumption is alcoholism, a very serious and common disease in our country. *Other reasons not to drink alcohol...*

•**Cancer risk.** According to the American Cancer Society, men who have two alcoholic drinks a day and women who have one alcoholic drink a day increase their risk of certain cancers—of the esophagus, pharynx, mouth, liver, breast and colon. If you enjoy drinking each day, limit consumption to half a drink for women and one drink for men so as not to increase cancer risk.

•**Heart risk.** Paradoxically, the same amount of alcohol that has been shown to have a heart-protective effect—two drinks daily for men and one for women—also has been shown to raise triglyceride levels. High levels of these fats increase heart disease risk. Excessive drinking also raises the risk of high blood pressure, heart failure and stroke.

•**Obesity risk.** Alcohol contains simple carbohydrates. Consuming large amounts of simple carbs increases the risk of obesity and diabetes.

•**Fetal risk.** Mothers who drink alcohol during pregnancy predispose their babies to birth defects.

You can dramatically reduce your risk of heart disease without negative effects by not smoking, avoiding secondhand smoke, exercising regularly and consuming a Mediterranean-style diet. This diet is rich in fruits and vegetables, whole grains, nuts, seeds, legumes and olive oil—and has low to moderate amounts of dairy, fish and poultry, and little red meat. You also might take fish oil with a combined EPA and DHA total of 500 mg daily to get heart-healthy essential fatty acids.

Also drink purple grape juice. It makes arteries more flexible and reduces the susceptibility of LDL cholesterol to cause damage in patients with coronary artery disease. Purple grape juice has potent antioxidant activity and, like red wine, contains resveratrol. It is high in simple sugars, so drink only six ounces daily—with a meal to slow sugar absorption. If you have diabetes, have no more than four ounces daily with a meal.

Calcium, Vitamin D Supplements Build Bones Fast!

Orthopaedic Research Society.

Creighton University doctors regularly recommend that aging women taking calcium and vitamin D supplements to help reduce their risk of broken bones and osteoporosis. But even short periods of supplementation may reduce the risk of stress fractures in younger women.

So concludes a new study of 5,200 female US Navy recruits going through basic training. Half of the women—ages 17 to 35—were given daily vitamin supplements of 2,000 milligrams of calcium and 800 international units of vitamin D. The others received placebo pills.

SURPRISING RESULTS

After eight weeks, researchers noted stress fractures in 170 recruits. These overuse injuries were 25% more common in those taking the dummy pills. Not surprisingly, researchers also noted that smoking increased bone injury risk, while a history of exercise decreased the risk.

Vitamin D helps the body absorb calcium, which is vital to bone formation and repair.

"What really surprised us is that calcium/vitamin D supplements made a significant difference in such a short period of time," says study lead Joan Lappe, a professor of nursing and medicine at Creighton University in Omaha, Nebraska. "Frankly, we were not sure we would see any statistically significant results in only eight weeks."

Bottom line: Although these findings are preliminary, they could help reduce bone injuries in high school and other amateur athletes.

■ ■ ■ ■

Soy Foods Reduce Fracture Risk

A study of the soy intake of 24,403 postmenopausal women over four and a half years found that those who ate 13 g or more of soy protein daily were 37% less likely to break a bone than those who consumed less than 5 g daily.

Theory: Soy slows bone breakdown.

Self-defense: Postmenopausal women should aim to get at least 5 g of soy protein in their diets daily.

Sources: Soy milk (10 g per eight ounces) and tofu (13 g per four ounces).

Xianglan Zhang, MD, MPH, research instructor of medicine, Vanderbilt University School of Medicine, Nashville, TN.

■ ■ ■ ■

Tomato Juice: Great for Your Heart

Drinking tomato juice protects the heart, says new research from Australia.

New finding: People with type 2 diabetes or impaired glucose tolerance (a precursor to diabetes) who drank 8.5 ounces of tomato juice a day for three weeks experienced a 30% to 40% reduction in platelet aggression, a key to the clot formation that can trigger heart attack. This benefit is believed to apply to healthy people as well.

Bonus: Tomato juice also reduces risk for deep vein thrombosis (DVT), dangerous blood clots that can occur after sitting for long hours.

Helpful: Drink 8 ounces of low-sodium tomato juice each day.

Manohar L. Garg, PhD, associate professor of nutrition and dietetics, University of Newcastle, Australia.

Could Iron Help You Grow More Hair?

Journal of the American Academy of Dermatology.

After reviewing 40 years of medical literature, Cleveland Clinic researchers think they have discovered an often overlooked cause of baldness—iron deficiency.

"We believe that iron deficiency may be related to many forms of hair loss and that people may need higher levels of iron stores than previously thought to regrow hair," says Dr. Wilma Bergfeld, head of clinical research in the department of dermatology, who headed the data review. "If doctors can understand fully the relationship between iron deficiency and hair loss, then they can help people regrow hair more effectively."

However, she and others are still scratching their heads on specific recommendations.

Iron deficiency is the world's most common nutritional deficiency. It can be caused by inadequate dietary intake of iron, excessive menstrual bleeding, and other forms of blood loss. Treatment includes adequate dietary intake of iron and, when appropriate, iron supplements. However, use of supplements, especially in middle age and beyond, should be done under a doctor's supervision.

Doctors at the Cleveland Clinic routinely screen for iron deficiency in patients with hair loss. If iron deficiency is detected and treated in the early stages, patients may be able to grow hair more effectively, they say.

info Learn more about hair loss at the Web site of the American Hair Loss Association, *www.americanhairloss.org.*

■ ■ ■ ■

Hair-Raising Discovery!

Scientists have identified two mutations in a gene that lead to some cases of *trichotillomania,* or compulsive hair-pulling. Between 3% and 5% of Americans suffer from this condition, now thought to be caused by faulty connections between neurons—and not by negative life experiences.

Duke University Medical Center.

Folic Acid Sharpens Aging Minds

Richard Finnell, PhD, Regents Professor, Center for Environmental and Genetic Medicine, Texas A&M Health Science Center Institute of Biosciences and Technology at Houston.
Maria Carrillo, PhD, director of medical and scientific relations, Alzheimer's Association.
The Lancet.

Folic acid, the B vitamin perhaps best known for helping to prevent birth defects, can sharpen an aging mind, say Dutch researchers.

Their research is the latest to suggest that folic acid supplementation can improve memory and thinking ability in older adults—as well as provide other health benefits.

Folic acid supplements are considered especially helpful for people with high blood levels of the amino acid homocysteine. High levels of this dangerous substance, caused in part by low consumption of folic acid, are linked with increased risk for cardiovascular disease and stroke and possibly Alzheimer's disease.

THE STUDY

For this study, researchers randomly assigned 818 adults between ages 50 and 70 to receive either a daily 800-microgram folic acid supplement or a placebo for three years.

At the study's start, all participants had low levels of folic acid—also known as folate—as evidenced by elevated homocysteine concentrations.

Results: Those getting the vitamin supplements had actually improved—and not only maintained—their thinking ability, especially in the areas of memory and information processing speed. What's more, their blood concentrations of the nutrient increased 576% and their homocysteine levels fell 26%.

Previously, the same Dutch researchers found that people who took a folic acid supplement had less decline in hearing low-frequency sounds over time, compared with people who didn't take the supplement.

THE REACTION

"We can certainly take away that folate is going to be beneficial for cognitive improvement when you have high homocysteine levels," says Maria Carrillo, director of medical and scientific relations at the Alzheimer's Association.

Adds Richard Finnell, professor at Texas A&M's Health Science Center, "This underscores the importance of B vitamins. They do more than protect babies against birth defects."

Folic acid has several functions: It helps the body digest and utilize proteins and to synthesize new proteins when they are needed; it's essential for the production of red blood cells and the synthesis of DNA; it helps with tissue growth and cell function; it helps to increase appetite when needed; and it stimulates the formation of digestive acids.

Good food sources of folate include beans and legumes; citrus fruits and juices; wheat bran and other whole grains; dark, green leafy vegetables; poultry; pork; shellfish and liver.

info The US Library of Medicine has more information on folic acid at *http://www.nlm.nih.gov/medlineplus/folicacid.html.*

Folic Acid May Prevent Cancer of Larynx

Cancer.

Folic acid supplements commonly used to prevent birth defects and believed to lower risk of heart disease and stroke may soon be used to prevent cancer of the larynx.

In a small, preliminary study of people with precancerous lesions called leukoplakia, Italian researchers say that the lesions disappeared in about one in four given folic acid supplements, an over-the-counter B vitamin. Meanwhile, 44% of study participants experienced at least partial shrinking of lesions. Leukoplakia left unchecked can eventually turn into cancer.

All of the study participants took 5 milligrams of folic acid, three times a day for six months.

THE STUDY

For the study, the researchers recruited 43 people who had been diagnosed with laryngeal leukoplakia. Some 88% were smokers, and all but three were men.

Because prior studies had shown that people with head and neck cancers and laryngeal leukoplakia often have low blood levels of folate, the natural form of folic acid, the researchers wanted to learn if supplements of the nutrient could help prevent the progression of leukoplakia to cancer.

Blood tests were done periodically to ensure the volunteers were taking their supplements as requested. The researchers also measured the leukoplakias once a month.

About one-quarter of the group showed no response the folic acid regimen. Nearly half experienced a partial shrinkage of their leukoplakia. But 12 people—28%—had a "complete response," meaning their leukoplakia disappeared, say researchers.

Each year, nearly 40,000 Americans are diagnosed with head and neck cancers, including cancer of the larynx, according to the US National Cancer Institute. These types of cancer are most common in people older than 50, and tobacco use is the top risk factor.

The Vitamin That May Lower Risk Of Multiple Sclerosis

Alberto Ascherio, MD, associate professor of nutrition and epidemiology, Harvard School of Public Health, Boston.

Nicholas LaRocca, PhD, director of health care delivery and policy research, National Multiple Sclerosis Society, New York City.

Journal of the American Medical Association.

Could sunshine be the secret to preventing multiple sclerosis? Maybe, concludes new research—but only for white people.

Harvard researchers report that Caucasians with high circulating levels of vitamin D—a nutrient mainly produced by the body after sun exposure—had a lower risk of developing multiple sclerosis (MS) than those with lower D blood levels. However, no such association was found for blacks or Hispanics in this study.

THE STUDY

Using blood samples stored among a repository of more than 7 million samples maintained by the US Department of Defense, the researchers compared blood samples of 257 people with multiple sclerosis to 514 others, matched on age, sex and race. These samples came from 149 whites, 77 blacks and 32 Hispanics.

The samples were analyzed for levels of circulating vitamin D and separated the samples into five groups based on the vitamin D levels.

"The group [of whites] with the highest vitamin D levels had a 62% decreased risk compared to the group with the lowest levels," says study lead Dr. Alberto Ascherio.

However, no association between vitamin D levels and MS occurrence was noted in blacks and Hispanics—possibly because they had lower levels of circulating vitamin D, say researchers.

THE EXPLANATION

Ascherio says researchers don't know for sure whether vitamin D may play a role in causing MS, but they suspect that it probably does. "There is a pretty good convergence of evidence that vitamin D affects the immune system to lower the risk of MS," he says.

However, he cautions that it was too soon to recommend that anyone—even those at high risk of developing MS—begin taking vitamin D supplements or increasing their sun exposure with the hope of preventing MS. MS affects about 400,000 Americans and affects the central nervous system.

Symptoms include poor coordination, loss of balance, blurred vision, fatigue, cognitive problems, numbness and possible paralysis.

THE REACTION

"This is another piece of the puzzle, and it may help to explain why we see geographic difference in MS," says Dr. Nicholas LaRocca, associate vice president of health care delivery and policy research at the National Multiple Sclerosis Society.

But what does this association mean? "Is it an actual risk factor? How does it work? What can we do about it? In the future, if one could establish a causal relationship, it could present an opportunity for a partially preventive strategy," LaRocca adds. "Right now, the scientific community is not convinced that there's enough evidence to recommend taking vitamin D supplements, though."

info To learn more about multiple sclerosis, visit the National Multiple Sclerosis Society at *www.nmss.org.*

Ray of Hope: Sun May Protect Against Skin Cancer

Martin Weinstock, MD, PhD, chairman, skin cancer advisory group, American Cancer Society, and professor of dermatology and community health, Brown University, Providence, RI.

Marianne Berwick, PhD, professor of internal medicine and chief of epidemiology, University of New Mexico's Cancer Research and Treatment Center, Albuquerque.

Katharine Tallmadge, RD, dietitian, Washington, DC, and spokeswoman, American Dietetic Association.

Kathleen Egan, MA, BSN, professor of epidemiology, H. Lee Moffitt Cancer Center and Research Institute, Tampa, FL.

Nature Immunology.

It puzzles even scientists, but new research suggests that the main cause of deadly skin cancer—sunlight—might also protect against the disease.

The secret, say experts, is in the skin absorbing the right amount of ultraviolet B (UVB) light —enough to stimulate a healthy, vitamin D–linked immune response but not so much that it boosts skin cancer risk.

THE STUDY

In their study, a group led by immunologists at Stanford University worked with cells in the lab and discovered a biochemical chain of events that appears to link sunlight exposure to the skin's own immune defenses.

The researchers started from an old notion that an inactive precursor of vitamin D, called vitamin D3, is generated in the skin in response to sun exposure. Specifically, a short-wavelength form of UV light, called UVB, is responsible for D3 generation.

Through contact with various enzymes in the liver and kidneys, the body turns D3, usually inert and powerless, into an active compound called 1,25(OH)2D3. And that's where the immune-system connection kicks in, say the Stanford scientists.

THE RESULTS

They found that the new compound 1,25 (OH) 2D3 "signaled (immune) T-cells," pushing them to migrate back to specific sites in the skin's epidermis. Once there, these powerful immune system agents stand on guard against infection and even cancer, say the researchers.

Bottom line: "The same wavelengths of sunlight that are most potent in inducing skin cancer—UVB—are also the wavelengths that produce this vitamin D precursor, D3," says Dr. Martin Weinstock, chairman of the skin cancer advisory group at the American Cancer Society. And it's D3 that's the catalyst that gets the whole chain of events rolling.

Weinstock, also a professor of dermatology and community health at Brown University, says this finding is about to change the American Cancer Society's long-standing recommendation to avoid intense sunshine and always wearing sunscreen when outdoors.

PAST FINDINGS

But the Stanford study follows earlier research, published in 2005, that noted melanoma patients with higher levels of daily sun exposure actually had a better chance of survival than patients who spent less time in the sun.

"A little bit of sunlight is good for people, but I think that one of the problems that the American Cancer Society and dermatologists have is, how do you define what a little bit is?" says that study's lead, epidemiologist Marianne Berwick of the University of New Mexico's Cancer Research and Treatment Center. "How do you tell people that it's OK to have a little bit of sunlight but not too much?"

THE ROLE OF VITAMIN D

Nutritionists have known for decades that sunlight stimulates vitamin D production in the skin. In fact, this natural process is the body's major source of the nutrient. A proper amount of vitamin D is crucial to bone health, "and there's also a bunch of evidence that vitamin D may have a role in preventing colon cancer, although there's still some controversy about that," says Weinstock.

PROPER DEFENSE

So, how much sunlight is enough to get the ideal amount of vitamin D?

Katharine Tallmadge, a Washington, DC, dietitian and a spokeswoman for the American Dietetic Association, suggests that most people can probably get the US Department of Agriculture's recommended 400 daily IUs of vitamin D by spending 30 to 60 minutes outdoors each day.

EXPERT AGREES

Kathleen Egan, a professor of epidemiology at the H. Lee Moffitt Cancer Center and Research Institute in Tampa, Florida, agrees that it's not difficult for people to soak up the sun's goodness without boosting their cancer risk. "The skin actually creates an amazing amount of vitamin D," she says. "It doesn't take much exposure to make enough of the vitamin D that's certainly needed to preserve bone health, for example."

info For more information on skin cancer, visit the American Cancer Society Web site at *www.cancer.org,* or The Skin Cancer Foundation at *www.skincancer.org.*

■ ■ ■ ■

Can the Sun Stop Breast and Colon Cancer?

Sunlight may help protect against colon, breast and other cancers.

Theory: Ultraviolet (UVB) rays trigger production of vitamin D in the skin, which protects against cancer by reducing cell proliferation and angiogenesis (development of new blood vessels). Inadequate exposure to UVB rays has been blamed for about 45,000 premature cancer deaths.

Self-defense: Spend some time every day in the sun without sunscreen, but not enough time to cause reddening or burning of the skin.

Other vitamin D sources: Cold-water fish, such as sardines and salmon.

William B. Grant, PhD, founding director, Sunlight, Nutrition and Health Research Center, San Francisco. *www.sunarc.org.*

Natural Ways to Prevent 80% of Vision Problems

Dr. Mark Stengler is a licensed naturopathic medical doctor and a leading authority on the practice of alternative and integrated medicine. An associate clinical professor at the National College of Naturopathic Medicine in Portland, OR, Dr. Stengler has served on a medical advisory committee for the Yale University Complementary Medicine Outcomes Research Project and is the author or coauthor of 16 books, including two best sellers—*The Natural Physician's Healing Therapies* and *Prescription for Natural Cures.* (Both from Bottom Line Books). Dr. Stengler is the founder and director of the La Jolla Whole Health Clinic in La Jolla, CA. *www.DrStengler.com.*

Millions of Americans have lost some or all of their sight to cataracts, glaucoma, macular degeneration and other eye diseases. Medications and surgical procedures can help, but the results are rarely optimal.

Fact: Up to 80% of all diseases can be prevented with natural approaches—and there is evidence that nutritional treatments can halt or even reverse underlying vision problems.

Sun exposure is one of the main causes of vision loss. Everyone should wear sunglasses that block the sun's damaging ultraviolet (UV) rays.

Other measures to combat vision loss include eating certain foods and taking supplements. The antioxidants described below (lutein, zeaxanthin and the recommended vitamin supplements) help prevent and treat most eye conditions. The other remedies described can help specific problems. You can take all the supplements listed here (available at health-food stores), but it is always wise to consult with your physician before taking any supplement.

LUTEIN

Spinach, kale and other leafy greens contain an antioxidant called lutein, which reduces damage caused by unstable molecules known as free radicals. Smoking and exposure to UV light are two common sources of free radicals. Decreasing damage from free radicals can reduce the risk of cataracts and macular degeneration.

Recommended: One to two servings of leafy greens daily, or supplement with 15 mg of lutein daily. I usually have my patients take a daily supplement that combines lutein (15 mg) with zeaxanthin (3 mg), another antioxidant. A study of 876 older adults found that those with the highest levels of these antioxidants were less likely to develop age-related macular degeneration.

VITAMINS C & E

Individually, these vitamins are among the most potent antioxidants. Taken together, they're very effective at preventing vision loss. Vitamin E blocks free radicals in the fatty parts of cells, such as in the macula of the eye, while vitamin C fortifies the watery portions in the cornea and retina.

For optimal protection, I recommend to my patients supplements of vitamins C and E, along with zinc and beta-carotene. Patients who take this combination daily can reduce their risk of vision loss. In patients who have age-related macular degeneration, these supplements can slow the disease's progression.

Recommended: Daily supplements with 400 IU of mixed natural vitamin E (a mixture of tocopherols and tocotrienols), 500 mg of vitamin C, 80 mg of zinc and 15 mg of beta-carotene.

GINKGO BILOBA

The herb ginkgo biloba blocks free radicals and dilates blood vessels, increasing circulation to the optic nerve. There is some evidence that it can improve peripheral vision in patients with glaucoma.

Recommended: 120 mg of ginkgo daily. Choose an extract that is standardized to 24% flavone glycosides.

Caution: Do not take a supplement with ginkgo if you are taking a prescription blood-thinning medication, such as *warfarin* (Coumadin).

N-ACETYL CARNOSINE

This naturally occurring molecule is composed of two amino acids.

A recent study found that *N-acetyl carnosine* (NAC) eyedrops improved visual acuity and glare sensitivity in patients with cataracts. During the two-year study, 90% of the eyes treated with NAC had significant improvements in vision.

Recommended: Patients with cataracts should ask their doctors about using topical NAC drops.

FISH OIL

About half of the retina consists of *docosahexaenoic acid* (DHA), a component in fish oil that provides the main structural support in cell membranes. DHA causes a significant drop in intraocular pressure—important for patients with glaucoma. Another component in fish oil, *eicosapentaenoic acid* (EPA), has anti-inflammatory effects and is thought to play an important role in maintaining visual acuity.

Recommended: Eat fish twice a week. Avoid fish high in mercury, including shark, swordfish, tilefish, king mackerel and large tuna, such as albacore, yellow-fin, bigeye and bluefin. Or take a fish-oil formula daily that includes 600 mg of EPA and 400 mg of DHA. Check with your doctor if you are on a blood thinner, such as warfarin.

MAGNESIUM AND CHROMIUM

Each of these minerals dilates blood vessels in the eye and reduces pressure from glaucoma. Chromium is particularly important for patients with diabetes, a common cause of vision loss. Chromium supplements help maintain an optimal blood-sugar balance and reduce the risk of glaucoma.

Recommended: Take 250 mg of magnesium (citrate or chelate) and 200 mcg of chromium (polynicotinate or picolinate) twice daily.

DIGESTIVE ENZYMES

Cells in the retina have an extremely high rate of metabolism. They require high levels of nutrients (along with blood and oxygen) for optimal function and to repair normal damage. Older adults often get insufficient nutrients, in part because levels of stomach acid decline with age and impair normal digestion.

Supplements that contain *betaine hydrochloride* mimic the *hydrochloric acid* normally produced by the stomach and can improve the digestion/absorption of eye-protecting nutrients, which are particularly helpful in the prevention and treatment of macular degeneration.

Recommended: One or two capsules of betaine hydrochloride with each meal.

Also helpful: One or two capsules of a full-spectrum plant-based enzyme (such as Longevity Science Total Gest) during or at the end of meals.

Caution: Patients who have active ulcers should not take digestive enzymes.

Natural Therapies That Help Heal Ulcers

James N. Dillard, MD, DC, assistant clinical professor at Columbia University College of Physicians and Surgeons and clinical director of Columbia's Rosenthal Center for Complementary and Alternative Medicine, both in New York City.

If you've got an ulcer, chances are you're taking an over-the-counter (OTC) antacid and/or prescription medication to neutralize gastric acid or inhibit its production. These medications include proton pump inhibitors (PPIs), such as *esomeprazole* (Nexium) and *lansoprazole* (Prevacid), and H2-blocking drugs, such as *cimetidine* (Tagamet) and *ranitidine* (Zantac).

What most people don't realize: There are several natural, complementary remedies that help reduce ulcer symptoms and promote healing while conventional treatment is under way. Some of these treatments also can help prevent ulcers in some patients.

WHAT CAUSES ULCERS

It's been more than 20 years since doctors learned that an infectious disease—rather than emotional stress—was the primary cause of most ulcers.

A screw-shaped bacterium, *Helicobacter pylori*, or *H. pylori*, burrows through the protective mucous lining in the small intestine and/or stomach, allowing harsh digestive fluids to accumulate and ulcerate the lining. About 50% of Americans over age 60 are infected with H. pylori. The bacterium doesn't always cause ulcers—but about 60% of patients with ulcers harbor H. pylori.

The remainder of ulcers are caused by regular use of stomach-damaging nonsteroidal anti-inflammatory drugs (NSAIDs), such as aspirin, *ibuprofen* (Advil) and *naproxen* (Aleve)…alcohol …and/or smoking. Excessive alcohol wears down the lining of the stomach and intestines. Nicotine causes the stomach to produce more acid.

Best complementary treatments…*

*Check with your doctor before taking supplements. They can interact with prescription medications.

NONDRUG THERAPIES

•**Probiotics.** The intestine contains up to four pounds of "friendly" bacteria, which aid digestion. There's some evidence that maintaining adequate levels of beneficial bacteria helps create an inhospitable environment for H. pylori and makes it harder for this ulcer-causing bacterium to thrive.

Self-defense: Take a probiotic supplement that contains *Lactobacillus acidophilus* and *Bifidobacterium bifidus*. These organisms create a healthful mix of bacteria and can inhibit the growth of harmful organisms. Probiotics are helpful if you've taken antibiotics, which can kill off some beneficial bacteria.

The optimal dose for probiotics hasn't been determined. Preliminary research cites a daily dose of up to 10 billion organisms—the amount usually included in one to two capsules. Probiotics are available at health-food stores.

•**Cabbage juice.** This folk remedy has some evidence to support it. Cabbage is high in vitamin C, which seems to inhibit growth of H. pylori. It also contains *glutamine*, an amino acid that may strengthen the protective lining in the stomach.

A small Stanford University School of Medicine study found that ulcer patients who drank about a quart of cabbage juice daily healed significantly faster than those who didn't drink it.

Self-defense: If you have an active ulcer, consider drinking a quart of cabbage juice (about the amount in half a head of cabbage) once daily for up to two weeks.

•**Deglycyrrhizinated licorice (DGL).** Herbalists often recommend fresh licorice root to heal ulcers. Licorice contains mucin, a substance that protects the stomach lining, and antioxidants that may inhibit H. pylori growth.

However, natural licorice can increase the effects of *aldosterone*, a hormone that promotes water retention and can increase blood pressure in some people. DGL supplements (available at health-food stores) are a better option, because the substances that increase blood pressure have been removed.

Self-defense: Take one DGL tablet before meals, and another before bed. DGL may be effective for people with ulcers whose H. pylori has been successfully treated with antibiotics but who still have some stomach irritation.

•**Vitamin A.** Vitamin A helps repair damaged mucous membranes. A report in the British medical journal *The Lancet* suggests that ulcers heal more quickly in patients given supplemental vitamin A.

Caution: High-dose vitamin A therapy can be toxic, so get your vitamin A from dietary sources along with a daily multivitamin—not from a separate vitamin A supplement.

Self-defense: Get 10,000 international units (IU) of vitamin A daily if you're undergoing ulcer treatment. (A multivitamin typically contains 3,500 IU to 5,000 IU of vitamin A.)

Good food sources: Beef liver (one-and-one-half ounces contains 13,593 IU)...carrots (one raw carrot contains 8,666 IU)...and spinach (one cup of raw spinach contains 2,813 IU).

•**Zinc.** Like vitamin A, zinc is involved in tissue healing. In Europe, a drug compound made with zinc plus an anti-inflammatory is often used for treating ulcers. Early studies indicate that zinc alone can speed ulcer healing and possibly even help prevent some ulcers.

Self-defense: Don't exceed the recommended daily intake (15 mg) of zinc. Take a daily multivitamin that includes zinc...and get adequate intake from dietary sources (five medium oysters, 13 mg...¾ cup fortified breakfast cereal, 15 mg...three-ounces lean beef tenderloin, 5 mg).

ANOTHER WAY TO FIGHT ULCERS

NSAIDs alleviate pain by inhibiting the production of pain-causing chemicals called *prostaglandins.* However, the body produces several kinds of prostaglandins, including some that protect the stomach lining. That's why NSAIDs, which block the production of pain-causing and stomach-protecting prostaglandins, make people who regularly use the drugs more susceptible to ulcers.

Self-defense: If you require regular pain relief, start with *acetaminophen* (Tylenol). It relieves pain without depleting stomach-protecting prostaglandins.

Caution: Taking more than the recommended dosage or drinking alcohol with acetaminophen can cause liver damage.

Also helpful: Ask your doctor about taking Arthrotec, a prescription drug combination that includes the NSAID *diclofenac* along with misoprostol, which protects the stomach and intestinal lining. One study found that patients taking Arthrotec experienced up to 80% fewer ulcers than those taking an NSAID alone.

Natural Remedies For Constipation

Dr. Mark Stengler is a licensed naturopathic medical doctor and a leading authority on the practice of alternative and integrated medicine. An associate clinical professor at the National College of Naturopathic Medicine in Portland, OR, Dr. Stengler has served on a medical advisory committee for the Yale University Complementary Medicine Outcomes Research Project and is the author or coauthor of 16 books, including two best sellers—*The Natural Physician's Healing Therapies* and *Prescription for Natural Cures.* (Both from Bottom Line Books). Dr. Stengler is the founder and director of the La Jolla Whole Health Clinic in La Jolla, CA. *www.DrStengler.com.*

Constipation is one of the most common digestive complaints, accounting for about 2.5 million doctor visits every year. But it occurs much more frequently than this number indicates because the majority of people with constipation treat it at home with over-the-counter laxatives.

Big mistake: Regular use of certain laxatives can make constipation worse by damaging the large intestine, making it "lazier" and even less efficient.

Most patients who experience constipation can prevent it permanently with dietary changes and other natural approaches. Even patients who have had constipation for years often can restore normal bowel function within two weeks.

WHAT'S NORMAL?

In a healthy body, waste travels through the digestive tract in a predictable, regular cycle, over a period of six to 24 hours. Most people have one to three bowel movements daily. Others have as few as three bowel movements a week. There's a lot of individual variability—what's normal for you might not be normal for someone else.

Red flag: Any change in your normal bowel habits. See a doctor if the frequency of bowel movements changes…you have blood in your stool…or you are experiencing intense abdominal pain. Constipation by itself is rarely dangerous, but it may be a sign of other problems, including colon cancer.

Stool in the intestine contains bacteria, fungi and metabolic by-products of digestion. If it remains in the colon for too long, these harmful substances cause a number of uncomfortable symptoms, such as bloating, painfully hard stools and a general sense of fatigue.

SUPPLEMENTS & FOODS

The right diet and supplements can relieve constipation. *Best choices…*

•**High-fiber foods,** including brown rice, whole-wheat bread, oatmeal, fruits, vegetables and legumes, such as beans and lentils. Fiber absorbs water in the intestine, which makes the stool bulkier. This triggers the intestinal contractions that cause bowel movements. Fiber also makes the stool softer, so it is easier to pass.

•**Psyllium.** If you don't eat a lot of plant foods, you can supplement with an over-the-counter product containing *psyllium* (such as Metamucil), following the directions on the label. Or take one teaspoon of ground psyllium seed husks twice daily. Psyllium acts as a bulking agent and increases the frequency—and comfort—of bowel movements. Be sure to drink plenty of water or juice to avoid making constipation worse.

•**Ground flaxseed** also works. It's a highly concentrated source of fiber, with the added benefit of supplying healthful omega-3 fatty acids. Have one to two tablespoons of ground flaxseed daily. You can sprinkle it on yogurt or cereal or just eat it plain. Be sure to drink at least 10 ounces of water with it. Don't eat whole flaxseed. It has a tough outer coating that is not broken down during digestion.

•**Stool softeners.** Common ones, such as *docusate* (Colace), are not laxatives and not habit forming, but you can get similar results with flaxseed oil. Take one to two tablespoons daily. The oil can go in a shake or on a salad.

•**Magnesium.** People with constipation often are deficient in this mineral. Magnesium helps in three ways—it increases the strength and regularity of the intestine's muscular contractions…it relaxes the nervous system…and at higher doses, it promotes the accumulation of water in the intestine, which boosts bowel function.

Foods high in magnesium: Green, leafy vegetables (such as spinach), brown rice, avocado, berries, cabbage, broccoli and bananas.

If you have acute constipation, take 250 mg of magnesium two to four times daily. Don't take supplemental magnesium for more than about a week. It can lead to dependence—reducing the colon's natural ability to contract—and can interfere with the normal absorption of nutrients. Don't take supplemental magnesium if you are pregnant unless authorized by your doctor.

•**Fermented foods.** People who eat sauerkraut, live-culture yogurt and/or kefir (a fermented milk) are less likely to experience constipation because fermented foods contain probiotics. These beneficial organisms crowd out harmful microbes that may impair digestion and elimination.

Eat fermented foods daily, or take a probiotic supplement. Look for a product that provides at least four billion active organisms, preferably a combination of *Lactobacillus acidophilus* and bifidus bacteria.

•**Milk thistle (Silybum marianum).** A traditional remedy for hepatitis, milk thistle improves the flow of bile, a digestive juice that breaks down fats in the intestinal tract. Bile improves the colon's motility (the ability of the colon to contract and eliminate wastes).

Dose: 200 mg to 250 mg of a product standardized to 80% silymarin (the active ingredient) with meals twice daily for six to eight weeks. Don't take it if you are pregnant or breastfeeding.

HOMEOPATHY

In homeopathy, individuals are given very small amounts of substances that would produce the same or similar symptoms of an illness in a healthy person if given in larger doses. These remedies stimulate the body's defenses to prevent or treat an illness.

It can be a challenge to find the right homeopathic remedy for constipation—but when it works, the results can be impressive. It's safe to self-medicate with homeopathy, but people tend to have better results when they work with a trained practitioner who can match specific remedies with symptoms. *Remedies to try...*

•**Alumina** is recommended for patients who typically go several days without having a bowel movement.

•**Calcarea carbonica** is for patients with chronic constipation who often feel cold, have clammy hands and/or feet and experience a lot of stress.

•**Lycopodium** is helpful for patients who experience gas and bloating along with constipation.

For each remedy, take two pellets of 30C potency twice daily for two weeks (or follow directions on the label).

GIVE UP DAIRY

A *New England Journal of Medicine* study of 65 children with chronic constipation reported that cow's milk was the cause in two-thirds of cases. It contains the protein casein, which has been shown to cause constipation.

Also, reduce the amount of saturated fats in your diet. A diet high in saturated fat slows motility—and the longer the stool stays in the intestine, the more likely it is to harden and interfere with normal bowel movements.

DAILY EXERCISE

Mild-to-moderate aerobic exercise—a 30-minute brisk walk, for example—helps stimulate intestinal contractions. It also reduces stress and relaxes the nervous system, which improves muscle movements in the intestine and helps prevent or treat constipation.

STRESS CONTROL

Yoga, Pilates, meditation and other stress-reducing activities can reduce constipation. Studies show that people who experience high levels of stress often have reduced intestinal efficiency. In addition, people with high stress levels often have hectic lifestyles and don't take the time for regular bowel movements. Every day, set aside time for mental and physical relaxation.

How to Avoid Dangerous Herb-Drug Interactions

Catherine Ulbricht, PharmD, is the senior attending pharmacist at Massachusetts General Hospital in Boston. She is editor-in-chief of *Journal of Herbal Pharmacotherapy* and cofounder of Natural Standard (*www.naturalstandard.com*), a Web site dedicated to the scientific study of integrated medicine. She is coeditor of *Natural Standard Herb & Supplement Handbook: The Clinical Bottom Line.* C.V. Mosby.

An increasing number of American adults now take herbs or nutritional supplements for a wide range of ailments, including arthritis, depression and nausea.

Problem: Unlike prescription drugs, herbal supplements are not regulated by the FDA, so there are no labeling requirements regarding potential interactions with prescription or over-the-counter (OTC) drugs.

Whether they are used in capsules, extracts, liquid, cream or tea, many herbal products can be harmful when combined with prescription or OTC medication.

What happens: Some herbs can interact with medications by affecting their absorption, metabolism or by other mechanisms. As a result, drug levels may become too high or too low.

Catherine Ulbricht, PharmD, is a pharmacist at Massachusetts General Hospital and one of the country's leading experts on herb-drug interactions. *Her advice on commonly used herbs...* *

CAYENNE

Cayenne is also known as chili or red pepper. Cayenne's active component, capsaicin, which is used as a spice in food, is commonly used as a pain reliever in prescription medicine, often for osteoarthritis, rheumatoid arthritis and diabetic neuropathy (nerve pain resulting from diabetes).

Possible interactions: When combined with aspirin, *ibuprofen* (Advil) or any other nonsteroidal anti-inflammatory drug (NSAID), cayenne may increase these drugs' side effects, especially gastrointestinal (GI) upset. In some people, cayenne also may enhance the pain-relieving action of NSAIDs.

Like NSAIDs, cayenne can have a blood-thinning effect, increasing the risk for bleeding.

*Check with your doctor or pharmacist before taking any herbal product.

(When used topically, this risk is lessened because lower doses of cayenne are absorbed.) Do not use cayenne if you take a *monoamine oxidase* (MAO) inhibitor antidepressant, such as *phenelzine* (Nardil).

Caution: Avoid getting cayenne (in any form) in your eyes, nose, etc., where it can cause burning or stinging.

GINGER

Ginger is a popular antidote for nausea and/or vomiting. Research suggests that ginger also may help prevent blood clotting and reduce blood sugar levels.

Possible interactions: If you take an NSAID or antiplatelet drug, such as *clopidogrel* (Plavix), ginger may further increase bleeding risk.

Caution: Although there's strong evidence that it is particularly effective for nausea and/or vomiting in pregnant women, high-dose supplemental ginger (more than 1 g daily) is not recommended during pregnancy because of possible fetal damage and/or increased bleeding risk. Because of the lack of long-term studies on ginger, consult your doctor before taking it for an extended period of time.

GREEN TEA

As scientific evidence has revealed the disease-fighting benefits of antioxidant-rich green tea, an increasing number of Americans have begun drinking it—or, in some cases, taking it in capsules or extracts. Although new research questions the health benefits of green tea, some studies have found that it may help prevent cancer, especially malignancies of the GI tract, breast and lung. More investigation is needed to confirm these findings. To read more about clinical trials on green tea, go to the National Institutes of Health's Web site, *www.clinicaltrials.gov.*

Possible interactions: Most forms of green tea contain caffeine, which may intensify the effect of any medication that increases blood pressure and/or heart rate, such as the decongestant *pseudoephedrine* (Sudafed). Decaffeinated green tea is available, but this form still contains some caffeine and may not have the same health benefits.

Caution: People with arrhythmia (abnormal heart rhythm) should consume no more than moderate amounts of green tea, determined by their personal sensitivity to caffeine.

LICORICE

Licorice contains a compound known as glycyrrhizin, which has antiviral properties. For this reason, licorice is often used to treat the common cold and herpes infections (including cold sores). However, some studies have shown that topical licorice cream does not help genital herpes.

Possible interactions: Licorice can interact with diuretics, such as *chlorothiazide* (Diuril) and *furosemide* (Lasix), and any medication that affects hormone levels, such as birth control pills.

Caution: It also may increase blood pressure and bleeding risk.

MILK THISTLE

This popular herb is used for liver problems, including cirrhosis and hepatitis. These benefits are well documented by research.

Possible interactions: Milk thistle may interfere with how the liver breaks down certain drugs, such as antibiotics and antifungals. Milk thistle also may interact with the anticonvulsant *phenytoin* (Dilantin). The herb may lower blood sugar and cause heartburn, nausea and vomiting or other GI upset.

Caution: If you take diabetes medication, do not use milk thistle unless you are supervised by a health-care professional.

ST. JOHN'S WORT

St. John's wort is commonly used for depression. Several studies show that it may work as well as a prescription antidepressant, such as *paroxetine* (Paxil), for mild to moderate depressive disorders. More research is needed before St. John's wort can be recommended for severe depression.

Possible interactions: St. John's wort may interact with drugs that are broken down by the liver, including birth control pills, the blood thinner *warfarin* (Coumadin) and migraine medications. People who take St. John's wort may experience stomach upset, fatigue, sexual dysfunction, dizziness or headaches.

Caution: St. John's wort should not be taken with prescription antidepressant medication.

Stop Pain Without Drugs

Donna Finando, a Roslyn Heights, NY–based licensed acupuncturist (LAc) and massage therapist (LMT). She is the author of the *Trigger Point Self-Care Manual for Pain-Free Movement*. Inner Traditions.

Most over-the-counter and prescription pain relievers temporarily ease aches and pains, but these medications do not address the root cause of the problem. In a surprising number of cases, muscular tightness is responsible for common types of pain.

Here's what happens: When any one of the more than 200 muscles in your body suffers from overuse or an injury, it can develop a trigger point—a tiny knot in which a strand of the muscle becomes constricted, making the muscle stiff and weak.

Left untreated, this condition can persist for years, causing pain to recur repeatedly. Fortunately, you can relieve this type of pain with a simple technique known as trigger-point therapy. It involves locating the associated trigger points and compressing them for 20 to 30 seconds several times a day. Press only hard enough to feel the tightness of the muscle and the soreness of the trigger point. Stretches for each condition (as shown) also should be repeated several times daily.

Helpful: Whenever possible, also apply 20 minutes of moist heat once or twice a day to the affected muscle. Moist heat brings blood and body fluids to the muscle, increasing circulation. (Moist heating pads by Cara, Sunbeam or Thermophore can be purchased at most drugstores for $20 to $50.)

If you've worked on your muscles for several days and felt little or no relief, check with your doctor to make sure there is no other source of pain, such as arthritis.

Conditions often caused by trigger points—and how to treat them...

STIFF NECK

Stiff neck frequently occurs after sleeping with your head turned all the way to one side, or as a result of holding a phone between your ear and shoulder. The condition is often due to a trigger point in the levator scapulae muscle, which runs from the inner edge of the shoulder blade to the neck.

To find the trigger point: Reach the hand that is on your pain-free side over to touch your shoulder on the painful side. Locate the inside edge of the shoulder blade, then move your hand a bit closer to your spine, feeling for a hard band the size of a pencil running up toward your neck. While bending your neck toward your pain-free side, use your fingers to locate a tender spot along this band, then press it for 20 to 30 seconds.

Helpful stretch: Turn your chin 30 degrees away from the affected side, then drop your chin down slightly toward your chest. Hold for a slow count of 20.

HIP, BUTTOCK AND LEG PAIN

Pain in the hips, buttocks or legs is often diagnosed as sciatica (pain in your back that radiates into your buttocks and legs) when it actually may be caused by trigger points in the muscles of the back and buttocks. One of these muscles, the gluteus medius, lies midway between the top of your pelvis and the top of your thighbone.

To find the trigger point: Lie on the floor on your pain-free side with your knees slightly bent, and use your fingers to massage your hip under the top of your pelvis and down toward the top of your thighbone. If trigger points are present, you'll feel taut bands and tender spots. Once you've located a tender spot, roll onto your painful side and place a tennis ball between this spot and the floor. Then let your weight press the ball into the tender area for 20 to 30 seconds.

Helpful stretch: Stand facing a wall with your arms raised and the backs of your hands pressed against your forehead. Cross your pain-free leg in front of your other leg. Bend the knee of your rear leg into the back of your pain-free leg while shifting your weight onto your painful hip. This should create a stretch between your pelvis and the top of your thighbone. Hold for a slow count of 20.

CALF PAIN

If you're experiencing pain or soreness in your calf or the back of your knee, it may be caused by trigger points in the gastrocnemius muscle (the large muscle that gives the calf its characteristic shape).

To find the trigger point: Sit in a chair and place the sole of the foot of your affected leg on a footstool or coffee table in front of you. Place one hand on the outer side of this leg and the other on the inner side of this leg—in both cases, just above the ankle. Run your fingers along your Achilles tendon (the large tendon at the back of your heel) and work your way to the middle of the calf, feeling for tender spots. Continue upward, toward the back of the knee. When you find a tender spot, compress it with your fingers for 20 to 30 seconds.

Helpful stretch: While standing about 12 inches from a wall, facing the wall, place your hands on the wall at chest level. Keeping your feet hip-width apart and the toes of both feet facing the wall, move your painful leg 18 inches behind the other leg. Bend your front knee, keeping your rear leg straight. Your weight should remain on the front leg. Hold for a slow count of 20.

TENNIS ELBOW

Inflammation of the tendon on the outside of the elbow, known as "tennis elbow," can cause sharp pain down the back of the forearm into the wrist, making it hard to grip objects. However, sometimes the condition may not be an inflammation but a result of trigger points in the extensor muscles of the hand and fingers, which can be caused by repeated or forceful gripping, such as when holding a tennis racket—or even a coffee cup.

To find the trigger point: Rest the elbow and forearm of your sore arm on a table, with your palm facing up. Use your opposite hand to feel along the muscle on the outside (thumb side) of your elbow crease, then follow this muscle down toward your hand. When you find a tender spot, press down and hold for 20 to 30 seconds.

Helpful stretch: Sit on a chair, and keeping your elbow straight, place the back of the hand on the affected arm flat on the seat beside you, palm up, feeling a stretch in your forearm. Hold for a slow count of 20.

Illustrations by Shawn Banner.

Echinacea Warning: Could It Increase Colon Cancer?

Journal of Clinical Pharmacy and Therapeutics.

The popular herbal cold remedy Echinacea may increase concentrations of gastrointestinal bacteria linked with colon cancer, say University of Arkansas researchers.

In their study, daily doses of Echinacea purpurea, a commonly used variety of the popular supplement, were given to 15 healthy adults for 10 days. Then researchers analyzed their stool samples.

The researchers found increased concentrations of anaerobic Bacteroides bacteria in general and of Bacteroides fragilis in particular. Bacteroides play a role in the normal functioning of the colon but, under certain conditions, they can also act as cancer-causing pathogens. This is especially true of B. fragilis strains, say the researchers.

Worth noting: Increased Bacterioides concentrations have been reported in people at high risk for colon cancer. And previous research shows that B. fragilis may contribute to inflammatory bowel disease and diarrhea.

■ ■ ■ ■

Another Opinion: Echinacea Is Effective

The herb echinacea does boost the immune system and helps to fight upper-respiratory tract infections, despite a recent study indicating the contrary, says Mark A. Stengler, ND. The study dosages (1 gram daily) was too low. During acute illnesses, such as colds, flu, bronchitis and ear infections, echinacea should be taken in high doses of 2 milliliters of liquid extract or two 300-mg capsules every two waking hours for the first 24 hours and every three hours after that. It is helpful as a skin ointment for wounds, eczema and burns. It also may be effective for sore throats and as a cream for rheumatoid arthritis. Check with your doctor before starting treatment.

Dr. Mark Stengler is a licensed naturopathic medical doctor and a leading authority on the practice of alternative and integrated medicine. An associate clinical professor at the National College of Naturopathic Medicine in Portland, OR, Dr. Stengler has served on a medical advisory committee for the Yale University Complementary Medicine Outcomes Research Project and is the author or coauthor of 16 books, including two best sellers—*The Natural Physician's Healing Therapies* and *Prescription for Natural Cures.* (Both from Bottom Line Books). Dr. Stengler is the founder and director of the La Jolla Whole Health Clinic in La Jolla, CA. *www.DrStengler.com.*

Easing Depression Without a Prescription

Nadia Marsh, MD, chief, division of geriatrics, Cabrini Medical Center, New York City.

James Blumenthal, PhD, professor of psychology, Duke University, Durham, NC.

You can treat depression without drugs. Studies show for some patients, effective relief may result from activities such as exercise and spending time with friends.

"These are things that are certainly worth trying and are generally healthy, anyway," says Dr. Nadia Marsh, an expert in treating depression and chief of the division of geriatrics at Cabrini Medical Center in New York City.

People with mild depression will likely benefit most from such natural remedies; those with major depression typically need medication such as serotonin reuptake inhibitors (SSRIs) like Prozac or Zoloft, she says. *Here's what some research reveals...*

THE EFFECT OF EXERCISE

"Exercise, at least when performed in a group setting, seems to be at least as effective as standard antidepressant medications in reducing symptoms in patients with major depression," says researcher James Blumenthal, a professor of medical psychology at Duke University. In his study, 10 months of regular, moderate exercise reduced depressive symptoms at a rate equal to that of Zoloft.

Explanation: In addition to boosting "feel-good" hormones that boost mood and help ease stress, "people who exercise also tend to feel that they have more control over their life," notes Marsh. That's important, since a persistent feeling of helplessness is a hallmark of depression.

In another study, researchers at the University of Texas Southwestern Medical Center at Dallas note that 30-minute workouts, done three to five times a week, cut depressive symptoms in half in young adults.

THE POWER OF PALS

It's clear that social interaction—contact with friends, family, clubs and group activities—can boost mood and help ease depression.

"If you're socially isolated, especially, just reaching out can help," Marsh says. "It can have a huge impact on how people see themselves and help them to 'reorient.'"

SHORT-TERM STRATEGIES

Interventions such as massage therapy, acupuncture or aromatherapy are also being explored as alternatives—or additions—to medication in treating depression. So far, the evidence suggests they are great at easing short-term stress. "But the real issue, when it comes to depression, is what is the effect over the long term?" Marsh asks. "Right now, nobody really knows."

What is known: There's little evidence to support the use of folate or other B vitamins to ward off the blues. And the popular herbal remedy St. John's wort seems to be ineffective for moderate-to-severe depression. For milder cases, "it's unclear what the correct dose should be; the studies have been all over the map," says Marsh.

In fact, she warns that taking St. John's wort while on SSRIs can hurt the effectiveness of the prescription medication and raises the risk of dangerous side effects. St. John's wort can be especially dangerous for cancer patients on chemotherapy. Always let your doctor know what over-the-counter medications, herbal or otherwise, you might be taking she adds.

info To learn more about depression, visit the US National Institute of Mental Health's Web site at *www.nimh.nih.gov.*

Talk Away Depression

Journal of Consulting and Clinical Psychology.

Adding a little telephone-based counseling talk to the typical treatment for depression—medication—goes a long way in helping to overcome the illness, concludes the largest study of phone-based counseling to date.

Among the 400 patients studied, those who received brief phone-based psychotherapy soon after they started taking antidepressants fared better than those getting meds alone.

Researchers say those getting talk time reported better improvement in symptoms, higher satisfaction with their treatment, and were more likely to continue taking their drugs than those getting meds alone.

And these positive effects continued for up to 18 months after the first telephone consult, says lead researcher Evette J. Ludman of the Group Health Center for Health Studies in Seattle. She notes the benefits were more pronounced in patients with moderate to severe depression than those with milder forms of the disease.

The secret may be in what is said: During these phone sessions, therapists encouraged patients to identify and counter their negative thoughts, to pursue activities they had enjoyed in the past, and to develop a plan to care for themselves.

Take a Deep Breath —Anger May Be Tough on Lungs

Rosalind Wright, MD, assistant professor of medicine, Harvard Medical School, and assistant professor of society, human development and health, Harvard School of Public Health, Boston.

Norman Edelman, MD, chief medical officer, American Lung Association.

Thorax.

Keeping your temper in check may do more than help your heart—it may also prolong lung health.

New research shows that long-term hostility could damage lung function and speed the natural age-related decline in lung power.

"Psychological stress and distress and negative emotional states like hostility can disrupt immune function and trigger inflammatory processes, much like allergens in the environment," says study author Dr. Rosalind Wright, assistant professor of medicine at Harvard Medical School.

Hostility and anger is already linked with many other health problems in older adults, including heart disease and asthma. But until now, there had been little specific research into how these types of psychological factors affect lung function decline.

THE FINDINGS

To see if there was any link between anger and hostility and the way the lungs work, Wright and her colleagues examined 670 men aged 45 to 86.

Levels of hostility, measured at the beginning of the study, averaged 18.5 points on a standard scale, with values ranging from seven to 37 points. Lung function appeared to decline as anger numbers rose, and vice-versa.

The association held steady even after adjusting for smoking, educational attainment and other factors.

THE THEORY

How might anger be linked to lung function? "A person who tends to be more hostile might be more likely to adopt negative coping strategies, such as smoking," says Wright. "But that didn't seem to be the case. We controlled for smoking."

Interestingly, those with higher levels of hostility also had a faster rate of natural decline in lung function, say researchers.

Because all of the participants were older, white men, the results cannot be extrapolated to other groups. The findings also can't be taken to suggest that there is a cause-and-effect relationship between hostility and anger and declining lung function, add the scientists. For now, they are noting an association.

Dr. Norman Edelman, chief medical officer at the American Lung Association, says he's not surprised by Wright's study. "There's lots of biological plausibility, lots of mechanisms by which this could take place."

The bottom line: Wright hopes her findings provide more incentive for people to manage their mood for better health.

"Psychological stress seems to trigger similar types of biological disruptions," she says. "When you have something throwing the system out of balance, that might put you in a state of chronic inflammation. If you raise someone's awareness about their emotional state or personality disposition or level of stress, they can modify their lifestyle or use interventions like cognitive behavioral therapy."

info For more information about lung heath, visit the American Lung Association at *www.lungusa.org.*

Foods Fight Headaches

Elaine Magee, MPH, RD, registered dietitian, Pleasant Hill, CA, and author of 25 books on nutrition, including *Tell Me What to Eat If I Have Headaches and Migraines.* New Page.

More than 45 million Americans annually seek medical treatment for frequent or severe headaches. Doctors have identified dozens of headache triggers, including stress, air pollution and weather changes, but one of the main triggers—especially for migraines—is diet.

At least 30% of migraine patients have one or more food triggers. In some cases, a single food may be responsible. Most patients have combination triggers—for example, red wine plus a high level of stress plus an extra cup of coffee in the morning.

Everyone who experiences migraines and other types of headaches should keep a food and lifestyle diary. Write down the foods and beverages you consume. Also note patterns that precede headaches—exercise activities, changes in sleep, stress level, menstrual cycle, etc. After a few weeks, review your diary and identify likely connections.

WHAT TO AVOID

•**Caffeine** is one of the main headache triggers. Some people get headaches when they consume any caffeine. Others get headaches when they consume less than they usually do and then need caffeine to relieve the headache.

If you drink coffee or other caffeinated beverages regularly, blood vessels in the brain become sensitized to the caffeine's effects. Eliminating or cutting back on caffeine causes rebound headaches in about half of patients.

People with chronic headaches often are advised to eliminate caffeine completely. Instead of quitting abruptly, gradually taper off. If you're used to drinking three cups of coffee a day, drink only two cups daily for a week. For several days after that, substitute decaf for one of your daily servings. Then dilute your regular coffee with decaf until you quit entirely.

•**High-fat foods.** Significantly reducing dietary fat decreases the frequency and intensity of headaches. Try to limit total fat intake to 20% of total calories. In particular, avoid saturated fats (mainly found in meats, fast food and full-fat dairy products) and trans fats (often called "partially hydrogenated oils" on labels and found in margarines, snack foods and packaged baked goods).

Tyramine is a natural by-product of the amino acid tyrosine. Foods that are aged or fermented tend to be high in tyramine, which can cause vascular spasms that result in migraines.

Main offenders: Red wine, aged cheeses including blue and cheddar, deli meats and overripe bananas.

Stick with fresh meats and cheeses such as cottage cheese, ricotta and fresh mozzarella. White wine and beer have less tyramine than red wine—but any alcohol can trigger headaches.

•**Food additives,** including monosodium glutamate (MSG), nitrates and nitrites, dilate blood vessels and trigger migraines in people who are sensitive to these additives. Nitrates and nitrites are found mainly in processed meats, such as hot dogs, bacon and salami. MSG is added to literally thousands of processed foods. Check food labels, and avoid products that contain any of these additives.

FOODS THAT HELP

•**Omega-3 fatty acids.** The healthful fats in fish, flaxseeds and olive oil can reduce migraines by stimulating the production of body chemicals that inhibit inflammation in blood vessels in the brain.

Recommended: Two to three servings of fish weekly. Also, have one tablespoon daily of ground flaxseed (you can add it to cereal or smoothies or sprinkle on salads or yogurt). Cook with olive oil or canola oil, which contain more omega-3s than other vegetable oils.

•**Magnesium.** There is some evidence that adequate magnesium intake can help women prevent headaches (including migraines) associated with menstruation. The recommended daily intake for most women is 320 milligrams (mg). High-magnesium foods include whole grains, nuts, seeds, soy foods, legumes and dark green vegetables.

Examples: Almonds, two tablespoons (86 mg of magnesium)…artichoke, one medium (180 mg)…brown rice, two-thirds cup (57 mg)…peanut butter, two tablespoons (51 mg)…pumpkin seeds, two tablespoons (152 mg)…cooked spinach, one-half cup (78 mg)…tofu, one-half cup (118 mg).

•**Water helps prevent dehydration**—a common cause of headaches. Try to drink eight eight-ounce glasses every day.

■ ■ ■ ■

Natural Remedies for Heartburn

Many people who suffer from heartburn take over-the-counter antacids or expensive prescription medication, such as *esomeprazole* (Nexium) and *lansoprazole* (Prevacid). These treatments can help but often cause side effects, such as diarrhea and dry mouth.

Heartburn, a sharp, burning pain under the rib cage, occurs when stomach contents "back up" (reflux) into the esophagus.

Chamomile, ginger and deglycyrrhizinated licorice have long been used (in tea, extract and tincture) to relieve heartburn as well as indigestion and intestinal irritation. Their effectiveness is supported by anecdotal evidence.

For relief proven in clinical studies, try pectin, a substance found in the outer skin and rind of fruits and vegetables. Apples and bananas are among the best sources of pectin. If you suffer from heartburn, try eating an apple (do not choose green or other tart varieties) or a banana to see if it relieves your symptoms.

Pectin supplements, which are available at most health-food stores, are another option. Take at the onset of heartburn until it subsides. For dosage, follow label instructions. Pectin supplements are generally safe but may interfere with the absorption of some medications, so check with your doctor before trying this supplement.

Caution: Chronic heartburn (more than twice a week) may indicate gastroesophageal reflux disease (GERD), a condition that should be treated by a gastroenterologist.

Ara DerMarderosian, PhD, is professor of pharmacognosy (the study of natural products used in medicine) and Roth chair of natural products at the University of the Sciences in Philadelphia. He also is the scientific director of the university's Complementary and Alternative Medicines Institute.

11

Nutrition, Diet & Fitness

Gain Weight, Lose Brain Power?

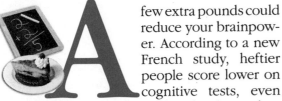

A few extra pounds could reduce your brainpower. According to a new French study, heftier people score lower on cognitive tests, even when factors such as education level are taken into account.

"These tests are sensitive enough to detect small variations in scientific studies. However, in a middle-aged, healthy, active population, these differences in the cognitive performances may be hardly perceived by individuals," said study author Dr. Maxime Cournot, a researcher with the Toulouse University Hospital and the National Institute of Health and Medical Research in France.

THE STUDY

Following up on previous studies linking weight and cognition, the new study aimed to find out if there is a connection in middle-aged healthy people.

To do so, the researchers analyzed statistics from a survey of 2,223 salaried French workers in 1996 and 2001. The workers were between 32 and 62 years old when the study began.

The study authors first calculated each participant's body-mass index (BMI), a ratio of weight and height. For reference, a 5-foot-5-inch woman weighing 139 pounds has a BMI of 23, which is considered normal. Statistical overweight begins at a BMI of 25, and obesity starts at a BMI of 30.

The team then compared BMI to the results of cognitive tests.

RESULTS

People with higher BMIs scored lower on cognitive tests that examined memory, attention

Maxime Cournot, MD, assistant professor, clinical epidemiology & preventive cardiology, department of epidemiology, Toulouse University Hospital and the National Institute of Health and Medical Research, Toulouse, France.

David Knopman, MD, professor, neurology, Mayo Clinic College of Medicine, Rochester, MN.

American Academy of Neurology news release. *Neurology.*

and thought-processing. For example, people on the thin side—with a BMI of 20—remembered an average of nine of 16 words in a memory test. On the other hand, those with a BMI of 30 remembered an average of seven words.

Those with higher BMIs also scored lower on the tests five years later.

The differences held up even when the numbers were adjusted for the possible influences of education level, age, gender and other factors.

EXPLANATION

How might obesity affect the brain? It's possible that excess weight could help clog the arteries in the brain just as it does in the heart, according to Dr. Cournot. It's also possible, she added, that obesity could disrupt hormones, such as insulin, that affect brain cells.

Dr. David Knopman, a professor of neurology at Mayo Clinic College of Medicine, is familiar with the findings. He said the real culprits could be diabetes and high blood pressure, both of which are "more strongly and consistently linked to both cognitive decline and dementia risk."

The study results need to be confirmed by other researchers, Cournot said, but they still support the general recommendation that people eat right and exercise to avoid obesity.

Knopman agreed. The study findings suggest that "obesity in midlife may have long-term consequences for the brain, not just for the heart," he said.

MORE INFORMATION

info To learn more about weight, visit the Obesity Society at *www.obesity.org*.

■ ■ ■ ■

Obesity Increases Dementia Risk

Obese people are twice as likely to develop dementia.

Theory: Obesity is associated with cardiovascular disease, which may impair blood flow to the brain and lead to dementia. Obesity is defined as a body mass index (BMI) of 30 or greater. Go to the CDC's Web site, *www.cdc. gov/nccdphp/dnpa/bmi*.

If your BMI is 30 or greater: Lose weight to reduce your dementia risk.

Miia Kivipelto, MD, PhD, postdoctoral fellow in geriatric epidemiology, the Karolinska Institutet, Stockholm, Sweden.

Exercise Reverses Damage from A High-Fat Meal

Janet P. Wallace, PhD, professor, kinesiology, Indiana University, Bloomington.

Jeannie Moloo, RD, PhD, spokeswoman, American Dietetic Association, and registered dietitian, Sacramento, CA.
European Journal of Applied Physiology.

So, you've just polished off a meal high in fat, and now you're feeling guilty? Wait an hour or two, then get a little exercise, and you can reverse the potential damage to your arteries, a new study suggests.

And you don't even have to head to the gym for that exercise. "We're talking about a walk, we're not talking about changing your clothes and sweating," said Janet P. Wallace, a professor of kinesiology at Indiana University, and lead investigator for the study.

BACKGROUND

According to Wallace, after a fatty meal, arteries lose their ability to expand in response to an increase in blood flow. The effect peaks four to six hours after eating—usually just in time for your next meal. So, four hours after a fatty meal, your arteries look like those of a person with heart disease, she said.

"That post-meal period is a hot topic among all the researchers in heart disease, diabetes and obesity," Wallace said. "That period sets up the environment for the artery to be unhealthy."

THE STUDY

Wallace and her colleagues studied eight healthy 25-year-olds. Each of the participants—five men and three women—completed three scenarios. They ate a low-fat breakfast, a high-fat breakfast and a high-fat breakfast followed two hours later by a 45-minute walk on a treadmill at a moderate pace. Each meal totaled 940 calories and the high-fat meal contained about 48 grams of fat and the low-fat meal actually contained no fat.

The researchers used a blood pressure cuff to measure blood flow in the brachial artery, the major blood vessel of the upper arm, before and after each scenario.

RESULTS

"The brachial artery represents what is going on in the arteries of the heart," Wallace said. "The ideal range is about 6% to 10%," she said.

After the high-fat meal alone, the brachial artery dilation dropped from 6% to 4%, Wallace said. "A range of 3% to 5% is not good."

After the low-fat meal, dilation went from 6% to 6.5%, a slight improvement. After the high-fat meal and exercise, it went from 6% (before the meal) to 8.5%.

"Exercise does great things, and this obviously shows exercise is very effective in counteracting that high-fat meal," Wallace added.

MORE RESEARCH

Next, Wallace hopes to study the effect of exercise *before* a high-fat meal. "I think we will find it works as well." She emphasized that her research isn't meant to encourage people to indulge in high-fat fare. But she's realistic. "There are people who are going to eat high-fat meals," she said.

Jeannie Moloo, a Sacramento, California, registered dietitian and a spokeswoman for the American Dietetic Association, offered a caveat about the study. "We need to keep in mind the results apply only to the population investigated and that was young, healthy and physically active adults. The small number of subjects, only eight, makes it difficult to tell if there are differences in responses between men and women."

info To learn more about a healthy diet, visit the Web site of the American Dietetic Association at *www.eatright.org.*

■ ■ ■ ■

Exercise Controls Triglyceride Levels

Eating high-fat foods, such as whipped cream and chocolate, causes triglyceride levels to spike, increasing heart disease risk.

Recent study: Triglyceride levels of all participants who ate high-fat foods rose, but the levels of those who exercised for 90 minutes before eating were 25% lower than the levels of nonexercisers.

Jason M.R. Gill, PhD, researcher, department of vascular biochemistry, University of Glasgow, Glasgow Royal Infirmary, Scotland, and leader of a study of triglycerides, published in *Journal of the American College of Cardiology.*

Hair Analysis May Help Detect Eating Disorders

Kent Hatch, PhD, assistant professor, integrative biology, Brigham Young University, Provo, UT.

Cynthia M. Bulik, PhD, William and Jeanne Jordan Distinguished Professor of Eating Disorders, and director, eating disorders program, University of North Carolina at Chapel Hill.

Rapid Communications in Mass Spectrometry.

Eating disorders can be difficult to diagnose, often because patients don't realize they have a problem or they try to hide it. But researchers at Brigham Young University (BYU) say they've developed a new test that can determine whether someone is struggling with conditions such as anorexia nervosa and bulimia.

"Your body records your eating habits in the hair. So, we can use that to tell the nutritional health of an individual." As hair grows, new proteins are added to the base of each strand, pushing the strand up and out of the hair follicle. These proteins are influenced by what you eat. So, each strand of hair is a chemical "diary" that is a record of day-to-day nutrition, said lead researcher Kent Hatch, an assistant professor of integrative biology at BYU.

HOW IT WORKS

The new test analyzes two molecules, carbon and nitrogen. Based on the makeup of these molecules, the researchers said they've been able to diagnose eating disorders.

"By taking some hairs from an individual and analyzing it for carbon and nitrogen, we can tell with 80% accuracy whether someone has anorexia or bulimia," Hatch said. "The test provides an objective way of discerning whether they have an eating disorder."

The goal of the study was to see if the molecular patterns differed between people with eating disorders and those with normal eating behaviors. The test was so powerful that it required only five strands of hair, Hatch said.

"With further work, we hope to not only use the test as a diagnostic tool but be able to use it to help monitor a person's recovery," he said.

"This test might be an auxiliary test, because right now we don't have good biological markers of anorexia nervosa," said Cynthia M. Bulik, the William and Jeanne Jordan Distinguished Professor of Eating Disorders and director of the eating disorders program at the University of North Carolina School of Medicine.

info To learn more, visit the National Eating Disorders Association's Web site at *www.nationaleatingdisorders.org*.

■ ■ ■ ■

Anorexia and Dopamine

Anorexia may be caused by dopamine over-activity in the brain.

Recent finding: Anorexia nervosa sufferers may have increased chemical activity in their dopamine receptors, which control reward and reinforcement. Dopamine affects how individuals respond to stimuli and how positive and negative reinforcement are viewed. This may explain why women with anorexia don't get any pleasure from losing weight.

Walter H. Kaye, MD, professor of psychiatry, University of Pittsburgh Medical Center, Western Psychiatric Institute and Clinic, Pittsburgh, and leader of a study of brain imaging, published in *Biological Psychiatry*.

Anti-Fat Protein to Keep You Slim May Be Coming Soon

Alessandro Bartolomucci, PhD, Institute of Neuroscience, Consiglio Nazionale delle Ricerche, Rome.

Cathy Nonas, RD, director, obesity and diabetes programs, North General Hospital, New York City, and spokeswoman, American Dietetic Association.

Proceedings of the National Academy of Sciences.

Eating all you want without gaining weight seems like a dream come true—and it did, at least for some lab mice. Mice gorging on high-calorie, high-fat diets for two weeks stayed slender, thanks to an "antiobesity" protein injected into their brains, Italian researchers report.

"Whether this translates to humans and whether it translates to humans without tremendous side effects is another story," said Cathy Nonas, director of the obesity and diabetes programs at North General Hospital in New York City, and a spokeswoman for the American Dietetic Association.

According to Nonas, a "wonder drug" that wards off obesity while allowing people to eat all they want has long been the goal of pharmaceutical companies worldwide. So far, most research efforts have focused on agents that "rev up" metabolism to burn off excess calories.

THE STUDY

This latest research, led by Alessandro Bartolomucci of the Consiglio Nazionale delle Ricerche, in Rome, focused on a protein byproduct of the VGF gene, which has long been linked to metabolism.

Bartolomucci's group first identified this protein, a peptide called TLQP-21, in the brains of rats. "It was an unproved assumption that VGF-derived peptides could regulate metabolism," the Italian team noted.

The researchers isolated TLQP-21 and injected it into the brains of lab mice every day for 14 days. At the same time, the mice were given high-fat diets that would normally trigger weight gain.

In this case, however, that didn't happen.

According to the researchers, the mice stayed slim because the peptide boosted their metabolic rate.

The peptide also affected key factors in metabolism and calorie-burning, he said. These included a rise in blood levels of the hormone epinephrine, as well as changes in locomotor and thyroid function.

LIMITATIONS

Bartolomucci believes TLQP-21 has potential as an antiobesity agent for use in humans. But he stressed that, "we are in an early stage of research. Indeed, this is the first study where the peptide is identified and the first study where its role in metabolic function has been tested."

"You can only do brain injections to a rat and a mouse," pointed out Nonas. "You'd have to go a long way before you could take that and turn it into something that would work in a pill form or be injected into fat tissue."

info Information on healthy dieting can be found at the American Dietetic Association Web site at *www.eatright.org*.

■ ■ ■ ■

Serve Snacks in Small Bowls

Using smaller serving bowls and plates is key for portion control and cutting calories.

New finding: People offered peanuts and a pretzel-and-chip mix from four-liter bowls ate 56% more than those offered the same snacks from two-liter bowls.

Theory: Serving-bowl size suggests how much food is appropriate to eat.

Brian Wansink, PhD, professor of marketing, applied economics and management, Cornell University, Ithaca, NY.

Low-Cal Diets Put Athletes at Risk for Stress Fractures

Saint Louis University Medical Center news release.

Another danger of dieting in young women may be seen on the playing fields. Female college athletes who restrict their calorie intake may be putting themselves at risk for stress fractures, new research finds.

THE STUDY

Researchers from Saint Louis University investigated possible causes of exercise-related leg pain, including stress fractures, in 76 female college athletes playing soccer, field hockey, cross-country running or volleyball.

The athletes who developed stress fractures were more likely to have "disordered eating," which included insufficient calorie intake due to eating disorders and other nutritional deficiencies.

"When people expend more calories than they consume, they release fewer hormones, which slows down menstrual cycles. This decreases estrogen in the body, which is responsible for bone development," said Mark Reinking, chairman of the department of physical therapy at Saint Louis University's Doisy College of Health Sciences.

Risk fractures for exercise-related leg pain overall were a prior history of leg pain, disordered eating, and excessive pronation (rolling inward) of the foot.

info For more on stress fractures, visit the Web site of the American Academy of Orthopaedic Surgeons at *http://orthoinfo.aaos.org*.

■ ■ ■ ■

Run Backward?

Running backward works the lungs more efficiently than running forward, burns more calories and lets bones absorb shock more effectively. Backward running also helps recovery from sprained ankles, pulled hamstrings and other leg and knee injuries, because it puts less impact on joints.

Best: Start slowly, until you build confidence.

Dean Karnazes, San Francisco–based ultra-marathoner and author of *Ultra-Marathon Man: Confessions of an All-Night Runner.* Tarcher.

Potassium Test May Improve Your Diet

American Society of Nephrology news release.

Diet plays a key role in overall health, especially when it comes to risks for heart disease, stroke and cancer. But there is no simple, objective and inexpensive way for physicians to assess a patient's diet, according to researchers. Now, a Canadian study finds that a simple test to check potassium levels in urine may help doctors assess and improve patients' eating habits.

THE STUDY

Researchers focused on urinary potassium as a potentially useful marker of a healthy diet. Evidence suggests that a diet high in potassium reduces the risk of developing a number of health problems.

The researchers collected urine samples from 220 people, ages 18 to 50, who also provided information about their eating habits over the previous year. The participants' blood pressure, heart rate, weight and height were also checked.

The study found a link between increased levels of potassium in the urine, a healthier diet, and lower weight, blood pressure and heart rate.

IMPLICATION

"These findings suggest, for the first time, that the amount of potassium in the urine is a valid, objective indicator of diet quality," said researcher Dr. Andrew Mente, of the Prosserman Center for Health Research in Toronto.

"This urinary marker is a simple, objective, universally available measure of diet quality that may aid physicians in providing effective dietary counseling. Physicians can now establish targets for therapy, monitor the effectiveness of dietary interventions over time, and provide effective dietary counseling to patients at risk because of poor food choices," Mente said.

Cool! Warm Watermelon Is Healthier

Penelope Perkins-Veazie, PhD, plant physiologist, South Central Agricultural Research Laboratory, USDA Agricultural Research Service, Lane, OK.
Lona Sandon, RD, assistant professor, clinical nutrition, University of Texas Southwestern Medical Center, Dallas.
Journal of Agriculture and Food Chemistry.

For many Americans, nothing is better on a hot day than biting into an ice-cold slice of watermelon. But scientists now say the juicy summer fruit is most nutritious when stored and served at room temperature.

THE STUDY

Researchers compared the levels of key antioxidants in whole watermelons that were either refrigerated or stored at room temperature for two weeks. Ripening watermelon at room temperature increases its nutritional value.

"The amount of lycopene in watermelons increased an average of 20% when we left them out uncut at room temperature, while beta carotene actually doubled," said study author Penelope Perkins-Veazie, a plant physiologist at the South Central Agricultural Research Laboratory with the USDA Agricultural Research Service in Lane, Oklahoma.

Perkins-Veazie noted that, like tomatoes, the red flesh of watermelons owes its coloring to an abundance of the antioxidant lycopene, an organic pigment from the carotenoid family that ranges in shade from pale yellow to deep red. Beta carotene—another carotenoid—is also present in watermelons, although at far lower levels.

Researchers realized that little was known about the impact storage can have after harvesting and packaging and once the heavy fruit is in the kitchen.

THE RESULTS

After two weeks, the researchers found that lycopene levels were dependent on storage temperature. Ripening at room temperature increases nutritional value.

Compared with measurements taken at picking, carotenoid levels in melons stored at room temperature (70 degrees F) increased by 11% to 40%, depending on the variety.

The carotenoid level of melons stored at below room temperature, by contrast, did not increase. The researchers posited that a drop in carotenoid activity at the colder temperatures might have halted a ripening process that continues the buildup of beneficial antioxidants.

FOOD SAFETY

"But we don't want people to think they can take cut watermelon and just leave it out in room temperature, because that's a safety issue," cautioned Perkins-Veazie.

"If it's cut, you want to leave it in the fridge," she advised. "If it's uncut, it's perfectly all right to leave it on the counter for a day or two."

Lona Sandon, an assistant professor of clinical nutrition at the University of Texas Southwestern Medical Center at Dallas, agreed that food safety takes precedence over antioxidant concerns.

"But you can leave certain fruits sitting out," she added. "In fact, there are several fruits that ripen better when left out—peaches, bananas —that not only end up having better nutrient quality but also perhaps better taste."

info For more information on fruit safety, visit the US Food and Drug Administration Web site at *www.fda.gov.*

■ ■ ■ ■

No-Guilt Watermelon Cake

Who thought of watermelons in a cake? Here's a show-stopping dessert perfect for special occasions.

Ingredients:
1 watermelon
½ container (8 ounces) fat-free frozen whipped topping, thawed
1 container (8 ounces) nonfat light lemon yogurt
Fresh fruit to decorate cake (strawberries, kiwi fruit, grapes, blueberries)

Instructions:
Select a symmetrical watermelon approximately 7 to 9 inches in diameter. Cut a 3-inch-thick cross section from the watermelon. Cut 4 slits through rind without cutting flesh. Cut between white rind portion and red flesh to remove rind. Fold together whipped topping

and yogurt. Pat watermelon cake dry with paper towel.

Place watermelon cake on flat serving plate. Frost top and sides with whipped topping mixture. Decorate as desired with fresh fruit. Refrigerate until ready to serve. Can be stored several hours or overnight. Cut in wedges to serve.

Servings: Serves 10

 For more recipes, visit the Web site *www. recipegoldmine.com.*

New Medicines Stop Dementia, Diabetes And More

Mark Hyman, MD, a board-certified family medicine physician in private practice in Lenox, MA, and coauthor of *Ultraprevention* and the author of *Ultrametabolism*. Scribner. He is editor-in-chief of *Alternative Therapies in Health and Medicine*, a peer-reviewed journal in alternative medicine.

When most Americans go to a medical doctor, they leave with a prescription for medication or a recommendation for surgery or radiation therapy. Few people are aware of an entirely different approach known as functional medicine, which treats the causes of disease rather than the symptoms.

Functional medicine is supported by new discoveries in "systems biology," which maintains that disease is caused by imbalances in core systems of the body, such as the digestive system. Systems biology is so important that the National Institutes of Health (NIH) is spending hundreds of millions of dollars to incorporate these principles into the current body of scientific research.

How I have used functional medicine to treat the following conditions...

DEMENTIA

John, a 70-year-old businessman, consulted me after he was diagnosed with dementia and had begun to decline rapidly. He had become irritable, was unable to interact with his family or run his business, and had short-term-memory problems.

In conventional medicine, doctors wait until dementia-like symptoms develop, then they prescribe medication that does little to improve those symptoms.

Functional medicine approach: Common causes of dementia-like symptoms, such as blood sugar irregularities, inflammation, elevated levels of the amino acid homocysteine and mercury toxicity, are addressed.

John had extraordinarily high levels of mercury (as determined by urine tests)...insulin resistance (an inability of the body's cells to efficiently use blood glucose)...and severe gastrointestinal problems. For 40 years, he had taken drugs, such as the tranquilizer *trifluoperazine* (Stelazine), because his doctor had believed that John's irritable bowel syndrome (IBS), a condition that causes abdominal pain, constipation and/or diarrhea, had stemmed from psychological problems. He also was deficient in vitamin B-12 and folic acid, which are essential for cognitive functioning.

Solution: I prescribed dietary changes to correct John's insulin resistance and various nutritional supplements, including vitamin B-12, folic acid and fish oil, to improve brain function. I treated his mercury toxicity—caused in part by eating mercury-tainted fish—with chelating agents, which remove metals from the body. Within a year, he no longer displayed symptoms of dementia.

DIABETES

Edward, 62, had been diagnosed with diabetes, heart failure, angina, sleep apnea (a sleep disorder that causes people to repeatedly stop breathing), acid reflux, sinus problems and fatigue.

Most medical doctors do not diagnose diabetes until a patient's fasting blood sugar (glucose) level is elevated (126 or above)—at which point, medication is prescribed. Conventional medicine takes a similar approach to treating the other health problems with which Edward had been diagnosed.

Functional medicine approach: I worked with Edward to correct the insulin resistance that

had triggered his diabetes. With blood tests, we can detect insulin imbalances decades before glucose rises to dangerous levels and intervene to prevent diabetes. Edward's insulin resistance was largely due to a diet that was high in refined flour and sugar as well as saturated fat. In addition, he got virtually no exercise.

Solution: I advised Edward to eat protein (such as lean poultry, fish, eggs, legumes, nuts, seeds and tofu) in the morning to help regulate his insulin levels and curb his appetite and sugar cravings. I also increased his intake of omega-3 fatty acids to reduce his blood sugar levels and control inflammation...recommended that he eat more fiber (50 g daily) to slow down his body's absorption of sugar...and suggested that he eat three meals and two snacks a day for better blood sugar and hormonal control.

I also asked Edward to perform aerobic exercise 30 minutes daily and strength training for 20 minutes three times a week, and to take supplements that help curb blood sugar—alpha lipoic acid, the mineral chromium and glucomannan, a soluble, highly viscous fiber derived from konjac root.

Result? He lost 140 pounds in 18 months and has no signs of diabetes.

IRRITABLE BOWEL SYNDROME

Alexis, 45, had suffered from the gastrointestinal disorder IBS since she was a teenager. Her primary symptom was sudden, painful, cramping diarrhea as well as bloating after every meal, especially if she ate starchy foods. She also suffered from rectal itching, which is often a sign of yeast infection, and food allergies.

Functional medicine approach: IBS can be caused by a number of factors, such as a disruption in the balance of "good" and "bad" bacteria in the digestive tract, yeast infection and food sensitivities—especially to gluten, dairy products or eggs.

A special breath test showed that Alexis had too much bacteria in her digestive system as a result of a diet that was high in sugar and low in fiber. In her small intestine, the bacteria fermented the food she was digesting, particularly sugar or starchy foods. This led to bloating after meals and diarrhea attacks.

Solution: I prescribed an antifungal drug, *fluconazole* (Diflucan), to treat her yeast problem…asked Alexis to stop eating foods to which she was allergic (dairy and wheat) for a period of three months…and recommended that she take probiotic supplements, "good" bacteria to normalize her gut, as well as zinc to help activate enzymes in her digestive system.

I advised Alexis to consume extra fiber as well as fish oil and turmeric to reduce gut inflammation, and vitamin B-6, magnesium and a traditional Chinese herbal formula to balance her estrogen and progesterone levels (which are greatly affected by abnormal gut bacteria).

When Alexis returned two months later, her IBS symptoms had been eliminated, and she had lost 20 pounds. She looked and said she felt 10 years younger.

info To find a doctor who practices functional medicine, contact The Institute for Functional Medicine at 800-228-0622 or *www.functionalmedicine.org*.

■ ■ ■ ■

Delicious Ways to Fill Up On Healthy Omega-3s

The three major sources of omega-3 fatty acids, which reduce inflammation in the body and protect against heart disease, are flaxseed, walnuts and fatty fish, such as salmon and mackerel. Of these sources, flaxseed has the lowest number of calories ounce for ounce. Each of the following provides 1,000 mg of omega-3s—two teaspoons of ground flaxseed, which has about 25 calories…five walnut halves, with approximately 70 calories…and two ounces of cooked salmon (wild Atlantic salmon contains about 100 calories, and farmed Atlantic salmon has about 115). To get the anti-inflammatory benefits of omega-3 fatty acids, I recommend consuming 2,000 mg of omega-3s daily—from flaxseed or other sources.

Vijay Vad, MD, assistant professor of rehabilitation medicine, Weill Cornell Medical College, New York City.

■ ■ ■ ■

Nutty Ways to Protect Your Heart

Pecans and walnuts are high in a form of vitamin E called gamma tocopherol…almonds are high in alpha tocopherol. These powerful antioxidants help reduce risk of hardening of the arteries and heart disease. They also lower total and LDL (bad) cholesterol and raise HDL (good) cholesterol.

Best: Eat a moderate-sized handful of nuts every day.

Ella Haddad, DrPH, associate professor, department of nutrition, School of Public Health, Loma Linda University, Loma Linda, CA, and leader of a study published in Nutrition Research.

Weight Loss Pills That Work

Harry G. Preuss, MD, CNS, FACN, professor of physiology, medicine and pathology at Georgetown University Medical Center, Washington, DC. He is a certified nutrition specialist, fellow of the American College of Nutrition and author of more than 300 scientific studies. He is coauthor of The Natural Fat-Loss Pharmacy. *Broadway.*

Weight-loss "pills" often are viewed with skepticism and for good reason. Many are ineffective…some even are dangerous. But a few nutritional and herbal supplements do work. Some offer bonus health benefits, too. These natural substances have been scientifically shown to aid weight loss by helping the body burn more calories and fat…reducing appetite…improving how the body handles blood sugar…and blocking absorption of fat and carbohydrates.

Laboratory, toxicological and clinical studies—and years of everyday use by millions of people—demonstrate that these supplements are safe. However, it is prudent to take any supplement under the guidance of a qualified health professional. All of the following are available in health-food stores unless otherwise noted.

GREEN TEA EXTRACT

Green tea contains catechins, a class of powerful antioxidants. EGCG is short for epigallocatechin gallate, the most abundant catechin in green tea.

THE RESEARCH

In a study published in *British Journal of Nutrition*, Canadian researchers gave one group of men a supplement containing EGCG and caffeine and another group a placebo. Those who took the supplement burned 180 more calories a day—a level that could help a person shed 22 pounds in a year. For those already at their normal weight, studies show an EGCG/caffeine supplement can help maintain weight. (Previous studies had shown that an EGCG/caffeine combination burns more calories than either EGCG or caffeine alone.)

The combination works by stimulating the sympathetic nervous system, which helps regulate appetite, temperature and many other metabolic processes, including calorie-burning and fat-burning. However, unlike potentially heart-damaging weight-loss herbs, such as ephedra, which also stimulate the sympathetic nervous system, a therapeutic dose of EGCG/caffeine doesn't increase heart rate or significantly boost blood pressure.

Dose: 575 milligrams (mg) of green tea catechins (with 325 mg from EGCG) and 100 mg of caffeine a day. Supplements with this mixture include Schiff-Natural Green Tea Diet and Universal Nutrition-Thermo Green Tea Caps.

Bonus: EGCG may be neuroprotective in humans—it has reduced the severity of Alzheimer's disease in laboratory animals genetically programmed to develop the disease.

CLA

Conjugated linoleic acid (CLA) is a type of fatty acid—a building block of fat. It is found in small quantities in meat and milk. CLA can help the body lose fat and build muscle.

THE RESEARCH

In a study conducted in Norway and published in *The American Journal of Clinical Nutrition*, 149 women and 31 men received either CLA or a placebo daily. Within three months, the CLA group lost an average of five pounds of body fat and gained two pounds of firming muscle—without dieting or exercise. The placebo group had no change in body composition.

In a study published in the *International Journal of Obesity,* people who took CLA for six months—from August 2004 through February 2005—experienced no weight gain during the November–December holiday period. People who didn't take CLA gained an average of 1.5 pounds during the holidays.

Researchers don't yet know exactly how CLA works, but it may stop dietary fat from entering fat cells.

Dose: 3.4 grams a day.

Bonus: In a study conducted at the University of British Columbia, people with mild-to-moderate asthma experienced a complete normalization of their airways when they took CLA, which decreases inflammation.

MCTS

Medium-chain triglycerides (MCTs) are a type of fat. Triglyceride molecules are typically arranged in chains, with carbon atoms as the links. Most triglycerides you eat are long-chain triglycerides, with up to 24 carbon links. MCTs have only six to 12 carbon links. During digestion, long-chain triglycerides combine with transport molecules and travel in the circulatory system, where they're deposited in fat cells. Because of their unique length, MCTs don't require transport molecules —they move directly from the stomach to the liver, where most are instantly incinerated for fuel (and very few are stored as fat). This unusual digestive process increases calorie burning.

THE RESEARCH

In a study conducted at the University of Manitoba in Canada and published in *The American Journal of Clinical Nutrition*, 24 men who took MCT supplements burned an average of 100 more calories per day, compared with men who took a placebo.

Dose: MCT is derived from coconut oil, a saturated fat. There have been concerns that MCT supplements could increase cholesterol levels. The MCT formulation used in the study above includes cholesterol-lowering plant sterols —and lowered total cholesterol by 13% and LDL (bad) cholesterol by 14%. This supplement, Slim

Smart (*www.nfh.ca*), is available for sale only through health professionals.

CHROMIUM

The trace mineral chromium increases the number of insulin receptors on muscle and fat cells, helping those cells utilize blood sugar more effectively. The body uses blood sugar to build muscle, storing less of it as fat.

THE RESEARCH

In a study of overweight women, those who took chromium supplements while on a diet and exercise program lost weight the healthy way—84% as fat, 16% as muscle. Those who didn't take chromium lost weight but 8% as fat and 92% as muscle.

Losing muscle rather than fat is the sad fate of many dieters. (Evolutionarily, your hunter-gatherer body is programmed to lose muscle, to preserve fat stores in case of famine.) Muscle burns many more calories a day than fat, so you end up with a body that burns fewer calories. Postdiet, you return to a normal level of eating but gain weight. Chromium can help prevent this common metabolic problem.

Dose: 600 micrograms (mcg) daily, until you reach your weight-loss goal. The maintenance dose—for lifelong blood sugar balance—is 200 mcg a day.

Caution: Too much chromium can cause major side effects, such as anemia, kidney failure and liver damage. Ask your doctor if chromium is right for you.

Bonus: Because it regulates blood sugar, chromium can help prevent or normalize type 2 diabetes.

STARCH-BLOCKER

An extract of white kidney beans, a starch-blocker limits the action of *alpha-amylase*, the digestive enzyme that breaks down starch in the intestines. In a study conducted in Italy, 60 overweight but healthy people received either a starch-blocker or a placebo for 30 days while on a diet of 2,000 to 2,200 calories per day that included lots of starch, such as bread and pasta. Those taking the starch-blocker lost an average of seven pounds...those taking the placebo didn't lose weight.

Dose: A dose of 300 mg, taken right before each meal, with eight ounces of water. Look for a product with Phase 2 as the starch-blocker. It's the most widely studied starch-blocker.

HOW TO CHOOSE

With a health professional's guidance, choose one or two supplements that fit your weight-loss goals and lifestyle.

Example: A person eating a lot of carbohydrates might take a starch-blocker to cut absorption and chromium to balance blood sugar.

If after two months or so the selection doesn't seem to be working, stop taking those and try another one or two supplements.

'Eat Less, Lose More'... And Other Diet Myths

Mark Hyman, MD, a board-certified family medicine physician in private practice in Lenox, MA, and coauthor of *Ultraprevention* and the author of *Ultrametabolism.* Scribner. He is editor-in-chief of *Alternative Therapies in Health and Medicine*, a peer-reviewed journal in alternative medicine.

Losing weight can be hard work. People feel they have to count calories, endure hunger pangs and work up a sweat. It's no wonder so many give up and regain their hard-lost pounds. It doesn't have to be that way. The reason we are losing the battle of the bulge is that we have bought into some common myths about weight loss. *Here, six of those myths and what to do instead...*

Myth 1: The less you eat, the more weight you'll lose.

Our bodies are made up of hundreds of genes that protect us from starvation. That's why we end up gaining weight if we start out eating too few calories. You can starve yourself for only so long before your body engages a primitive response that compensates for starvation by making you overeat. In my experience, the average person who goes on a diet actually gains five pounds.

What to do: Never go on a diet. Instead, eat foods that turn on your metabolism. These are whole foods that come from nature, such as vegetables, fruits, whole grains, nuts, seeds, beans and lean animal protein. If you eat only these foods, you won't have trouble with your appetite—it will self-regulate, and the triggers that drive overeating will be under control.

Myth 2: It doesn't matter what kind of exercise you do, as long as you exercise.

It's true that any kind of exercise is better than no exercise, but interval training is the most effective for weight loss. Interval training consists of short bursts of intense activity followed by longer periods of lighter activity. This kind of training tunes up your metabolism so you burn more calories all day and while you sleep, not just when you are exercising.

What to do: Aim for 20 to 30 minutes of interval training two to three days a week. Exercise as vigorously as you can for 30 to 60 seconds, and then slow your pace for three minutes, repeating this pattern for about a half hour.

If you are over 30, have a physical before you start interval training. If you are out of shape, ease into a regular exercise routine first—you might start by walking for 30 minutes five times a week.

Myth 3: You can control your weight by counting calories.

Many people believe that all calories are the same when it comes to weight control—that if you substitute 100 calories' worth of, say, cookies for 100 calories of carrots, you'll come out even. But food isn't just about calories. Everything that you eat contains "instructions" for your DNA, your hormones and your metabolism. Different foods contain different information.

For instance, the sugar in soda enters your blood rapidly, increasing insulin levels. Insulin is a hormone that promotes more fat storage around the middle and raises inflammation levels in the body, which in turn promotes more weight gain.

On the other hand, the same amount of sugar from kidney beans enters your blood slowly. Because the sugar is absorbed over time, your insulin levels remain stable and more of the calories are burned and fewer are stored.

What to do: Don't focus on the number of calories you are consuming. Losing weight is not about counting calories—it's about eating the right calories.

Myth 4: Eating fat makes you fat.

Dietary fat does not correlate with excess body fat. Any weight-loss resulting from a low-fat diet is usually modest and temporary. The amount of fat Americans eat has dropped from 42% to 34% of total calories on average, but we still are getting fatter. That's because all fats are not created equal. There are good fats, bad fats and ugly fats. Good fats actually can help you lose weight, but many of us have nearly eliminated them from our diet.

Two examples of good fats are omega-3s and monounsaturated fats. Omega-3s are found in fish, flaxseed and flax oil, and nuts and seeds, such as walnuts and pumpkin seeds. Monounsaturated fats are found in olive oil, avocados and nuts.

Bad fats include refined polyunsaturated vegetable oil—such as corn and safflower—and most saturated fat, found in meat and animal products, such as butter.

The ugly fats are trans fats, often found in snack foods and packaged baked goods. Trans fat comes from adding hydrogen to vegetable oil through a process called hydrogenation.

What to do: Eat good fats. These improve your metabolism by activating genes that help you burn fats. Saturated and trans fats turn off fat-burning genes. The Inuit people of Greenland used to eat a diet that was very high in fat—primarily omega-3 and monounsaturated fat—and they were thin and healthy. Now they have shifted to a diet that is lower in fat and high in carbohydrates from junk food, and many are obese, with higher rates of heart disease and other illnesses.

Myth 5: Going low-carb will make you thin.

Carbohydrates are the single most important food you can eat for long-term health and weight loss. They are the source of most of the vitamins, minerals and fiber in our diet—and all the phytonutrients, plant compounds that are key regulators of our health. Phytonutrients turn on the genes that help us burn fat and age slowly. They contain disease-fighting nutrients. Some examples are the isoflavones in soy foods, polyphenols in cocoa and glucosinolates in broccoli.

However, just as there are different fats, there are different types of carbohydrates.

What to do: Eat complex carbohydrates—vegetables, fruits, nuts, seeds, beans and whole grains. These tend to have low glycemic loads, which means they are absorbed slowly and don't raise blood sugar quickly, so you feel full longer. Refined carbs, such as white flour, rice and pasta, along with sugary foods, make your blood sugar spike so that you feel hungry sooner.

Myth 6: **It doesn't matter what time you eat.**

Sumo wrestlers look the way they do because they fast during the day, then overeat at night and go to bed. Like Sumo wrestlers, we eat most of our calories late in the day. When you eat late, calories are stored instead of burned.

What to do: Don't eat within two to three hours of going to bed, because you need to give your body time to digest and burn off your food. Also, eat throughout the day to keep blood sugar levels stable. Breakfast is important. I can't tell you how many people I have helped to lose weight by having them eat breakfast. The National Weight Control Registry, which is tracking long-term weight-loss maintenance in more than 5,000 people, has found that 96% of those who have maintained weight loss for six years eat breakfast regularly.

Are You Getting Too Much Salt?

Mark Houston, MD, clinical professor of medicine at Vanderbilt University Medical School and medical director at the Hypertension and Vascular Biology Institute and the Life Extension Institute at Saint Thomas Hospital and Medical Center, all in Nashville, TN. Dr. Houston is the editor-in-chief of the *Journal of the American Nutraceutical Society* and the author of *What Your Doctor May Not Tell You About Hypertension: The Revolutionary Nutrition and Lifestyle Program to Help Fight High Blood Pressure.* Warner.

For years, Americans have been warned that excessive use of salt (sodium chloride) can elevate blood pressure in some people.

Now: Doctors are becoming increasingly concerned about the amount of salt consumed by Americans and fear that it is contributing to even more health problems than previously believed.

Latest development: The American Medical Association has recommended that the FDA require food manufacturers to place warning labels on high-sodium foods.

SOURCES OF SODIUM

Sodium is a mineral that is found naturally in most foods. Everyone is aware of high-sodium foods, such as soy sauce, pickles, potato chips, most canned foods, frozen dinners and lunch meats.

However, few people realize that sodium is found in most carbonated drinks, including many diet sodas. Many brands of tomato juice contain significant amounts of sodium.

Example: Campbell's V8 contains 590 mg of sodium (more than one-quarter of the recommended daily total) per eight-ounce serving. Small amounts of sodium are even found in the tap water of many US municipalities.

Healthful foods, including poultry, dairy products and vegetables, also contain sodium.

Caution: Sodium is found in many over-the-counter medications.

Examples: Alka Seltzer (567 mg per tablet) …and Bromo Seltzer (959 mg per packet).

Our bodies require sodium to help regulate fluid balance. The mineral also is essential for nerve and muscle function. Sodium works with the mineral potassium, which counters the adverse effects of sodium, to keep the proper amount of liquid and electrolytes (minerals needed for proper functioning of the body) inside the body's cells. These minerals are excreted via sweat and urine. Imbalances can occur when too much sodium remains in the body in relation to potassium.

DANGERS OF TOO MUCH SODIUM

Even though high blood pressure (hypertension) is the most commonly recognized health risk associated with excessive sodium intake, there are other potentially serious conditions that can result.

Even in someone who does not have hypertension, excessive sodium intake increases risk for congestive heart failure (inadequate pumping action of the heart)…kidney disease…hardening of the arteries (arteriosclerosis)…swelling of the lower legs, ankles and feet (edema)…and ischemic stroke (impaired blood flow to the brain) as well as hemorrhagic stroke (bleeding into or around the brain).

Consuming too much sodium also may increase your risk for osteoporosis. That's because sodium and bone-strengthening calcium metabolism are linked. High sodium intake may increase the excretion of calcium, which is removed from the body—along with excess sodium—via urine. Over time, calcium stores in the bones will be reduced. This can lead to a calcium deficiency that often results in osteoporosis.

SAFE SODIUM LEVELS

The average American consumes at least 4,000 mg of sodium daily, but research shows that this is far too much. Our bodies require only about 500 mg of sodium daily to maintain normal functioning.

To avoid potential dangers, healthy adults should limit their sodium intake to 2,300 mg (approximately one teaspoon) daily, according to the American Heart Association (AHA).

In my opinion, everyone should limit sodium intake to 1,500 mg daily—especially older adults (age 65 or older), people with hypertension (blood pressure of 140/90 or above) or prehypertension (blood pressure of 120/80 to 139/89), diabetics, obese patients and people with kidney disease or a history of heart failure.

SALT SENSITIVITY

Salt sensitivity is a measure of how blood pressure responds to changes in salt intake. An estimated 60% of Americans with high blood pressure—and 25% of Americans with normal blood pressure—are salt sensitive.

In a recent study, salt sensitivity was found to increase a person's risk for death as much as high blood pressure, regardless of whether blood pressure actually was elevated.

In the study, salt sensitivity was measured by giving study participants a saline solution followed by a diuretic (a water- and salt-excreting drug) and testing blood pressure volume (the fluid content within blood vessels) over a two-day period as salt in the body was increased and then decreased. Unfortunately, there is no test available to the public for salt sensitivity.

Simply putting away the salt shaker is not the full solution.

Salt added to food by the eaters themselves accounts for only about 15% of the average American's total daily sodium intake. About 75% comes from sodium in processed and restaurant food, while the remaining 10% of a person's total sodium intake comes from the natural sodium content of food.

Cutting back on canned and processed foods, including fast food, while increasing your intake of fresh fruits and vegetables can substantially lower your sodium intake—most produce contains small amounts of sodium and increases levels of sodium-balancing potassium. To reduce sodium intake when dining in a restaurant, ask that no salt be added to your food.

SALT SUBSTITUTES

Our bodies function most efficiently when we maintain a five-to-one ratio of potassium to sodium. In addition to fruits and vegetables, most unprocessed natural foods, including whole grains and legumes, contain more potassium than sodium. Maintaining this dietary ratio promotes healthy blood pressure.

Some salt substitutes, such as Nu-Salt and NoSalt, contain potassium chloride rather than sodium chloride. These substitutes, available at most grocery stores, taste much like table salt and can be used without potential health risks by most people.

Caution: Potassium chloride–based salt substitutes can be harmful to people who have kidney disease, which can inhibit the proper excretion of potassium and lead to heart and nerve problems. In addition, if you're taking drugs that cause potassium retention, including those for high blood pressure or congestive heart failure, consult your doctor before using a salt substitute.

Good alternative: A seasoning blend such as Mrs. Dash, which does not contain potassium chloride.

Herbs and spices also add flavor to food. Instead of mimicking the taste of sodium with salt substitutes, try using garlic, lemon juice, flavored vinegar, cumin, pepper, tarragon and/or oregano in food. After a few weeks of reducing salt intake, most people no longer miss it.

Strength Training Is The Best Exercise for Your Health...Really!

Wayne Westcott, PhD, fitness research director for the South Shore YMCA in Quincy, MA. He is the author or coauthor of 20 books, including *Strength Training Past 50*. Human Kinetics.

Thirty minutes of aerobic exercise, such as walking or cycling, three to five days per week has long been known to help prevent cardiovascular disease.

Latest development: A recent study published in *Circulation,* the journal of the American Heart Association, concluded that strength training is equally important for maintaining healthy cholesterol levels and blood pressure —and even more critical for preventing diabetes and boosting the body's metabolism, which helps burn calories and prevent weight gain.

Why is this type of exercise so important? Researchers have found that regular strength training is the only way to prevent the five- to seven-pound loss in muscle mass that all adults —except trained athletes—experience each decade beginning in their mid-20s.

That's why the American College of Sports Medicine (ACSM) now recommends that, in addition to regular aerobic workouts, all adults perform two or three strength-training sessions per week. Each workout should last 20 to 40 minutes and consist of eight or more exercises that work all the major muscle groups of the body.

There's just one problem: If you walk into a health club or local YMCA, you're likely to encounter a bewildering array of strength-training classes that claim to "firm and tone your body," "build lean muscle mass" or some combination of the above. Which type of class is right for you?*

Any class you're considering should be supervised by a trainer who has been certified by a national fitness organization, such as the ACSM or the American Council on Exercise. When properly supervised, strength training is one of the safest forms of exercise there is—even among elderly and frail adults.

Caution: Your muscles require 48 to 72 hours to recover from each strength-training workout. Adults age 50 or older should strength train every three days.

What you need to know about strength-training classes...

BODY SCULPTING

What it does: Tones muscles, while moderately increasing strength and muscle tissue.

These classes include a variety of strength-building exercises, using elastic resistance bands, dumbbells, medicine balls (handheld, weighted exercise balls) and calisthenics. A typical body-sculpting class consists of eight to 15 different exercises that work all the body's major muscle groups. Each exercise should involve 20 repetitions or less, and take no more than two minutes.

While body-sculpting classes don't produce as much gain in strength and muscle mass as other types of strength-training exercises, they will increase lean muscle tissue somewhat, and are highly effective at increasing functional muscle strength (used for lifting and carrying).

PILATES

What it does: Strengthens the "core" muscles of the low back, front abdominal muscles and oblique muscles that run from the back of the abdomen to the front.

Pilates classes use slow-moving stretches and resistance exercises to increase flexibility and strength. These moves are performed using Pilates equipment (pulleys and weights set on a frame) or without equipment on a floor mat.

*If you prefer at-home exercise, Tufts University and the Centers for Disease Control and Prevention (CDC) have created a strength-training program called "Growing Stronger." It can be downloaded for free from the CDC Web site, *www.cdc.gov/nccdhph/dnpa/physical/growing_stronger/.* Click on "Resources." Or you can purchase it at *www.tuftsbooks.com.*

Caution: If you have back pain, check with a doctor before taking Pilates classes to be sure you have no structural abnormalities that might be exacerbated.

Note: Core-training classes offer benefits that are similar to those of Pilates and typically consist of a variety of resistance exercises using calisthenics, medicine balls, lightweight dumbbells, resistance bands and inflated stability balls (which you sit on while exercising)—all designed to activate and strengthen the low-back and abdominal muscles.

WEIGHT TRAINING

What it does: Builds strength and muscle mass.

When it comes to increasing strength and muscle mass, no other form of strength training comes close to matching standard weight training. Weight training typically involves about 10 different resistance exercises covering all the major muscle groups. They can be performed with weight machines (such as those made by Nautilus or Cybex) or free weights (barbells and dumbbells). In each exercise, a weight is lifted eight to 12 times in a slow, controlled fashion.

Research has found that weight training increases the glucose uptake of the body's muscles by nearly 25% (reducing the risk for diabetes), and lowers blood pressure by an average of 4 mmHg systolic (top number) and 2 mmHg diastolic (bottom number) over periods of two to four months. By stimulating the skeletal system, it also can help maintain bone density.

CIRCUIT TRAINING

What it does: Combines the maximum strength- and muscle-building benefits of weight training with an aerobic workout that benefits the cardiovascular system.

In a circuit-training class, exercisers perform about 10 weight-training exercises for one minute each. Between these strength exercises, a minute or two of aerobic activity (such as riding a stationary bicycle or walking/jogging on a treadmill) is performed.

These classes are excellent time-savers, since they offer the benefits of weight training and an aerobic workout in a single session of 30 to 45 minutes. Due to the aerobic component, circuit training also burns about 50% more calories per workout session than standard strength-training classes.

Yoga Exercises Anyone Can Do

Susan Winter Ward, a Pagosa Springs, Colorado–based yoga instructor and the author of *Yoga for the Young at Heart: Accessible Yoga for Every Body.* New World Library. She has taught yoga for 14 years and is the creator of the Yoga for the Young at Heart video series, which can be ordered on her Web site, *www.yogaheart.com.*

Many people assume that they could never practice yoga because it requires so much flexibility. The truth is, inflexibility is actually one of the best reasons to do yoga.

Traditional yoga can be more challenging for people who suffer joint stiffness due to osteoarthritis or inactivity—the stretching as well as getting up and down from the floor, where some yoga poses are performed, can be difficult. But there is an alternative.

I've created a series of yoga exercises designed to be performed while seated in a chair.* These poses are accessible for people with physical handicaps, such as multiple sclerosis or muscular dystrophy. Chair yoga also can be done at your desk, or while traveling on a plane or a train.

The following series of exercises require little space and no equipment other than a firm, steady chair. When combined with cardiovascular exercise, such as brisk walking, and strength training, such as weight-lifting, chair yoga helps create a well-balanced exercise program. All inhalations and exhalations for these exercises should be done through the nose for a count of five.

For maximum benefits, practice the following exercises daily...

•**Breathing for relaxation.** Deep breathing brings extra oxygen into the lungs and bloodstream, both relaxing and energizing the body, and calming the mind.

*Check with your doctor before starting this—or any—exercise program.

What to do: Sit up straight. Place your right hand over your heart and your left hand over your stomach. Close your eyes and breathe in deeply. Exhale, then breathe in again, while focusing on lifting your chest and expanding your ribs. Inhale, then exhale while maintaining a straight spine. Repeat five to 10 times.

•**Butterfly curls.** These stretch the back of the neck, the spine, rib cage and arms.

What to do: Sitting toward the front of your chair, straighten your back and clasp your hands behind your head. Breathe in deeply and lengthen your spine while pulling your elbows back and letting your rib cage expand. Keeping your back flat, exhale and curl your head forward, pulling your elbows gently toward each other. Take a few deep breaths, lifting your chest toward your chin as you inhale and dropping your chin toward your chest as you exhale. Repeat five times.

•**Windmill.** This relaxes the shoulders, neck and arms.

What to do: Sitting up straight, inhale as you raise your right arm overhead. Bend your right elbow so that it points upward and your fingers touch your upper spine or neck. Exhale, then inhale again.

Next, stretch your left arm out to your left side and bend your elbow, bringing the back of your left hand to your spine. Exhale, pressing your hands gently toward each other while keeping your back and shoulder blades flat. Inhale, lifting your chest and gently pressing your hands toward each other as you exhale. If you like, you can hold a belt or strap between your hands. Repeat three to five times.

•**Expand your heart.** This pose relaxes the back, shoulders and chest, and aids breathing by creating space in the rib cage for the lungs to expand.

What to do: Sitting toward the front of your chair, clasp your hands behind you at the waist. With your elbows bent, press your shoulder blades together, lifting your chest. Inhale, drawing your elbows toward each other. Lengthen your spine as you inhale and lift your ribs away from your hips. Exhale as you press your knuckles down toward the chair seat. Repeat three to five times, taking long, deep breaths.

•**Seated push-ups.** This exercise strengthens the arms, back and shoulders.

What to do: Sit near the front of your chair and put your hands on the front corners of the seat. Inhaling deeply, with your elbows in toward your sides, straighten your elbows and lift yourself off the seat of the chair. Keep your legs and shoulders relaxed and avoid pushing with your feet. Exhale as you slowly lower yourself. Repeat at least five times.

•**Spinal twist.** This stretches the rib cage and spine and eases back strain. It also aids digestion by massaging the stomach and intestines.

What to do: Sitting up straight, cross your right leg over your left and place your left hand on the inside of your left knee. Inhale deeply as you twist to the right, pulling your right elbow and shoulder around toward the back of the chair. Keeping your back straight, take three to five deep breaths as you hold the pose. Lengthen your spine by lifting through the top of your head with each inhalation, and twist a bit farther to the right with each exhalation. Return to center, then repeat on the opposite side.

•**Cervical stretch.** This pose stretches and relaxes the arms, wrists, hands, shoulders, back and chest. It counteracts the effects of typing and eases headaches due to shoulder tension.

What to do: Sitting near the front of your chair, inhale deeply and raise your arms overhead. Interlace your fingers, palms facing the ceiling. Exhale, pressing through the heels of your hands. Inhale again, tucking your chin in toward your throat. While holding this position, exhale and let your chin drop toward your chest. Breathe deeply three to five times, feeling the stretch down to your shoulder blades with each exhalation.

•**Hamstring stretch.** This stretches the backs of the thighs, releases low-back tension, strengthens the back and abdomen, and improves digestion.

What to do: Sitting toward the front of your chair, place both feet flat on the floor. While keeping your back flat and chest lifted, clasp your left knee just below the kneecap with both hands and pull your thigh toward your rib cage. Hold for three to five breaths. Switch legs and repeat.

Illustrations by Shawn Banner.

Erase Years from Your Age by Walking

Michael F. Roizen, MD, chair of the division of anesthesiology, critical care medicine and comprehensive pain management at The Cleveland Clinic. He created the RealAge concept and wrote the best-selling RealAge: Are You As Young As You Can Be? *Collins. He is author, with Tracy Hafen and Lawrence A. Armour, of* The RealAge Workout: Maximum Health, Minimum Work. *Collins. www.realage.com.*

Walking is the single best thing you can do for your health. I view it as the fountain of youth. In my RealAge book, I showed how aging has little to do with calendar years. A 50-year-old man could have the arteries and immune system of a 75-year-old. Someone else might be 75 but have a RealAge—measured by the risk of disease, disability or death—of a 52-year-old. Exercise is a key factor in reducing your RealAge—and just 30 minutes of walking a day can make you healthier, more energetic and, in a real sense, younger.

HEALTH BENEFITS

Walking is easy to do, doesn't require any special equipment (except walking shoes) and conveys many of the same health benefits as more strenuous exercise.

Walking helps prevent fatty buildup in the arteries. When your arteries are clogged with fatty buildup, your cardiovascular system ages more quickly, and so does your entire body. Aging of the arteries brings on cardiovascular disease, the major cause of heart attacks and strokes. It also leads to loss of energy, memory loss and, in men, impotence. Walking can help keep arteries young and healthy.

Walking every day also decreases the risk of such conditions as macular degeneration (the leading cause of blindness in people over age 50) and arthritis. The long-running Framingham Heart Study found that people with arthritis who walked daily for 30 minutes and supplemented their diets with vitamins C and D and calcium were able to stop the progression of joint damage. Walking also prevented osteoarthritis in patients who didn't already have it.

Walking can even reduce the risk of some forms of cancer by as much as 50%.

GET READY

Studies show that people who walk as little as 10 minutes a day—or even just once a week—on a regular basis have less risk of dying prematurely than those who are sedentary. For optimal health gains, you should walk for at least 30 minutes daily. People who take three 10-minute walks each day have about the same health gains as those who walk for 30 minutes straight. *Helpful…*

•**Warm up before walking.** Walk more slowly than usual for the first several minutes. This warm-up heats the muscles and makes them more flexible and efficient and less prone to injury. It also increases circulation in the joints.

•**Wear a watch.** Measure time rather than distance. Time is easy to count, and you can walk for 30 minutes at a comfortable pace. You don't need to follow a track or a premeasured route—and you won't try to force yourself to go a certain distance.

•**Don't miss a day.** Make 30 minutes a day of walking a priority. Things like yard work and housecleaning help, too, but they can't take the place of your daily walks.

Malls are terrific places to walk if the weather is bad, and most YMCAs have walking tracks and treadmills. If your budget permits, buy a treadmill so you can walk any time of the day or night without leaving home.

POSTWALKING STRETCH

Once your routine becomes ingrained, set aside two to three minutes to stretch after you're done walking. Stretching improves joint range of motion. Without a normal range of motion in the joints, daily activities become more difficult and the risk of musculoskeletal injury increases. Some people find that stretching also reduces soreness, though I can't find hard evidence to support that claim.

To perform a stretch, move slowly into the stretch position until you feel a gentle pulling sensation, not pain. Hold the stretch for 10 to 30 seconds without bouncing. Repeat each stretch two or three times.

Here is a sample postwalking stretch for each key muscle group...

•**Hamstring.** Sit on the floor with both feet straight out in front of you. Keep your left leg extended, and bend the right so that the sole of your right foot is against the inner thigh of your left leg. Lean forward over the left leg until you feel a gentle stretch along the back of your extended thigh, keeping your back as straight as possible. Repeat with the right leg extended.

•**Quadricep.** Stand on your right leg, and bend the left so that your left knee is pointed toward the floor. Then reach your left hand behind you and take hold of your left ankle. Your hips should be pressed forward so that you feel a gentle stretch along the front of your left thigh. (You may need to stand near a wall for balance.) Repeat, standing on your left leg with the right leg bent.

•**Buttock.** Lie on your back, and bend both legs, keeping your feet flat on the floor. Cross the ankle of your right foot just above your left knee. Lift your left foot off the floor, and bring both legs toward your chest. Hold on to your left thigh to help pull your legs closer to your chest until you feel a gentle stretch near your right hip and buttock. Repeat with the other leg.

•**Adductor.** Lie on your back, and bend both knees. Open your knees out to the sides, and place the soles of your feet together. Pull your feet in toward you, allowing your knees to drop toward the floor until you feel a gentle stretch in the groin and inner-thigh area.

•**Hip flexor.** Stand with the left foot in front of the right, with your weight centered evenly between both feet. Keeping your back straight, bend your knees slightly, lowering yourself toward the floor and tucking your hips under. You should feel a gentle stretch along the front

of your right hip. Repeat with the right foot in front of the left.

•**Calf.** Sit on the floor with both feet extended in front of you. Keeping your back as straight as possible, flex your toes toward you until you feel a gentle stretch in the back of both legs.

•**Lower back.** Sit on the floor cross-legged. Keeping your head in line with your spine, lean forward with your upper body and reach your arms out in front of you until you feel a gentle stretch in your lower back.

What to Do When You Don't Feel Like Exercising

Gabe Mirkin, MD, a physician with a specialty in sports medicine in private practice in Chevy Chase, MD, and an associate professor of pediatrics at the Georgetown University School of Medicine in Washington, DC. He is the author of eight books, including *The Healthy Heart Miracle: Your Roadmap to Lifelong Health.* HarperCollins.

We all know that regular physical activity is crucial for good health—it reduces our risk for heart disease, diabetes, stroke, certain types of cancer, mental disorders, including depression and anxiety, and even premature death.

Problem: Nearly nine out of every 10 people who start an exercise program drop out within six weeks, typically due to injuries and/or lack of social reinforcement. But these aren't the only reasons that people give for skipping workouts.

In my 46 years as a practicing sports medicine physician, I've heard all kinds of excuses for not exercising. Here are the most common excuses and the rebuttals I give my patients to get them back on track...

Excuse: I'm so out of shape that I wouldn't know where to begin.

My rebuttal: No matter how out of shape you might be, you'll immediately begin getting fitter once you engage in any regular physical activity. If you haven't exercised in a long time, start by simply getting a bit more physical activity each day and gradually increasing it.

The most popular recommendations are to park a block from where you're heading and walk the rest of the way and/or to take the stairs instead of the elevator.

Other possibilities: Do gardening or yard work...vacuum and wash your car...walk around the inside and/or outside of your house...tackle a cleaning project you've been putting off...ride a bike to nearby destinations instead of driving ...and/or stroll around a park or mall.

When you're ready to start a more formal exercise program, don't choose an activity that requires a great deal of skill or strength you don't yet have, such as in-line skating, jumping rope or rock climbing. Instead, try a low-risk activity that you already know how to do. Walking is great for most people.

Other good choices: Swimming, cycling, jogging and/or dancing (aerobic or ballroom).

Start with just a few minutes a day. Begin very slowly and continue until your muscles start to hurt or you feel uncomfortable, then quit for the day. Do this every day until you can exercise continuously for 30 minutes daily without feeling sore. You can always add more challenging activities to your program later.

Excuse: I'm afraid that I'll strain my heart.

My rebuttal: It's true that heart rate and blood pressure rise during exercise, but this doesn't pose a danger for most people. A recently published Johns Hopkins study of healthy older people with mild hypertension (130–159 mmHg/85–99 mmHg) found that the short-term spike in blood pressure they experienced during moderate exercise (the equivalent of brisk walking plus weight training) didn't harm their hearts in any way. Since regular physical activity helps lower your heart rate and blood pressure when you're not exercising, being physically fit actually results in less overall strain on your heart.

Important: Always check with your doctor before starting any exercise program. If you ever develop chest pain, shortness of breath or dizziness during exercise, stop at once. If your symptoms go away as soon as you stop, check with your doctor as soon as possible. If symptoms continue, consult a doctor immediately.

Excuse: I can't find time in my schedule to exercise.

My rebuttal: There's no "best" time to exercise. The ideal time is any time that you will do it. It really doesn't matter whether you exercise first thing in the morning, during your lunch break or sometime in the early evening. And you don't have to exercise for long stretches at a time to get tremendous benefits. Multiple short bouts of exercise can be as effective as long sessions in strengthening your heart. Perform longer workouts (one hour or more) on the weekends, when you are more likely to have the time.

For some people, keeping an exercise diary is helpful. Use a calendar to schedule your workouts. After every workout, jot down what you did, how long you did it and how much distance you covered, if applicable. Tracking your progress will give you a sense of accomplishment and keeps you focused on your goals.

Excuse: I started to exercise once but got injured.

My rebuttal: It's true that almost two-thirds of people who start an exercise program end up dropping out because of an injury. Jogging is especially hard on your knees, hips and other joints because your feet hit the ground with a force greater than twice your body weight. However, the more slowly you run, the lower the shock. If you approach your exercise prudently, you probably won't get injured.

Here are some examples of exercises that are not likely to injure you—and that you may enjoy...

•**Take up swimming or tai chi.** These activities put little or no stress on your joints—while delivering significant fitness benefits. Swimming improves cardiovascular health, while tai chi strengthens muscles.

•**If you enjoy cycling, consider buying**— or getting your gym to buy—a recumbent stationary bike, which provides back support while you pedal.

Typical cost: $500. You can use it year-round indoors, and it's considered one of the safest types of exercise equipment available. This type of exercise is ideal for most people with back problems.

Excuse: I get bored.

My rebuttal: Exercise can be a great social activity itself—and can lead to a more interesting social life in general. Studies have shown that the people who stick to their exercise programs are more likely to meet regularly with other exercisers in some formalized way.

You don't have to exercise with others every day—but try to meet one or more people at least once a week. Join a walking, running or cycling club that has regular weekend events…agree to meet with one or more friends at a regular time each week for a group walk, swim, bike ride or gym workout…or set up a weekly session with a personal trainer. You won't be bored.

MY FAVORITES

Ballroom dancing and cycling are both great activities for couples. My wife and I like to ride bikes together, but we cycle at different speeds. So we bought a tandem bike that lets us ride together—each of us pedaling at our own level of effort—and joined a club that holds group tandem rides on the weekend.

10 Surprising Ways to Stay Healthy and Control Your Weight

Mehmet C. Oz, MD, medical director of the Integrated Medical Center and director of the Cardiovascular Institute at NewYork–Presbyterian Medical Center and professor and vice chairman of surgery at Columbia University, both in New York City. He is coauthor, with Michael F. Roizen, MD, of *You on a Diet: The Owner's Manual for Waist Management*. Free Press.

Whether you're trying to lose weight or simply find a healthful eating plan you can stick with, you're bound to fail if you try to stay on a diet. Invariably, people on diets end up depriving themselves of certain foods and/or scrupulously counting calories.

Problem: Virtually no one can maintain long-term deprivation because our bodies are programmed to avoid this type of ongoing discomfort. And calorie restriction causes your metabolism to slow down in order to preserve energy, often resulting in more stored fat.

The secret is to work with your body's chemistry rather than against it, so healthful eating becomes automatic, not forced.

Recent development: Body weight used to be considered one of the best indicators of overall health.

Now: Research has shown that your waist measurement (at or just below your navel) may be more reliable. That's because abdominal fat is especially harmful due to its proximity to your vital organs, where it can lead to harmful increases in cholesterol and triglyceride levels. Fat in this area has been linked to heart disease, cancer and diabetes. Studies have found that men should strive for a waist measurement of 35 inches or less, while women should aim for 32½ inches or less. When these measurements are exceeded, health risks increase. For example, risk for metabolic syndrome (a group of conditions, including hypertension and abdominal obesity, that raises diabetes and cardiovascular disease risk) increases by 40% at 40 inches for men and 37 inches for women.

Important: Even if your weight is ideal, you still can benefit from some of the strategies described below because they promote healthy cholesterol and blood pressure levels. *My recommendations…*

1. Spice up your morning eggs. Cayenne and other forms of red pepper contain capsaicin, a substance that suppresses appetite signals, increases metabolism and decreases the desire for food later in the day. In addition, eggs are high in protein, which tends to induce feelings of fullness.

2. Consume fiber early in the day. Fiber increases levels of appetite-suppressing signals in the small intestine. Eating fiber early in the day makes people less hungry in the afternoon— the time when most of us tend to eat snacks and other calorie-dense foods. Consume about 30 g of fiber daily in the form of high-fiber cereals, fruits and vegetables, and 100% whole grains.

3. Eat nuts. The monounsaturated fat in nuts stimulates the production of cholecystokinin (CCK), a chemical messenger that slows the rate at which the stomach empties and reduces appetite without putting your body into starvation mode—that is, the point at which it starts conserving calories, rather than burning them. Before lunch and/or dinner, have about six walnuts, 12 almonds or 12 hazelnuts.

4. Drink coffee instead of soft drinks. Coffee (caffeinated and decaffeinated) is a rich source of antioxidants, and Americans consume more of it than any other antioxidant-rich food. Coffee is much lower in calories (if you don't add a lot of sugar and/or creamer) than sugary soft drinks.

Bonus: Caffeine stimulates the release of norepinephrine, a hormone that suppresses appetite and promotes calorie burning by increasing heart rate and metabolism. Green tea also is a rich source of antioxidants and caffeine.

5. Supplement with 5-hydroxytryptophan (5-HTP). Related to the amino acid tryptophan and sold as a weight-loss supplement, 5-HTP increases brain levels of serotonin, a neurotransmitter that controls appetite. In one study, people taking 5-HTP for six weeks lost an average of 12 pounds, compared with only four pounds in a control group.

Recommended dose: 300 mg daily.

Bonus: 5-HTP has mood-enhancing benefits.

6. Turn up the thermostat. One reason that people tend to eat more during the cold months is that cold temperatures stimulate appetite. Also, people with naturally low body temperatures tend to have a slower metabolism and are more prone to weight gain. Staying warm may be a natural form of appetite control, particularly if you increase body temperature with exercise. Every one degree increase in body temperature increases metabolism by 14%.

7. Ask your doctor about Tagamet. The active ingredient (cimetidine) in this heartburn drug is thought to activate appetite-suppressing CCK. One 12-week study found that people taking a prescription form of Tagamet (400 mg, three times daily) had about a 5% decrease in waist size.

Important: Tagamet is unlikely to cause significant side effects, but should be taken to aid weight loss only if you have heartburn symptoms.

8. Consider using nicotine. It's common for people who quit smoking to gain weight, probably because the nicotine in tobacco suppresses appetite, increases metabolism and damages taste buds, which makes food less appealing. Studies have shown that nicotine—in the form of patches and gum, not from cigarettes—when combined with small amounts of caffeine, can help some people lose weight.

If you've hit a weight plateau: Talk to your doctor about combining a nicotine patch with two cups of coffee daily. Even for non-smokers, this approach can be used temporarily (to avoid possible addiction risk) to jump-start weight-loss efforts.

9. Smell grapefruit. Grapefruit oil, available from aromatherapy shops, emits an aroma that is thought to affect liver enzymes and help promote weight loss. In preliminary research, animals exposed to grapefruit scent for 15 minutes, three times weekly, had a reduction in appetite and body weight.

10. Control emotional stress. People who live with chronic stress (due to family pressures, a fast-paced job, etc.) produce high levels of cortisol, a stress hormone that increases the propensity for the omentum—a structure located near the stomach—to store fat. Excessive fat in the omentum can significantly increase waist size.

Important: Exercise is among the best ways to lower stress—and curb accumulations of omentum fat.

Recommended: A 30-minute walk and five minutes' worth of stretching daily…and three weekly sessions that include basic exercises, such as push-ups, shoulder shrugs, abdominal crunches, etc.

■ **More from Dr. Oz…**

What Type of Taster Are You?

Everyone likes some foods more than others, but genetic factors also determine whether we eat—or avoid—the foods that play a key role in weight management.

Supertasters tend to avoid fruits and vegetables because these foods may taste very bitter to them. Low intake of produce may put these people at greater risk for certain diseases and colon polyps. To ensure adequate nutritional intake, supertasters should take a daily multivitamin.

Undertasters, on the other hand, often eat too many sweets because they require a lot of sweet foods to feel satisfied. Therefore, undertasters should carefully monitor their intake of sweets.

To determine your type…

Mix a 1 g-sized pack of *saccharin* (Sweet'N Low) in two-thirds of a cup of water, then sip. If it tastes mostly bitter, you're probably a supertaster. If the taste seems more sweet than bitter, you're probably an undertaster.

Whole Grains Fight Serious Illnesses

Joanne Slavin, RD, PhD, food science and nutrition professor at the University of Minnesota in St. Paul. She is the author of dozens of medical articles on dietary fiber.

Everyone knows that eating ample amounts of fruits and vegetables can lower cholesterol, promote weight control and help prevent heart attack, stroke, diabetes and some types of cancer. But few people realize that whole grains are just as good as fruits and vegetables—and sometimes even better—at fighting many of these serious illnesses.

Fiber gets most of the credit for the healthful properties of whole grains, but studies have found that the phytochemicals, antioxidants, vitamins and minerals found in whole grains, which contain all parts of the grain, are just as important. *The whole grains described below can be found at most health-food stores and many grocery stores…*

AMARANTH

What it's good for: This tiny grain with an earthy, faintly grassy taste may protect against heart disease and cancer. It is also an excellent source of complete protein—that is, one that contains all eight essential amino acids.

Major effective ingredients: Vitamins E and B. Amaranth is also rich in calcium, phosphorus and iron.

How to add it to your diet: As it cooks, amaranth releases a glutinous starch that adds body to soups and stews.

*For recipes using whole grains, read *Whole Grains Every Day Every Way*, Clarkson Potter, by Lorna Sass or visit the Web site of the Whole Grains Council, *www. wholegrainscouncil.org*.

BROWN RICE

What it's good for: Helps fight eye disease (macular degeneration) and certain cancers, including lung cancer.

Major effective ingredients: Vitamin E and other antioxidants.

How to add it to your diet: Season brown rice as you would white rice, or it can be added to soups, casseroles, stir-fry dishes and salads.

CORN

What it's good for: Helps fight heart disease and cancer…and may guard against cataracts.

Major effective ingredients: Of all the grains, whole-grain corn is the richest source of antioxidants. It's also a good source of insoluble fiber, which cannot be digested but adds bulk to the stool.

How to add it to your diet: Choose whole-grain corn-based cereals, whole-grain cornmeal breads and cornmeal tortillas.

OATS AND BARLEY

What they are good for: Lowering cholesterol.

Major effective ingredient: Soluble fiber. When soluble fiber is digested, it changes to a gummy consistency that lowers blood cholesterol. The exact mechanism of this effect is not yet known.

How to add oats to your diet: Choose an oat cereal or oatmeal or make oatmeal cookies.

How to add barley to your diet: Use it to thicken soups and make creamy risottos, or cook it with carrots.

RYE

What it's good for: Protects against heart disease and hormone-dependent cancers, such as breast and prostate malignancies.

Major effective ingredient: Rye is a rich source of lignans, a class of phytoestrogens (plant compounds that help protect against the harmful effects of excess estrogen).

How to add it to your diet: Use whole-grain rye bread or whole-grain rye crackers.

WHEAT

What it's good for: It has a laxative effect that aids digestion and also is high in vitamins, minerals and antioxidants.

Major effective ingredient: Insoluble fiber.

How to add it to your diet: Replace white bread with whole-wheat bread…and highly processed cereals with whole-grain cereals.

Helpful: To ensure that a bread product contains whole grain, the label must include the word "whole."

Example: For whole wheat, look for whole-wheat flour or whole-wheat grain. Breads that contain seven, 12 or even 15 grains are not necessarily whole-grain breads.

Tricks to Make Yourself Eat Less

Lisa R. Young, PhD, RD, adjunct professor of nutrition at New York University and a nutritionist in private practice, both in New York City. She is the author of *The Portion Teller Plan: The No-Diet Reality Guide to Eating, Cheating and Losing Weight Permanently.* Morgan Road.

The food industry knows a powerful truth about one of your human weaknesses—the more food that is put in front of you, the more you will eat. This is generally true even for people who are weight-conscious, or who just feel better when they eat less.

It's easy to spot the "supersize" portion trend at a restaurant when you receive a giant bowl of pasta or a six-inch-high pile of onion rings—less easy to escape the same mindset when you eat at home.

Problem: Because Americans are eating more food than ever before, 66% of them are overweight or obese.* Being overweight or obese increases risk for diabetes, heart disease, high blood pressure, joint problems and even some types of cancer.

Childhood admonitions to "clean your plate!" …the desire to get what you pay for…and the time lapse between eating and feeling full (about 20 minutes) are some of the factors that

*Overweight is defined as a body mass index, or BMI, above 25…obesity is a BMI above 30. To determine your BMI, multiply your weight in pounds by 704.5. Divide that number by your height in inches squared. For a BMI calculator, visit the National Heart, Lung and Blood Institute Web site (*http://nhlbisupport.com/bmi*).

make most people eat whatever food is in front of them.

Even worse: The degree to which typical portion sizes have increased over the years is astounding. For example, fountain sodas during the 1950s and 1960s were about seven ounces, compared with 12 to 64 ounces these days. A typical bag of popcorn at the movies was once about five to six cups. Now a large bucket with butter flavor contains up to 20 cups and 1,640 calories. A pasta entrée at a restaurant? Double what it used to be. Eating at home? Standard plates, bowls and glasses are bigger, too—so we fill them up with more food.

HOW MUCH ARE YOU EATING?

The first step toward eating sensibly is to know how much you're consuming. This is much harder than it sounds. In one informal experiment conducted by a food writer in New York City, four expert nutritionists were given heaping plates of food (including pasta, risotto and sandwiches) and asked to estimate calorie and fat content. No one came even remotely close.

Nutritional guidelines generally suggest eating a set number of "servings" of meats, vegetables and other food groups. But a serving, which is usually defined in ounces, tablespoons or cups, is not the same as a portion, which is the actual amount of food served—at home or at a restaurant.

Examples: For grain products, a "serving" equals one slice of bread, one cup of ready-to-eat cold cereal or one-half cup of pasta. A restaurant order of linguine is likely to be three cups—nearly a whole day's recommended intake of grain! And a single bagel, in today's standard size of five ounces, equals *five* slices of bread.

DEVELOP PORTION AWARENESS

The problem with dietary guidelines is that measurements, such as cups, ounces and tablespoons, aren't easy to eyeball.

Helpful: Measure out the portion you ordinarily take. Then measure out a standard serving of meat, vegetables, pasta, etc. See what each looks like in comparison.

Important: If your usual portion of meat is actually two servings, you don't necessarily have to cut back during that meal—just know that you have consumed nearly a day's allocation of meat and adjust the rest of the day's intake accordingly.

RESTAURANT SMARTS

Portion inflation is most out of control in restaurants—where the average American eats four times a week. *To defend yourself against today's supersize restaurant meals, follow these steps...*

•**Have a snack at home.** About an hour before eating out, eat some fruit, low-fat yogurt or vegetable-based soup (made without milk or cream), so you won't arrive at the restaurant famished.

•**Have the right appetizer.** Many people skip the appetizer in an attempt to cut down on the size of their meal. That's a mistake. Order a soup, salad or a vegetable appetizer to fill up, and tell the waiter not to bring the bread basket. A Pennsylvania State University study found that starting lunch with a low-calorie salad cuts the total caloric intake of the meal by as much as 12% because the fiber contained in the salad is filling.

•**Order small entrées.** Or order a half-size portion, if available. Or share a full-size entrée with your dining companion—in most restaurants, it will be enough (especially if you add a salad or a side order of vegetables).

•**Eat only half of the meal.** When you order an entrée for yourself, eat half and ask the waiter to wrap up the rest to take home. This way, you'll be eating about as much as restaurant-goers did 20 years ago.

Helpful: Don't rely on willpower alone—when the entrée first arrives, set aside what you plan to eat and ask the waiter to wrap up the rest.

•**Slow down!** Eat at a leisurely pace to give your body time to catch up with your appetite, and stop before you're full—no matter how much is left. If you're tempted to finish off the plate or go back for seconds, stop and wait 20 minutes. That's usually all it takes to feel satiated.

PORTION CONTROL AT HOME

Portion sizes are set not only by restaurants, but also by food and even dinnerware manufacturers. *Here's how to protect yourself...*

•**Choose smaller dinnerware.** We're conditioned to think that a meal-size portion is what fills a plate. That's why you should set your table with eight- to 10-ounce (not 20-ounce) glasses ...10-inch (rather than 12-inch) dinner plates... and bowls that hold two cups rather than four.

Helpful: One woman I know found a simple way to downsize her portions—she bought a charming set of 1950s dishes at a flea market.

•**Divide your plate.** Allocate space on your plate to meet healthful dietary recommendations —fill half with vegetables and fruit...one-fourth with meat, fish or another protein source...and one-fourth with grains or starchy vegetables.

Helpful: Plates marked with portion reminders for adults and children are available from BeBetter Networks, 304-345-6800, *www.the portionplate.com.*

Cost: About $10 per plate.

•**Create your own snack portions.** To control your consumption of pretzels, chips and other snack foods, read the label to see how many servings the package contains—and portion it out into that number of plastic, resealable bags. Do the same with three-ounce portions of deli meats.

•**Substitute foods.** Three cups of popcorn is just as filling as three-quarters cup of pretzels —and popcorn is a healthful whole grain, while pretzels are typically refined. Three cups of puffed wheat go a lot further than one-quarter cup of granola. Fresh fruits typically leave you feeling more satisfied and with fewer calories than juices or dried fruit.

■ **More from Dr. Young...**

Serving-Size Guide

One serving looks like...

VEGETABLES AND FRUIT

Daily intake: Three or more servings of vegetables...two to four servings of fruits.

1 cup of raw fruit or vegetables = fist
1 medium fruit = baseball
½ cup of cooked fruit or vegetables = ½ baseball
¼ cup of raisins = large egg

GRAIN PRODUCTS

Daily intake: Four to eight servings of grains and starchy vegetables.

1 cup of cereal flakes = fist
½ cup of cooked rice, pasta or potato = ½ baseball
1 slice of bread = cassette tape

MEAT AND ALTERNATIVES

Daily intake: Two to three servings of meat, poultry, fish or a meat alternative.

3 oz. of meat, fish or poultry = deck of cards

Daily intake: Two to three servings of dairy products.

1 oz. of cheese = 4 dice

FATS

Daily intake: One to three servings of fats.

1 tsp. of butter or other spread = 1 die
1 Tbsp. of peanut butter = ½ Ping-Pong ball

■ ■ ■ ■

Sweet! Mandarin Oranges Lower Liver Cancer Risk

According to scientists at Kyoto Prefectural University of Medicine in Japan, mandarin oranges may reduce the risk of liver cancer in patients with chronic viral hepatitis. Thirty patients who drank one cup daily of a beverage containing mandarin orange juice for one year showed no signs of liver cancer. However, nearly 9% of 45 patients who did not drink the beverage developed liver cancer.

Further positive findings come from a team at the National Institute of Fruit Tree Science in Japan who surveyed 1,073 Japanese people who consumed large amounts of mandarin oranges. The researchers report that chemical markers in the subjects' blood were associated with a lower risk for liver disease, atherosclerosis, and insulin resistance, which can lead to diabetes.

Hoyoku Nishino, MD, PhD, researcher, Kyoto Prefectural University of Medicine, Kyoto, Japan. American Chemical Society annual meeting, San Francisco.

■ ■ ■ ■

If you are not a juice drinker, try this healthful recipe that includes mandarin oranges…

Mandarin Medallions Recipe

Ingredients:

1 (1-pound) pork tenderloin
1 tablespoon vegetable oil
½ cup orange juice
¼ cup orange marmalade
1 teaspoon prepared horseradish
½ teaspoon cinnamon
2 tablespoons lemon juice
1 tablespoon cornstarch
1 (10-ounce) can mandarin orange segments, drained

Instructions:

Slice tenderloin crosswise into eight pieces. Flatten slightly. Heat oil in large, heavy skillet over medium-high heat. Brown pork quickly, about one minute per side.

Mix thoroughly remaining ingredients except mandarin oranges; add to skillet, cook and stir until sauce thickens. Simmer 3 to 4 minutes. Remove to serving platter; garnish with mandarin oranges.

 For more recipes, visit the Web site *www. recipegoldmine.com.*

Eat Less and Boost Your Immune System

Janko Nikolich-Zugich, MD, PhD, senior scientist, Vaccine and Gene Therapy Institute, Oregon Health & Science University, Beaverton.
Proceedings of the National Academy of Sciences.

New research with rhesus monkeys sheds light on why restricting calories may extend your life span. Limiting consumption of calories seems to boost key infection-fighting cells in the immune system, the researchers say.

"The key finding is that in a primate species, which is very similar to ourselves, there is a very remarkable effect on the maintenance of the immune system with caloric restriction," said lead researcher Dr. Janko Nikolich-Zugich, a senior scientist at Oregon Health & Science University's Vaccine and Gene Therapy Institute.

THE STUDY

In the 42-month study, Nikolich-Zugich and his colleagues found that calorie restriction improved the maintenance and production of infection-fighting T-cells in 13 rhesus monkeys, 18 to 23 years of age, whose calories were restricted, compared with 28 monkeys who ate a normal diet.

The researchers found that calorie restriction improved T-cell function and reduced the production of inflammatory compounds. These findings suggest that limiting calories can delay immunological aging, and, in turn, life span may be increased by providing longer-term resistance to infectious diseases.

IMPLICATIONS

Nikolich-Zugich said that people who restrict the number of calories they take in also may live longer because their immune system is stronger. He said it may be possible to find a drug that mimics calorie restriction that could improve the immune system.

info For more information on the effects of calorie restriction, visit the Web site of the Calorie Restriction Society at *www.calorie restriction.org.*

A Biological Basis for Being a Couch Potato?

American Physiological Society news release.

B rain biology may explain why some people tend to be couch potatoes while others are more active. That's the conclusion of a US study that found some brains may naturally encourage restless behaviors that burn calories and help control weight.

THE STUDY

Researchers found that the brains of rats bred to be lean are more sensitive to a chemical produced in the brain called orexin A. This chemical stimulates appetite and spontaneous movement, such as fidgeting. The study also determined that compared with rats bred to be obese, the lean rats had a far greater expression of orexin receptors in an area of the brain called the hypothalamus.

IMPLICATION

"The greater expression of orexin receptors suggests the lean rats' brains were more sensitive to the orexin the brain produces. The results point to a biological basis for being a couch potato," said senior researcher Catherine M. Kotz of the VA Medical Center, University of Minnesota, and the Minnesota Obesity Center.

She said this research suggests that frequent unconscious movement, such as fidgeting, may burn calories and help control weight. It also could lead to the development of drugs to stimulate minor physical activity to promote weight loss.

info You can learn more about weight management by visiting *www.consumer.gov/ weightloss/setgoals.htm.*

■ ■ ■ ■

Weight Loss May Cut Prostate Cancer Risk

L osing weight may reduce the risk of prostate cancer, says an American Cancer Society study of nearly 70,000 men. The study also found that obesity increases the risk of more aggressive prostate cancer.

THE STUDY

The study participants reported their weight in 1982 and again 10 years later. The men were then followed until 2003. During that time, 5,000 of them were diagnosed with prostate cancer.

Men who lost at least 11 pounds between 1982 and 1992 were about half as likely as other men to be diagnosed with nonmetastatic, aggressive high-grade prostate cancer.

ADVICE

"Obesity is one of the most prevalent modifiable cancer risk factors. Previous studies have linked maintaining a healthy weight and weight loss to a decreasing risk of breast cancer," said study author Dr. Carmen Rodriguez.

"Our study linking obesity to aggressive prostate cancer adds to increasing evidence of the importance of maintaining a healthy weight through adult life. Although our study suggests that weight loss may lower the risk of aggressive prostate cancer, given the difficulty of losing weight, emphasis should be put on the importance of avoiding weight gain to reduce the risk of prostate cancer," Rodriguez said.

info Learn more about prostate cancer at the National Institutes of Health Web site at *http://nihseniorhealth.gov.*

American Cancer Society news release.

■ ■ ■ ■

Juicing for Health

Fruits and vegetables are chock-full of vitamins, minerals and phytonutrients, all of which play a crucial role in preventing cardiovascular disease, cancer and most other serious ailments. The most protective effect comes from having 10 daily servings of a wide variety of fruits and vegetables. Juicing can help you achieve this goal.

Making mostly vegetable juices, which contain much less of the naturally occurring sugar found in fruit juices, is recommended. People new to juicing can develop diarrhea, so begin slowly. Start with four ounces of fresh juice each morning (equivalent to one to two servings of fruits and vegetables). After a week, add four ounces in the evening.

Fresh is best, but juice can be stored for up to two days in a closed container or frozen. Juicing should not be a substitute for eating whole fruits and vegetables. You still need the fiber that most juicers remove. The Vita-Mix 5000 juicer (800-848-2649, *www.vitamix.com*) retains much of the fiber.

Vegetable Juice Recipe Ideas

Try these three-vegetable combinations for easy juicing.

The 3-C's (Carrot, Celery, Cabbage)

3–4 carrots

1–2 celery stalks

Small wedge cabbage

Sweet Drink

5 carrots

1 apple

½ beet

Muscle Beach

5 handfuls spinach

1 cucumber

2 carrots

For more recipes, consult *Juicing for Life* by Cherie Calbom (Avery).

Caution: If you have diabetes, check with your doctor before starting a juice program. The naturally occurring sugars, especially from fruit, may elevate blood glucose levels.

Dr. Mark Stengler is a licensed naturopathic medical doctor and a leading authority on the practice of alternative and integrated medicine. An associate clinical professor at the National College of Naturopathic Medicine in Portland, OR, Dr. Stengler has served on a medical advisory committee for the Yale University Complementary Medicine Outcomes Research Project and is the author or coauthor of 16 books, including two best sellers—*The Natural Physician's Healing Therapies* and *Prescription for Natural Cures.* (Both from Bottom Line Books). Dr. Stengler is the founder and director of the La Jolla Whole Health Clinic in La Jolla, CA. *www.DrStengler.com.*

Foods with Hidden Trans Fats

Dr. Mark Stengler is a licensed naturopathic medical doctor and a leading authority on the practice of alternative and integrated medicine. An associate clinical professor at the National College of Naturopathic Medicine in Portland, OR, Dr. Stengler has served on a medical advisory committee for the Yale University Complementary Medicine Outcomes Research Project and is the author or coauthor of 16 books, including two best sellers—*The Natural Physician's Healing Therapies* and *Prescription for Natural Cures.* (Both from Bottom Line Books). Dr. Stengler is the founder and director of the La Jolla Whole Health Clinic in La Jolla, CA. *www.DrStengler.com.*

Since the FDA has food producers to list trans fat content on food labels, many manufacturers have stopped using this harmful fat. However, not all foods are free of trans fat—and it may be "hidden" unless you know what to look for on food labels.

There's no question that trans fat is bad for your health. It raises LDL "bad" cholesterol and lowers HDL "good" cholesterol…and it increases inflammation in the body, a risk factor for heart disease, diabetes, cancer and other serious medical conditions.

THE EMERGENCE OF TRANS FAT

Trans fat (short for trans-fatty acids) has been used since the early 1900s, when food scientists discovered that if they pumped hydrogen through liquid vegetable oil, it turned into a viscous substance—known as partially hydrogenated oil. Trans fat not only created flaky crusts and the texture, or "mouth feel," of butter, but also extended the shelf life of foods when grocery stores began appearing in the US.

Because the fat served as an excellent substitute for lard, which spoiled easily, and butter, which was expensive, it became a mainstay in margarine, commercial baked goods, pastries, cookies, crackers and deep-fried foods as well as frozen dinners, chips and even some cereals.

WHERE TRANS FAT LURKS

According to the FDA trans fat labeling regulation, a food product can be made to appear to be free of trans fat even if it contains small amounts of the fat.

For example, the nutrition facts label of a food that contains trans fat, in an amount less than 0.5 g per serving, may claim "zero trans fat" —or it may omit a trans fat listing but include a footnote that reads, "Not a significant source of trans fat."

That's why it's important to look at the ingredient list as well as the nutrition facts label of all food products. If "partially hydrogenated oil," "shortening" or "vegetable shortening" appears in the ingredient list—but trans fat is not listed on the nutrition facts label—the food contains trans fat, but less than 0.5 g per serving.

Such small amounts of trans fat may, at first glance, seem insignificant, but that's not the case if you consume multiple daily servings of the food, as is common for many people.

Some snack foods, such as granola bars, tout "zero trans fat" per serving, while listing partially hydrogenated oil among the ingredients.

Example: Quaker Chewy Chocolate Chip Granola Bars state zero grams of trans fat per one-bar (24 g) serving but list partially hydrogenated soybean and/or cottonseed oil in the ingredient list. Aunt Jemima Complete Pancake & Waffle Mix also states zero grams of trans fat per serving (two four-inch pancakes), yet the ingredient list includes partially hydrogenated soybean oil.

Even some products promoted for their health benefits contain partially hydrogenated oil. For example, Benecol is a soft-spread substitute for margarine or butter that is advertised as having cholesterol-lowering effects, when two to three servings a day are consumed in place of other spreads. But Benecol's ingredient list includes partially hydrogenated soybean oil.

DANGERS OF SATURATED FAT

Although some meat and dairy products also contain small amounts of trans fat, in a naturally occurring form, their saturated fat content is a far more significant health concern.

Found primarily in whole milk, cheese, butter, ice cream and red meat, saturated fat has long been known to increase heart disease risk by raising cholesterol levels. Now, with the recent focus on the health dangers of trans fat, many experts fear that people will go too far in their efforts to avoid it—and end up eating more saturated fat as a result.

Scientific research has found that trans fat appears to be more harmful than saturated fat. However, according to the Institute of Medicine, a nonprofit organization that provides health advice to the public and private sectors, daily consumption of trans fat and saturated fat should be kept as low as possible.

Until more research is completed, I recommend treating saturated fat and trans fat as equal threats.

Wise idea: When evaluating a food product, add the grams of trans fat and saturated fat together. Limit your combined daily total intake of these fats to the daily recommended intake for saturated fat alone (20 g for people consuming 2,000 calories in a day).

Important: Polyunsaturated fat, found in corn, soybean and safflower oils...and mono-unsaturated fat, found in olives, avocados, nuts, and olive, canola and peanut oils...have the opposite effect—these fats reduce heart disease risk by lowering LDL and raising HDL levels.

Polyunsaturated and mono-unsaturated fats generally are found in foods of plant origin, and these fats remain liquid at room temperature. Most saturated fats come from animal sources and are solid at room temperature.

12

Pain Treatments

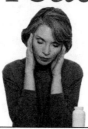

New Study Says Chondroitin Doesn't Work

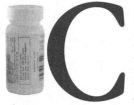

Chondroitin, an ingredient in arthritis supplements that sell in excess of $1 billion a year, does not relieve hip or knee pain stemming from osteoarthritis any better than a placebo, according to new research.

This cartilage extract is often combined with the amino sugar glucosamine, in capsules and pills specifically to ease arthritis pain and slow joint deterioration caused by the disease. Chondrotin-glucosamine products are among the most popular over-the-counter products sold at health-food stores, vitamin shops and pharmacies.

"Chondroitin is not efficacious for pain in osteoarthritis," says Dr. David T. Felson, a professor of medicine and epidemiology at Boston University. "I don't recommend that patients start taking glucosamine and chondroitin, because glucosamine also doesn't work."

However, he adds the supplements are not dangerous and may provide a placebo effect in which patients feel better because they believe the products work.

THE STUDIES

Felson's comments come after a close examination, by a team of Swiss researchers, on data on 20 previous studies involving more than 3,600 patients with osteoarthritis. In each of those studies, chondroitin was compared with a placebo or no treatment.

The researchers say that in people with advanced osteoarthritis, chondroitin is no more beneficial than a placebo. They also find no evidence showing any pain-relieving effect of chondroitin for early osteoarthritis.

Those researchers, like Felson, say that the use of chondroitin should be "discouraged" by doctors who treat the 21 million Americans with osteoarthritis.

David T. Felson, MD, MPH, professor of medicine and epidemiology, Boston University.
Annals of Internal Medicine.

info The American Academy of Orthopaedic Surgeons has more on osteoarthritis at *http://orthoinfo.aaos.org.*

Arthritis-Brain Link May Lead to New Treatments

Arthritis & Rheumatism.

It's scary having to deal with arthritis, with good reason. British scientists have discovered that pain signals of this common condition generate higher activity than other types of pain in the part of the brain that controls emotions and fear.

This suggests that arthritis pain may have more of an emotional impact and stronger association with fear and distress than other types of pain. This association may possibly lead to new ways of treating arthritis, says study lead author Professor A.K.P. Jones of the University of Manchester Rheumatic Diseases Centre.

In his small but significant study, 12 people with knee osteoarthritis underwent brain imaging scans as researchers monitored their brain activity under three circumstances—experiencing osteoarthritis pain; pain caused by heat application; and no pain.

Both the osteoarthritis and heat-induced pain activated a network of brain structures known as the pain matrix, which contains two parallel systems. One processes the emotional aspects of pain, including fear and stress; the other processes the pain's physical location, intensity and duration.

While both osteoarthritis and heat-induced pain activated both systems, the pain of arthritis caused heightened activity in the "fear" system, but not the heat-induced pain.

■ ■ ■ ■

Psoriasis Drug Stops Rheumatoid Arthritis

In an 18-month study of 110 people with an undetermined form of arthritis characterized by painful and stiff joints, those who took weekly doses of *methotrexate* (Rheumatrex) for 12 months were less likely to develop rheumatoid arthritis, one of the most debilitating forms of the disease—and more likely to go into remission—than those who took a placebo.

Theory: Methotrexate, a drug used to treat some cancers and severe psoriasis, works, in part, by curbing activation of white blood cells, which may play a role in causing rheumatoid arthritis.

Caution: For treatment of rheumatoid arthritis, methotrexate is taken once a week, not once a day, as it is for the treatment of cancer.

Thomas W. J. Huizinga, MD, PhD, professor and chairman, department of rheumatology, Leiden University Medical Center, The Netherlands.

■ ■ ■ ■

Smoking May Play Role in Knee Osteoarthritis

There is yet another reason to kick the smoking habit—it can help you kick more comfortably.

It appears that smoking may increase the risk for cartilage loss and lead to more severe pain in people with osteoarthritis of the knee, say researchers.

Researchers can't explain the specific cause-and-effect, but after following 159 men with knee osteoarthritis for 30 months, they found that across-the-board, smokers were at increased risk of cartilage loss and experienced more pain than men who did not smoke—even after adjusting for factors such as age, body weight and disease severity.

The greater pain seen in smokers isn't likely due to cartilage loss, since cartilage does not have pain fibers, explains study lead Dr. David Felson of Boston University School of Medicine. But smoking may affect other mechanisms in the body that control pain.

More research is currently under way.

David Felson, MD, director of the Clinical Epidemiology Research and Training Unit and professor of medicine and public health, Boston University School of Medicine.

Annals of the Rheumatic Diseases.

Arthritis Relief— Treatments That Work Very Well

John D. Clough, MD, rheumatologist in the department of rheumatic and immunologic disease at The Cleveland Clinic. He is author of *Arthritis: A Cleveland Clinic Guide.* The Cleveland Clinic.

More than 21 million Americans suffer from osteoarthritis, a degenerative joint disease. That's the bad news.

The good news—we know more about the disease now than ever before, including how to slow its progression.

CAUSES

There are many different forms of arthritis. Osteoarthritis is the most common form. When you have osteoarthritis, the cartilage that cushions the ends of the bones in your joints deteriorates. Over time, the cartilage may wear down completely, leaving bone rubbing on bone.

Osteoarthritis commonly affects the fingers, neck, lower back, hips and knees. *The exact cause of the disease isn't known, but the following are key risk factors...*

•**Advancing age.** People 45 years and older are at greater risk for the disease. In older people, the joint cartilage contains less fluid and may become brittle, which leads to deterioration.

•**Family history.** Heredity plays a role, especially in osteoarthritis of the hands. This particular type of osteoarthritis, which ultimately gives the fingers a gnarled appearance, is more common in women whose mothers also suffered from the condition.

•**Previous injury.** Not every joint injury causes a problem, but if you have had torn cartilage or a disruption of the ligaments in a major joint, then you are more likely to develop a problem in that area.

•**Obesity.** Being overweight puts unnecessary stress on weight-bearing joints—particularly hips and knees.

EARLY WARNINGS

Osteoarthritis often progresses slowly, but there can be early signs...

•**Joint pain** during or after use, after a period of inactivity or during a change in the weather.

•**Swelling and stiffness** in a joint, particularly after using it.

•**Joint instability,** especially noticeable in the knees, which can even take on a knock-kneed or bowlegged appearance as the cartilage deteriorates.

•**Bony lumps.** With osteoarthritis of the hands, these lumps (called Heberden's nodes and Bouchard's nodes) can appear on the middle or end joints of the fingers or at the base of your thumb.

PROTECT YOURSELF

There is no known cure for osteoarthritis, but lifestyle measures can help. *To prevent or slow progression of the disease...*

•**Lose weight.** While it's obvious that running and jumping can be hard on the joints, if you're overweight, even everyday tasks such as walking and climbing stairs can be problematic. Shed pounds, and you can ease the pressure on your weight-bearing joints.

•**Exercise.** Choose low-impact activities, such as walking, cycling and swimming, so that you don't put too much pressure on your joints.

If you've had a knee injury, it also pays to do quadriceps-strengthening and hamstring-stretching exercises so that those muscles can better stabilize and operate the knee.

New finding: A study recently published in *Arthritis & Rheumatism* shows that people with knee osteoarthritis who exercised regularly for as long as 18 months had less disability and were able to walk much greater distances than people who dropped out of the program.

Check with your doctor before beginning a regular exercise program. He/she may recommend working with a physical therapist who can design an exercise program to meet your specific needs.

MEDICATIONS

Osteoarthritis sufferers have a range of treatment options...

•**Oral medications.** The most commonly used drugs for osteoarthritis are pain relievers, such as *acetaminophen* (Tylenol) and non-steroidal anti-inflammatory drugs (NSAIDs), which fall into two categories...

•**Nonselective NSAIDs.** Drugs such as aspirin, *ibuprofen* (Advil), *diclofenac* (Voltaren) and *naproxen* (Aleve) are commonly used to treat the symptoms caused by inflammation (pain, swelling, redness, etc.), and they work very well for some people. However, long-term use of NSAIDs can cause problems ranging from stomach upset to gastrointestinal bleeding.

•**Injections.** In cases where a particular joint is acutely inflamed, a physician might opt to inject a corticosteroid preparation into the joint. This can provide rapid relief for up to several months, but long-term use of corticosteroids can be harmful to tissue and bones.

SUPPLEMENTS

Glucosamine and *chondroitin sulfate* play a role in the structure of cartilage and other connective tissue—and you can get them over-the-counter in supplement form. A massive study, known as the "Glucosamine/Chondroitin Arthritis Intervention Trial (GAIT)," coordinated by the University of Utah School of Medicine, found that in patients with moderate to severe pain, glucosamine and chondroitin provided statistically significant pain relief. However, the combination did not work any better than a placebo for the overall group of patients.

Also, a study conducted in 2002 suggests that glucosamine could potentially slow the progression of osteoarthritis of the knees, although not all studies of this supplement confirm this finding. More research is needed, but the supplements seem safe to use if you choose to try them.

Exception: People who are allergic to shellfish should steer clear of glucosamine, which is made from shellfish.

JOINT REPLACEMENT

In joint-replacement therapy (arthroplasty), the damaged joint is removed and replaced with a plastic or metal prosthesis. Joint replacement can be very effective, particularly for the major weight-bearing joints, such as the hips and knees, allowing you an active, pain-free life. Shoulder replacement also is effective, and the technology for smaller, more complex joints, such as the wrist and ankle, is improving.

Exercise Boosts Recovery For Arthritis Patients

Daniel Rooks, PhD, assistant professor, medicine, Division of Rheumatology and Center for the Study of Nutrition Medicine, Beth Israel Deaconess Medical Center, and Harvard Medical School, Boston.
"Effect of Preoperative Exercise on Measures of Functional Status in Men and Women Undergoing Total Hip and Knee Arthroplasty," an article that appeared in *Arthritis Care & Research.*

Weight training and cardiovascular exercise may be just the ticket for patients who are preparing for knee- or hip-replacement surgery, a new study suggests.

Those patients who took part in one-hour exercise regimens just three times a week were 73% less likely to be discharged to a rehabilitation center after their surgery, researchers found.

Only 12 of 36 patients who took part in the exercise had to enter the rehab centers, compared with 23 of 43 patients who didn't exercise, said study author Daniel Rooks, an assistant professor of medicine at Harvard Medical School, and Beth Israel Deaconess Medical Center in Boston.

While the study is small, Rooks said, "The benefits of exercise before surgery are very clear. The more you can do for yourself physically before surgery, the better off you are."

BACKGROUND

It's no secret that physically fit people are better able to tolerate osteoarthritis, Rooks said. "Their muscles and soft tissues are stronger and better conditioned, which helps stabilize the knee, protect the joints and allow people with arthritis to move with less discomfort." But it was unclear how much value exercise provides to people with severe arthritis who face surgery.

THE STUDY

Rooks and his colleagues enlisted patients who were preparing for either hip- or knee-replacement surgery and divided them into two groups. One group took part in one-hour group exercise regimens three times a week at a hospital-affiliated fitness center. At first, participants performed water exercises. Then they moved on to stationary bikes, weight lifting (with both machines and dumbbells) and abdominal strengthening exercises. They also stretched.

Even in a fairly brief time period—six weeks—the exercise paid benefits for the participants. "We saw that their level of function stabilized and their pain stabilized prior to surgery," Rooks said. "Those who did not exercise, their function and pain got worse."

IMPLICATIONS

Six weeks isn't enough time to boost muscle strength by major amounts, Rooks said. But, he added, it's possible that some of the benefits came because participants "were just feeling more confident and comfortable that they could exert themselves without hurting themselves."

Ultimately, the study shows that "just because you have arthritis doesn't mean you should not exercise, and if you have arthritis, it's another reason you should begin exercising or keep exercising," Rooks said.

info To learn more about arthritis and exercise, go to the National Institutes of Health Web site at *http://www.niams.nih.gov.* Click on "Health Information" and then scroll down to "Arthritis and Exercise."

Six Ways to Ease the Pain of Pinched Nerves

David Borenstein, MD, clinical professor of medicine at George Washington University Medical Center, Washington, DC. He maintains a private practice at Arthritis and Rheumatism Associates in Washington, DC, and is author of *Back in Control: Your Complete Prescription for Preventing, Treating, and Eliminating Back Pain from Your Life.* M. Evans and Company.

Nerve pain is one of the worst kinds of pain. People with a pinched nerve (sometimes called a "stinger") may experience sharp, burning pain for anywhere from a few seconds to a few days or longer. The pain usually comes on suddenly and may disappear just as fast—only to return. There also might be temporary numbness or slight weakness.

A nerve gets "pinched" when surrounding tissue presses against it and causes inflammation of the nerve. Causes include repetitive motions, traumatic injuries and joint diseases, such as rheumatoid arthritis. The most common

pinched nerves occur in the wrist, elbow, shoulder and foot. Nerve roots in the spinal canal also are vulnerable.

Red flag: Nerve pain that is accompanied by significant weakness or that doesn't improve within a few days needs to be checked by a physician. Excessive pressure on—or inflammation of—a nerve can result in loss of function and permanent damage.

SELF-HELP

To reduce the pain…

•**Stop repetitive movements.** A pinched nerve that's caused by performing the same movements over and over again usually will improve once the offending activity—leaning with your elbows on a counter, typing, working a cash register, etc.—is stopped for a few days. Avoiding these activities is also the best way to prevent a pinched nerve.

However, patients with job-related pain can't always afford to take time off. In that case, they should attempt to change their body position when doing the activity.

Example: Raising the back of a computer keyboard (most are adjustable) will enlarge the carpal tunnel in the wrist and reduce pressure on the nerve.

•**Ice the area.** Applying cold in the first 24 to 48 hours after nerve pain starts can reduce tissue swelling and nerve pressure. Use a cold pack or ice cubes wrapped in a towel. Hold cold against the affected area for about 15 minutes. Repeat every hour or two for a day or two.

•**Take an anti-inflammatory.** Over-the-counter analgesics that have anti-inflammatory properties, such as aspirin, ibuprofen and naproxen, reduce the body's production of chemicals that cause inflammation and swelling. Don't use *acetaminophen*. It will reduce pain but has little effect on inflammation.

•**Wear looser clothes.** It's fairly common for women to experience a pinched nerve in the outer thigh *(meralgia paresthetica)* from too-tight jeans or skirts…or foot pain *(tarsal tunnel syndrome)* from tight shoes.

MEDICAL CARE

Nerve pain that's severe or keeps coming back —or that's accompanied by other symptoms, such as a loss of bowel or bladder control—requires immediate medical care. Customized splints or braces can be used to minimize pressure on a nerve from repetitive movements. *Also helpful…*

•**An injection of a corticosteroid** into the painful area—or a short course of oral steroid therapy. These drugs reduce inflammation very quickly and provide short-term relief. The pain may disappear after a single treatment, but most patients need repeated courses. Sometimes, if pain is not relieved, acupuncture may be used in addition to medication and physical therapy.

•**Surgery is recommended** when the pain is severe or keeps coming back. The procedures vary depending on the part of the body affected.

Neck Pain? Quick Ways For Long-Lasting Relief

Gerard P. Varlotta, DO, an associate professor of rehabilitation medicine and director of sports rehabilitation at the Rusk Institute of Rehabilitation Medicine at New York University Medical Center in New York City.

There are very few upper-body movements that don't require use of the neck. That's why neck injury is one of the most common problems treated by orthopedists and physiatrists (doctors who specialize in rehabilitation medicine).

Most neck injuries are due to "onetime overload"—for example, putting too much strain on the neck by not keeping it in a neutral position while lifting a heavy object. Neck pain also can be caused by strain due to repetitive motions, such as twisting and turning the neck while exercising…muscle tension from stress…arthritic changes…or whiplash. Also, neck pain can be "referred" pain stemming from shoulder or elbow injuries or gallbladder disease.

Good news: Since neck pain usually includes muscle inflammation, it responds well to self-care. Even chronic pain usually can be relieved—and prevented—with simple exercises. Surgery is recommended in rare cases, such as those in which neck pain is accompanied by radiating arm pain and compression of a nerve.

REASONS FOR NECK PAIN

Severe neck pain usually comes on suddenly, but often there's an underlying irritation and/or weakness in the muscles. In most cases, the sufferer reports that the neck feels a little weak or sore, then suddenly worsens—after turning the head abruptly, for example.

When to get help: Neck pain that doesn't begin improving within 48 hours or is accompanied by neurological symptoms—tingling in the arms, hand weakness, loss of muscle strength, etc.—indicates a more serious problem. *Examples…*

•**Disk damage.** A herniated disk (the gelatinous material inside a disk pushes through the outer coating and presses against nearby nerves) can be excruciatingly painful and, in severe cases, cause permanent spinal cord damage.

Red flag: A loss of bowel and/or bladder control or any of the above neurological symptoms. See a doctor immediately.

•**Arthritic changes.** The joints in the neck can deteriorate or stiffen due to osteoarthritis or rheumatoid arthritis.

•**Whiplash.** Injury results when the head is jerked violently forward and backward, as can occur during a car accident.

The above problems are diagnosed during a physical exam, often in conjunction with an X-ray and/or magnetic resonance imaging (MRI) scan. Treatment involves controlling inflammation and restoring strength and range of motion.

RAPID PAIN RELIEF

In the absence of neurological symptoms, arthritis or traumatic injury, patients can assume that neck pain is probably due to muscle strain. *To reduce muscle inflammation and pain…*

•**Apply ice immediately.** It's the quickest way to reduce inflammation as well as pain—but only if you apply it within the first 24 to 48 hours. Hold a cold pack or ice cubes wrapped in a towel or washcloth to the painful area for 20 minutes once an hour throughout the day.

Important: Do *not* apply heat during the first two days after an injury. It relieves stiffness but can increase inflammation and pain.

•**Take the proper anti-inflammatory drug.** Over-the-counter *ibuprofen* (Advil) and *naproxen* (Aleve) are equally effective at relieving muscle pain and inflammation.

Main difference: Ibuprofen is a relatively short-acting drug—generally lasting four to six hours. Naproxen lasts eight to 12 hours. *Acetaminophen* (Tylenol) may help, but it mainly eases pain, not inflammation.

Caution: Ibuprofen and naproxen can cause stomach upset…*acetaminophen* can cause liver damage when combined with alcohol. Don't take any of these drugs for more than a week without consulting your doctor.

•**Stretch muscles often.** Stretching lengthens muscle fibers and reduces the tension caused by neck-related ergonomic problems, such as how you sit at a computer or hold a telephone. *Helpful…*

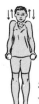 While standing or sitting, slowly lower your ear toward your shoulder. Stop when pain significantly increases. Hold the stretch for a few seconds, then relax. Switch to the other side. Repeat eight to 12 times, five times a day.

Bring your chin toward your shoulder, following the directions above.

Although chiropractic treatment can help alleviate pain that emanates from the neck joints, its effects are not long-lasting. Acupuncture also may be helpful but needs to be repeated until the pain dissipates.

LONG-TERM NECK CARE

Most people with chronic neck pain need to perform strengthening exercises (consult your doctor first) and change their posture.

Important: Don't sleep on your stomach—and don't raise your head too high with pillows. Both put excessive pressure on the neck.

Better: Sleep on your side with your head level—propped just high enough to keep your nose in line with your navel. The pillow (when compressed) should be just thick enough to support the side of your head without elevating it.

If you spend a great deal of time on the telephone, use a headset. Cradling a phone between the neck and shoulder is one of the most common causes of neck pain. Choose a headset that is comfortable for you. Good ones, such as those made by Plantronics, are available for $40 to $100 at electronics stores.

If you spend time at a desk, adjust your workstation. The center of a standard computer monitor should be directly at eye level (a bit lower if it's a large monitor)…your knees should be slightly lower than your hips…and use your chair's armrests when possible to avoid hunching forward.

Strengthen your neck and shoulders—they share some of the same muscles. Keeping these muscles strong makes them more flexible and less prone to injury. Perform eight to 12 repetitions of each of the following exercises three times, two to three days a week. Once you can do 12 repetitions easily, gradually increase the weight lifted.

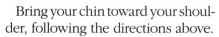 •**Shrugs.** While standing straight with your arms down at your sides, hold a two-pound dumbbell (or a household object, such as a can of soup) in each hand. With palms facing your thighs, shrug your shoulders as high as possible, keeping your head straight. Hold for five seconds, then return to the starting position.

•**Flies.** Lie on your back on an exercise bench, with a two-pound dumbbell in each hand. Hold your hands out to the sides so that the weights are about even with your chest. Keeping your back straight, raise your arms over your chest in a semicircular motion until the weights touch in the middle over your chest. Lower them back to chest level in the same semicircular motion.

•**Side deltoid raise.** While standing straight with your arms down at your sides, hold a two-pound dumbbell or other weight in each hand, with your palms facing your thighs. Keeping your elbows slightly bent, raise your arms up and out to your sides until they're shoulder level (your palms will be facing the floor in this position). Hold for five seconds, then slowly lower the weights.

Illustrations by Shawn Banner.

Rub Your Aches Away!

Beth E. Shubin Stein, MD, a sports medicine and shoulder surgeon with the Women's Sports Medicine Center at the Hospital for Special Surgery in New York City.

If you suffer from chronic arthritis pain or have aching muscle strains or spasms after exercising, chances are you regularly take aspirin or another nonsteroidal anti-inflammatory drug (NSAID), such as *ibuprofen* (Advil) or *naproxen* (Aleve).

There is another option. Over-the-counter (OTC) topical pain relievers can be very effective *without* causing the stomach upset or gastrointestinal bleeding that may accompany oral pain medication.

Latest development: A topical form of the oral prescription NSAID *diclofenac* (Voltaren) is expected to undergo FDA review within a year or so. It is already available in Europe and Canada.

Meanwhile, a variety of OTC topical pain relievers are available now. The products below relieve arthritis, backache and muscle strain. Most are used three to four times daily. Follow label instructions.

Helpful: If one type of topical pain reliever doesn't work for you, try one from another class until you find a product that provides relief.

Caution: Keep these products away from your eyes, nose and other mucous membranes.

SALICYLATES

These aspirin-based products dull pain and curb the inflammation that often accompanies and worsens pain.

How they work: Topical salicylates inhibit the production of *prostaglandins,* substances in the body that cause pain and swelling when they are released in response to strains, sprains and other injuries. *Salicylates include…*

- **BenGay Ultra Strength Pain Relieving Cream.**
- **Aspercreme Analgesic Creme Rub with Aloe.**
- **Sportscreme Deep Penetrating Pain Relieving Rub.**
- **Flexall Maximum Strength Pain Relieving Gel.**

Warning: Do not use salicylates if you are sensitive or allergic to aspirin or take blood-thinning medication that might interact with them. Consult a doctor before applying a salicylate to a large area several times a day.

COUNTERIRRITANTS

These pain relievers give the sensation of warmth or coolness to mask pain.

How they work: Creating a secondary stimulus to diminish the feeling of pain reduces physical discomfort. It's what you do instinctively when you stub your toe, then grab it to apply pressure. Both competing sensations travel to your brain at the same time—but because only a limited number of messages can be processed at one time, the initial feeling of pain is diminished. *Counterirritants include…*

- **Icy Hot Pain Relieving Balm, Extra Strength.**
- **Tiger Balm Extra Strength Pain Relieving Ointment.**
- **Therapeutic Mineral Ice.**

In most cases, coolness is beneficial for acute injuries, such as sprains, while warmth eases stiffness.

Caution: People sensitive to heat or cold should avoid counterirritants.

CAPSAICIN

These products, which are a type of counterirritant, contain *capsaicin,* an extract of hot peppers that causes a burning sensation.

How they work: Unlike most other counterirritants, capsaicin inhibits the production of substance P, a chemical that sends pain messages to the brain via the nervous system. *Capsaicins include…*

- **Zostrix Arthritis Pain Relief Cream.**
- **Capzasin HP Arthritis Pain Relief Creme.**

LIDOCAINE

Lidoderm is a prescription-only patch that contains *lidocaine,* a topical anesthetic similar to the novocaine that dentists often use to numb the gums.

How it works: Lidocaine blocks signals at the skin's nerve endings. The Lidoderm patch (lidocaine 5%) is worn for 12 hours a day over a period of days. It slowly releases medication, so it has longer-lasting effects than other pain relievers and helps with pain that emanates from nerves near the surface of your skin, such as that caused by shingles or diabetic neuropathy.

Caution: Side effects include dizziness, headache and nausea. Allergic reactions are rare but may occur.

Get Rid of Back Pain... For Good

Miriam E. Nelson, PhD, associate professor and director of John Hancock Center for Physical Activity and Nutrition at the Gerald J. and Dorothy R. Friedman School of Nutrition Science and Policy at Tufts University, Boston. A fellow of the American College of Sports Medicine, she is author, with Lawrence Lindner, of *Strong Women, Strong Backs.* Putnam.

As many as 90% of all adults suffer back pain at some point in their lives. Back pain—lower-back pain, in particular—ranks fifth among the most frequent reasons for hospitalizations.

Worse for women: Their musculoskeletal systems—ligaments, vertebrae, spinal disks, etc.—are more delicate than men's and more vulnerable to injury. Women also tend to be less active, on average, than men, and a sedentary lifestyle is a common cause of back pain.

Most back problems are caused by prolonged sitting or by lifting heavy objects the wrong way, but other factors contribute to back pain, including excess body weight, stress and depression. Even smoking is a factor for reasons that aren't exactly clear.

Simple lifestyle measures—maintaining a healthy weight, not smoking and controlling stress and depression—can prevent many cases of back pain. Most important, though, are exercises that strengthen muscles in the back, chest, abdomen, hips and sides. These are the core muscles—the scaffolding that supports the spine and enables the back to flex and twist without injury. Strengthening these muscles can relieve pain and also prevent it.

A FIVE-STEP PLAN

The following workout, which takes no more than 20 minutes, targets all of the core muscles. It can be done three to five times weekly (unlike most strength-training workouts, which should be done no more than three times a week, because muscles need time to recover between sessions). These exercises can be done more often because the intensity is lower—and they're less likely than traditional workouts to cause back pain or other injuries.

For each of the following exercises...

•**Complete 10 repetitions,** rest for one minute, then complete another 10 reps. If you can complete only five or six reps, the intensity is too high and you should do only what you can comfortably manage.

•**Work up to an advanced progression.** This is a way to increase the exercise intensity by making the movements more difficult.

•**Always warm up**—by taking a brisk walk around the block or stepping quickly in place—for five minutes before doing the exercises.

STEP 1: ABDOMINALS

Most people's abdominal muscles are weaker than they should be. Strengthening the abdominals is among the best ways to prevent back pain.

Starting position: Lie on your back on the floor with your knees bent and the soles of your feet flat on the floor. Lightly rest your hands on the lower part of the stomach.

The movement: Contract the abdominal muscles until you feel the small of the back pushing toward the floor. Imagine that you're pulling your belly button downward. Hold the "tense" position for three seconds, then relax.

Progression: Do almost the same exercise as above, with this difference. While the abdominal muscles are tight, raise the still-bent right leg a few inches off the floor and hold it up for three seconds, then place that leg down and raise the left leg for three seconds. The entire move will take 10 to 12 seconds.

STEP 2: CHEST MUSCLES

Along with abdominal exercises, chest workouts protect the back by strengthening the "front" of the core muscle groups.

Starting position: Stand facing a wall or a counter, about an arm's length away, with your feet hip-width apart and knees slightly bent. Put your palms on the wall (or lightly hold the edge of the counter).

The movement: Holding your body straight, bend at the elbows until you are leaning forward toward the wall or counter about 30 degrees. Pause in this position for a moment, then push with your arms until you're back in the starting position.

Progression: Work the same muscles with more intensity with a modified push-up. Lie facedown on the floor, with your palms directly next to your shoulders, elbows bent.

Keeping your knees on the floor, slowly push up only your chest. Keep your trunk in a straight line from your head to your knees. Push up until your shoulders are over your hands, but don't lock the elbows. Pause for a moment, then lower back down until your nose is about four inches from the floor. Keep your trunk in a straight line throughout the movements.

STEP 3: MIDBACK

Many exercises target the upper/lower back, but relatively few target the middle back—a common area for problems.

Starting position: Lie facedown on an exercise mat or carpet, with your arms straight out to 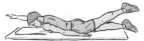 the sides, perpendicular to the body.

The movement: Contract your shoulder blades to lift the arms up and slightly back. Hold the arms in the lifted position, and make four figure eights with the hands. Then lower your arms to the starting position.

Progression: Make the figure eights with the thumbs down or up...or while holding a balled-up sock in each hand...or with the little finger up or down. Varying the movement works different parts of the muscles.

STEP 4: UPPER BACK

This exercise increases shoulder strength as well as back strength.

Starting position: Tie a knot in the middle of an elastic exercise band (available at sporting-goods stores for $2 to $3). Place the knot over the top of a door, and then close the door to anchor the band in place. The two ends

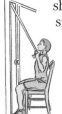

should be hanging down on the same side of the door. Sit in a chair facing the door, with your toes against the door. Hold one end of the band in each hand.

The movement: Slowly pull your hands down and in toward your chest. Keep your elbows pointed down and close to your body. Pause for a moment, then slowly let your arms extend back to the starting position.

Progression: When the exercise starts feeling easy, change to a higher-resistance band.

STEP 5: LOWER BACK

This is the area that gives most people problems.

Starting position: Lie facedown on an exercise mat or carpet. Reach your right hand in front of you, palm down. The left arm should be down alongside your body, with the palm up.

The movement: Slowly raise your right arm, chest and left leg about five inches off the floor. Keep your face down, so your spine is in a straight line. Keep your right leg and left hand on the ground. Pause for a moment, then return to the starting position.

Reverse the movement, raising your left arm, chest and right leg, and keeping the left leg and right hand on the floor.

Progression: Kneel on all fours. Raise your right arm straight in front of you while simultaneously raising the left leg straight behind. Keep the abdominal muscles contracted. Pause, return to the starting position. Then reverse the movement.

OPTIONAL EXERCISE: THIGHS, HIPS AND MORE

This optional exercise is a complex move that targets the upper legs as well as the trunk. It is good for improving stability and balance. The exercise requires the use of a stability ball, available at sporting-goods stores for about $20.

Starting position: Stand with your back to a wall, with the stability ball positioned between

271

your back and the wall. Lean back against the ball, with your feet a bit more than hip-width apart. Hold your arms straight in front of you or crossed over your chest.

The movement: While keeping light pressure on the ball with your lower back, bend at the knees and slowly squat down—the ball will roll with the movement. Squat down as far as you comfortably can. The ball will then be positioned at about the midback.

Keeping pressure on the ball, contract the buttocks and slowly "roll" yourself up and back to the starting position.

Illustrations by Shawn Banner.

Disk Transplant May Mean Long-Term Relief From Back Pain

Barth Green, MD, chairman of neurological surgery, University of Miami Miller Medical School, Miami.
Roger Hartl, MD, director, NewYork-Presbyterian/Weil Medical Center spine program, New York City.
The Lancet.

Long-term relief from the common problem of back pain can be achieved with transplanted spinal disks, according to Chinese surgeons.

Doctors at the University of Hong Kong and the Naval General Hospital in Bejing say this breakthrough treatment has been in the works for five years, when they first harvested spinal disks from human donors and transplanted them into five patients with chronic back pain caused by disk degeneration.

Since then, the doctors say, the patients who received the transplanted disks have all experienced improvement in symptoms, with no signs of immune rejection and only mild degeneration of the disks.

THE FUTURE?

Spinal disk transplants could have a real future because surgeons are not always happy with the results of current operations. When back pain

cannot be treated with medications, a surgical procedure called fusion is done, uniting the bones to relieve the pain.

"This is going in the right direction," says Dr. Roger Hartl, director of the spine program at NewYork Presbyterian/Weil Cornell Medical Center, referring to the new disk transplant technique.

Hartl is currently working with biomedical engineers at Cornell University's main campus in Ithaca, New York, trying to grow replacement disks using cell cultures.

"Biological replacement of a disk rather than fusion surgery or artificial disks is the way to go," says Hartl. "To me, the results are very promising. People have done this in animals, but the nice thing about this study is that it is the first time it has been done in humans."

"Very creative," is how Dr. Barth Green, chairman of neurological surgery at the University of Miami Miller School of Medicine, describes this cutting-edge technique. "But I think five patients are way too few to see whether this is going to be the answer for the long run."

PROCEED WITH CAUTION

Although back pain specialists are intrigued by reports of the new procedure, little is known about the patients who had the surgery or those who donated the disks. "It is hard to imagine that this will become standard treatment for people who have degenerative disk disease because of the problem of donation," notes Hartl.

"I don't think we're anywhere near ready to start doing it routinely because of the fact that a lot of important details have to be worked out," notes Green.

■ ■ ■ ■

What Is Sciatica?

Sciatica is a common form of low-back pain that radiates along one of the two sciatic nerves, each of which runs down the back of the thigh and calf and into the foot. Most cases of sciatica occur when one of the spinal disks—gel-filled pancakes of cartilage between the vertebrae—swells, tears (ruptures) or herniates (part of the interior of the disk bulges out), exerting painful pressure on a sciatic nerve. About 1 million Americans suffer from sciatica, and up to 300,000 a year have surgery to relieve the pain.

Eugene Carragee, MD, professor of orthopedic surgery and director of the Orthopedic Spine Center at Stanford University School of Medicine in Stanford, CA. He is the author of an editorial recently published in *The Journal of the American Medical Association*, discussing the new studies.

Popular Pain Treatments Bring Big Problems And Little Relief for Lower-Back Pain

Bridget A. Martell, MD, assistant clinical professor of medicine, Yale University School of Medicine, and associate director, Pfizer New Haven Clinical Research Unit, both in New Haven, CT.

Carmel Armon, MD, chief of neurology, Bayside Medical Center, Springfield, MA, and professor of neurology, Tufts University School of Medicine, Boston.

Neurology.

Annals of Internal Medicine.

Millions of Americans with lower-back pain may need to seek out alternatives for relief. Two popular types of treatments—potent opioid painkiller drugs and epidural steroid injections—are not being recommended for long-term care of this common source of pain.

Reason: Both treatments provide only short-term relief—and even then, with potential problems, according to new research.

PAINKILLER PROBLEMS

Although potent opioid drugs such as Oxycontin and Vicodin can treat back pain in the short term, it's not clear the drugs help in the long run and abuse may be common.

In fact, use of these highly addictive drugs can lead to abuse or dependency in one of every four cases, according to studies.

Even when the drugs aren't abused, there is no evidence they are effective in the long term,

says Dr. Bridget A. Martell, who reviewed 38 previous studies on the issue.

The bottom line: Over time, there is no evidence that opioids work any better than placebo, she notes.

INJECTION REJECTION

And despite their popularity, epidural steroid injections—best known for easing pain during childbirth—also strike out as a viable treatment for lower-back pain that radiates down a leg.

The use of epidurals to treat chronic back pain has grown in popularity. Recent figures show that some 40 million Medicare patients have received epidurals for lower-back pain.

But after reviewing various studies, researchers conclude that epidurals offer only minor, short-lived relief for back pain—lasting no more than two to six weeks.

"While some pain relief is a positive result in and of itself, the extent of leg- and back-pain relief from epidural steroid injections, on the average, fell short of the values typically viewed as clinically meaningful," notes guideline author Dr. Carmel Armon, chief of the division of neurology at Bayside Medical Center in Springfield, Massachusetts.

Because of this finding, the American Academy of Neurology is not recommending the use of epidurals for pain relief beyond three months. The academy also concludes this treatment does not help patients "buy time" to avoid surgery.

WHAT TO DO?

Lost hope in both treatments leave unanswered questions for the one in five Americans with chronic back pain, defined as discomfort lasting more than three months.

What does ease pain? Besides narcotic medication for the short term, doctors typically recommend exercise, nonsteroidal anti-inflammatory medicines (NSAIDs), tricyclic antidepressants, acupuncture and electrical stimulation.

info Learn more about back pain from the US National Institute of Neurological Disorders and Stroke at *http://www.ninds.nih.gov/disorders/backpain/*.

Shoulder Pain?

Jon J.P. Warner, MD, chief of the Harvard Shoulder Service and professor of orthopedic surgery at Harvard Medical School in Boston. He has published nearly 100 medical journal articles on treatment of the shoulder, and is coauthor of the medical textbook *Complex and Revision Problems in Shoulder Surgery.* Lippincott Williams & Wilkins.

Until recently, amateur and professional athletes were considered the primary recipients of surgery to repair an injured rotator cuff in the shoulder.

Now: As recent advances in technology have made the surgery safer and more effective than ever before, many people who have never stepped foot on a baseball field or tennis court are receiving the operation to repair ordinary wear and tear from heavy lifting and movements that require overhead extension of the arms.

Fortunately, many people can avoid rotator cuff surgery if they take the proper steps to prevent injury. If surgery is needed, most people are able to leave the hospital the same day as the procedure.

HOW DAMAGE OCCURS

A rotator cuff tear caused by a single traumatic injury, such as from a fall or lifting a heavy object, is rare. More commonly, years of minor wear and tear cause the tendons to become damaged and weak, much like a frayed rope. Doctors call this rotator cuff disease. With this condition, even a trivial trauma, such as one caused by swinging a golf club, can tear the tendon.

Rotator cuff disease is the third most common orthopedic complaint after low-back pain and knee pain. The condition usually is suspected when a patient feels pain when lifting an arm and/or during the night, when he/she may roll on to the injured shoulder, worsening the pain.

RISK FACTORS

Activities that can increase the wear-and-tear process of the rotator cuff include heavy lifting… performing overhead activities, such as assembly-line work…and overextending the shoulder during sports activities, such as tennis. *Other risk factors…*

•**Family history.** Genetics plays a role in the health of your body tissues, so if others in your family have had rotator cuff disease, your risk is increased.

•**Smoking.** Smoking has an effect on the blood supply everywhere in the body, including the tendons of the shoulder. Blood carries the cells that are necessary for healing minor injuries. Reduced blood flow slows healing and accelerates wear and tear on the rotator cuff.

•**Aging and overuse.** The more we use our shoulders, the greater the likelihood that the rotator cuff will "wear out." This happens through decades of normal use, or by intense overuse. That's why the risk increases as people get older…or if they engage in shoulder-heavy repetitive actions, such as swimming. Also vulnerable are people whose jobs involve heavy lifting, such as warehouse employees, or working with their arms overhead much of the time, such as electricians.

PREVENTING DAMAGE

If you have a family history of rotator cuff disease, you cannot change that fact. *However, there are steps you can take to minimize the effect of other risk factors…*

•**If you smoke, quit.** There are many reasons to avoid tobacco. Increased risk for rotator cuff disease can be added to the list.

•**Stretch the shoulder.** Do this before sports, such as tennis, golf, swimming and softball, or before lifting a heavy object—especially if you are age 45 or older. Many effective stretches are difficult to learn from a book and can increase the risk for injury if performed incorrectly. Ask an exercise trainer or physical therapist for hands-on guidance.

For a good basic stretch: With one hand, grasp the other arm above the elbow and pull it across your chest. Hold for a count of 10, then switch arms. Repeat 10 times.

•**Avoid certain shoulder movements.** At the gym, do not perform exercises that require the elbows to be pulled back behind the shoulder in an extreme extension position.

Example: Bench presses in which you bring the bar all the way down to your chest hyperextend the shoulder.

For proper form: Lie on the floor and practice a bench press by holding a broom handle instead of a bar. Your elbows will be stopped at the correct level by the floor.

If you work out with weights, avoid excess wear and tear by doing more repetitions at lower weights, rather than fewer repetitions at higher weights.

A general rule is to use weights that enable you to do 10 repetitions of an exercise. If you can do only five or six repetitions before feeling muscle fatigue, the weights are too heavy.

TELLTALE SYMPTOMS

The symptoms of rotator cuff disease vary, depending on the individual and the extent of damage. Some people experience agonizing pain, while others may have just a minor nagging ache. The pain usually is intermittent, but if it becomes constant, surgery is a reasonable treatment option.

Seek medical help for any shoulder pain that persists for longer than one week—or if you have pain while performing common tasks, such as reaching, dressing or playing your usual sports, or if the pain wakes you up at night.

Self-test: If you experience shoulder pain when pushing objects away from the body—but not when pulling objects toward you—your rotator cuff may be damaged.

WHEN TO TRY PHYSICAL THERAPY

If you think your rotator cuff may be damaged, see a doctor, preferably an orthopedist. If you get prompt attention, you may be able to avoid surgery by getting physical therapy.

Physical therapy can strengthen the rotator cuff and reduce pain by changing the shoulder mechanics. This means that both your flexibility and shoulder strength will be improved, allowing the shoulder to move in a way that doesn't irritate the rotator cuff.

A tear indicates advanced rotator cuff disease and usually is identified by a magnetic resonance imaging (MRI) scan. Once the tendon is torn, surgery is the only way to fix it—but the operation is not always recommended.

For example, if you are relatively inactive, with only mild pain and good function, you may do well with physical therapy and corticosteroid injections, which help reduce pain. Moreover, surgery has risks and entails a long recovery.

Some patients can modify their activities and experience minimal pain—without surgery.

IF YOU MUST HAVE SURGERY...

A year after rotator cuff surgery, 90% of patients report that they can participate in activities they could not do before surgery because of shoulder pain.

Whenever possible, choose arthroscopic surgery, in which the repair is performed through keyhole-sized incisions using surgical instruments, tiny lights and video cameras. During this procedure, the surgeon removes excess bone fragments from the shoulder to create more space for the rotator cuff. The alternative is open surgery, which carries a greater risk for infection as well as longer hospitalization.

If you need surgery, choose a surgeon who has performed arthroscopic rotator cuff repairs for at least three years, and who does at least two per week. (The surgery generally is covered by insurance.) Highly qualified surgeons are elected by their peers to American Shoulder and Elbow Surgeons, a professional society. To search the group's membership, call 847-698-1629 or check *www.ases-assn.org*.

Recovery from rotator cuff surgery can last a few months to a year. Physical therapy can be a prolonged and sometimes uncomfortable process, usually involving twice weekly sessions plus daily at-home therapy done by the patient. But if you are committed to the postoperative therapy program, you will have a more complete recovery.

■ **More from Dr. Warner...**

What Is the Rotator Cuff?

The rotator cuff consists of four muscles (and their tendons) that hold the upper arm in the shoulder joint. The rotator cuff compresses the ball (head of the humerus) into the socket so that shoulder rotation can occur. It acts like an intricate pulley mechanism, allowing the arm to move in every direction. Certain overhead arm movements can injure the rotator cuff by tearing fibers of the tendon.

■ ■ ■ ■

Three Great Ways to Help Stop Bruising

Apply ice to the sore spot—use an ice bag or a package of frozen vegetables wrapped in a towel. Don't leave it on for more than 15 minutes at a stretch.

•**Sit as much as possible** for the next few hours so that your body pumps less blood to the injured area.

•**If the injury is on a thigh,** put on support hose or spandex shorts—this applies mild pressure to broken blood vessels and further reduces the flow of blood.

•**If the injury is elsewhere,** wrap the area with a wide elastic bandage, but not too tightly —you should be able to slip a finger under the bandage.

Also: Applying Arnica Montana cream, available at health-food stores, has been shown in some studies to help reduce bruising.

Joan Wilen and Lydia Wilen, folk-remedy experts based in New York City and authors of many books, including most recently *Bottom Line's Healing Remedies.*

■ ■ ■ ■

Blood Test May Soon Prevent Carpal Tunnel Syndrome

A simple blood test may someday be the first step to preventing carpal tunnel syndrome, tendonitis and other painful overuse injuries. For the first time, researchers have detected that the human body pumps out certain chemicals that indicate early stages of these injuries.

That could be significant, because doctors currently have to rely on physical examinations and reported symptoms to diagnose repetitive motion injuries.

Problem: Most people don't suffer pain or other symptoms until the damage has already started and by then it may be too late.

In a small study, Temple University researchers analyzed blood samples in 22 people. They found that the body's immune system pumps out these biomarkers—specific substances—as the body begins to suffer damage due to repetitive stress.

"While not a diagnostic test, because the biomarkers could also indicate another type of injury, they do provide a red flag where before there was none," says Ann Barr, associate professor of physical therapy at Temple's College of Health Professions. This could lead to taking preventative measures before it becomes long-term or permanent damage and disability.

info The US National Institute of Neurological Disorders and Stroke has more on repetitive motion disorders at *www.ninds.nih.gov/disorders/.*

Ann Barr, associate professor of physical therapy, Temple University College of Health Professions, Philadelphia. *Clinical Science.*

New Way to Ease TMJ Pain—Works Better... Costs Less

Anna Stowell, MD, assistant professor of psychiatry, anesthesiology and pain management, University of Texas Southwestern Medical Center, Dallas.
Journal of the American Dental Association.

A new form of therapy that teaches patients pain-coping and relaxation techniques not only reduces pain for a common jaw disorder, which includes temporomandibular joint disorders (TMJD), as well if not better than standard medical care but also reduces its costs, finds new research.

The technique, called biopsychosocial intervention, mixes biofeedback with classroom-like education. Biofeedback is a widely used treatment technique in which people are trained to relax and improve their health by monitoring signals from their own bodies, assisted by a machine designed for that purpose. Biofeedback is often used to help people cope with pain.

But this new technique also relies on educating the patient about the mind-body relationship, the body's reaction to stress, and the importance of relaxation in everyday settings.

THE STUDY

In this study, researchers at the University of Texas Southwestern Medical Center in Dallas observed 81 women and 20 men, ages 18 to 70, with temporomandibular disorder (TMD).

This painful jaw disorder is caused by wear on the cartilage lining the jaw joint, resulting in pain from chewing, talking or clenching of the teeth. Affecting more than 10% of Americans, TMD is the second most common pain-causing muscular and skeletal condition after low-back pain.

Half of the study participants received six weeks of early biopsychosocial intervention, while the others received standard dental care.

One year later, those who received the biopsychosocial intervention had required less medical treatment for pain than those getting standard medical care. They also reported less pain, better mood, and proved to show better coping abilities than those getting standard care, say researchers.

They also saved money, because standard care for TMD—such as medication, physical therapy and surgery—can be expensive.

"The early intervention can reduce TMD-related pain levels, stave off chronic pain and save people money on costly treatments," notes study author Dr. Anna Stowell, assistant professor of psychiatry, anesthesiology and pain management at UT Southwestern.

info The American Academy of Otolaryngology—Head and Neck Surgery Web site explains temporomandibular joint dysfunction at *http://www.entnet.org/healthinfo/topics/tmj.cfm*.

Migraines? Two Meds Are Better Than One

Jan Lewis Brandes, MD, assistant clinical professor of neurology, Vanderbilt University School of Medicine, and neurologist, Nashville Neuroscience Group, Nashville.

Wade Cooper, DO, director, St. John's Health Chronic Headache and Migraine Institute, Madison Heights, MI.

Journal of the American Medical Association.

A new "combination" pill that combines two commonly used drugs for migraine pain provides faster and longer-lasting relief than using either medication alone.

So concludes new research of the experimental pill that combines *sumatriptan* (Imitrex) and *naproxen sodium* (Aleve).

Scientists say the new combo medication brought relief within 2 hours in 65% of study volunteers. About 55% reported pain relief from taking only sumatriptan and 44% from taking naproxen alone.

The FDA is currently considering approval of the combo drug, which would be sold under the brand name Trexima.

THE EXPLANATION

Why the better results from both drugs in one pill? "It really targets more of what's happening in the brain during migraine," explains study lead Dr. Jan Lewis Brandes, a neurologist at Vanderbilt University School of Medicine. "Sumatriptan works to constrict the blood vessels and interrupt pain, while naproxen works on the inflammatory process."

Although medications known as triptans—which include sumatriptan—have improved migraine management, some people still don't get relief, say experts. The new pill was developed because many headache experts already recommend a combination of medications to combat migraine pain.

But when you combine naproxen with sumatriptan, "it not only tends to help it be more effective," notes Dr. Wade Cooper, director of the St. John's Health Chronic Headache and Migraine Institute in Michigan, "it may help Imitrex work faster."

THE STUDY

For this study, 3,000 migraine sufferers between ages 18 and 65 were recruited at 118 clinics across the US. They were randomly assigned to one of four groups—the combination therapy (a single pill containing 85 milligrams sumatriptan and 500 milligrams naproxen sodium); 500 milligrams naproxen sodium alone; 85 milligrams sumatriptan alone; or a placebo.

They were told to take the medication when their migraine pain was moderate to severe in intensity.

More people reported short-term relief from headache pain and lessened sensitivity to lights and sounds on the combination therapy than on either drug alone or for the placebo. At 24 hours, results were similar, with more people on the combination therapy reporting sustained headache relief.

Because the combination drug would only be used on an as-needed basis, Lewis Brandes said she's not overly concerned that the medication would cause any of the gastrointestinal side effects, such as stomach bleeding, that can occur with long-term use of nonsteroidal anti-inflammatory medications such as *naproxen*.

Almost 30 million Americans suffer from migraines, according to the National Headache Foundation. Migraines may cause headache pain —often just on one side of the head, visual disturbances, sensitivity to light, and nausea and vomiting. Migraines may last hours or even days.

info Learn more about treating migraine from the American Academy of Family Physicians at *http://familydoctor.org/127.xml*.

■ ■ ■ ■

Migraines Can Trigger Depression

Women who get frequent headaches, particularly migraines, are four times more likely to suffer from major depression than those who only get them occasionally. Chronic pain from headaches can trigger depression…and depression may intensify the pain.

Medical News Today.

Common Painkillers May Cause Hypertension In Men

Gary Curhan, MD, ScD, physician and researcher, Brigham & Women's Hospital, Boston.
Suzanne Steinbaum, MD, director of women and heart disease, interventional cardiology and the Heart and Vascular Institute, Lenox Hill Hospital, New York City.
Archives of Internal Medicine.

The regular use of popular over-the-counter pain relievers has been shown in some studies to increase a woman's risk of developing high blood pressure.

Now, new research finds middle-aged men also face a higher hypertension risk from daily consumption of the three most commonly taken drugs in the US—*acetaminophen* such as Tylenol, *ibuprofen* such as Advil or Motrin, or aspirin.

It's suspected that all three types of painkillers may inhibit the effect of chemicals that would normally relax blood vessels and decrease blood pressure, say researchers.

"People should be aware that these drugs have potential adverse effects," says study lead Dr. Gary Curhan of Brigham & Women's Hospital in Boston. "I would recommend that individuals limit their use of these medications unless they are clearly indicated. If they have chronic symptoms requiring the use of these drugs, they should discuss alternative treatments with their health-care providers."

THE STUDY

In his study, Curhan's team tracked 16,031 male health professionals without a history of hypertension. The participants provided information about their use of these pain medications. The study participants were age 65 on average.

Bottom line: After four years of observation, researchers say that those who used *acetaminophen* six to seven days a week had a 34% higher risk of hypertension compared with men who did not use the drug. Similarly, men who took *ibuprofen* six or seven days a week had a 38% higher risk, while those taking aspirin had a 26% increased risk.

And compared with men who took no pills, those who took 15 or more pills each week— and other medication—had a 48% higher risk of hypertension.

ECHOES PAST FINDINGS

At least two large studies—involving only women—did find that similar use of analgesics might boost blood pressure risk in women.

"In fact, these classes of medications for pain are not as safe as we originally thought," notes Dr. Suzanne Steinbaum, director of the Heart and Vascular Institute at Lenox Hill Hospital in New York.

However, one previous study on men did not find a substantial increase in men's risk of hypertension from frequent use of these drugs.

Sleepless Nights Can Be a Real Pain For Women

Sleep.

Michael T. Smith, PhD, sleep researcher, Johns Hopkins University, Baltimore.

Sleepless nights can mean more painful days, according to the latest research done at Johns Hopkins University.

A new study finds that when people have sleep disturbances—insomnia, frequent awakenings from crying babies, or other interruptions to sound shut-eye—their pain threshold quickly decreases.

Explanation: So-called "fragmented sleep profiles" alter body systems that regulate and control pain, explains researcher Michael T. Smith of Johns Hopkins University.

THE STUDY

Smith tracked 32 healthy women whose sleep patterns were studied for seven nights. For the first two nights, the women slept undisturbed for eight hours. For the next few nights, the women were then assigned to one of three groups: a control group that continued to sleep undisturbed; a forced awakening (FA) group awakened once an hour (eight times) through the night; and a restricted sleep opportunity (RSO) group subjected to partial sleep deprivation by delaying their bedtime.

On the sixth night, the women in both the FA and RSO groups underwent 36 hours of total sleep deprivation, followed by an 11-hour recovery sleep.

Researchers then tested the women's pain thresholds and pain inhibition. Those with interrupted (FA) sleep showed an increase in spontaneous pain.

Bottom line: "Our research shows that disrupted sleep, marked by multiple prolonged awakenings, impairs natural pain-control mechanisms that are thought to play a key role in the development, maintenance, and exacerbation of chronic pain," says Smith.

info Learn more about sleep from the National Sleep Foundation at *http://www.sleep foundation.org.*

■ ■ ■ ■

Mental, Physical Torture Inflict Similar Pain

Which causes more pain—mental or physical torture?

After weighing the evidence—including interviews with 279 victims of either form of torture—British researchers conclude that it is too close to call: The resulting degree of mental distress and trauma is about the same from either form of torture.

Previously, some experts believed that physical torture was more devastating.

"Sham executions, witnessing the torture of close ones, threats of rape, fondling of genitals and isolation were associated with at least as much if not more distress than some of the physical torture stressors in terms of associated distress," note researchers from the University of London.

The team concludes that aggressive interrogation methods or detention involving deprivation of basic needs, being kept in uncomfortable conditions, hooding, isolation, forced nudity, forced stress positions, threats, humiliating treatment and other psychological abuse inflict as much mental harm as physical torture.

Archives of General Psychiatry.

■ ■ ■ ■

Meditation Lowers Brain's Pain Response Up to 50%

To boost your pain tolerance, say "ommm." Practicing transcendental meditation (TM) may reduce the brain's reaction to physical anguish.

So say scientists at the University of California, Irvine after using brain scans to monitor pain responses in those practicing this meditation program, which previous research suggests may improve high blood pressure and help ease other ailments.

"Prior research indicates that transcendental meditation creates a more balanced outlook on life and greater equanimity in reacting to stress," says meditation researcher David Orme-Johnson, who headed the NIH-funded study. "This study suggests that this is not just an attitudinal change, but a fundamental change in how the brain functions."

THE STUDY

First, his team used neuroimaging to study the brain's pain reaction centers in 12 healthy people who have been practicing TM for 30 years. They were compared with 12 others who never practiced TM, which involves meditating twice a day, for abut 20 minutes each time, with the use of a "mantra" word.

When exposed to the same pain, these long-time meditators had a 40% to 50% lower response to pain than 12 others who did not practice the program.

The kicker: After those nonmeditators had learned and practiced TM for five months, their brains were retested…and their pain response had also decreased by up to 50%.

info The National Center for Complementary and Alternative Medicine has more about meditation for health at *http://nccam.nih.gov/health/meditation/*.

David Orme-Johnson, meditation researcher, University of California, Irvine.
NeuroReport.

Ibuprofen Best for Kids' Pain

Eric Clark, MD, emergency medicine specialist, University of Ottawa School of Medicine, Ottawa, Canada.
Dennis Woo, MD, chairman of pediatrics, Santa Monica-UCLA and Orthopaedic Hospital, Santa Monica, CA.
Pediatrics.

The painkiller *ibuprofen*—found in over-the-counter Advil and Motrin—works better at relieving children's pain from musculoskeletal injuries such as sprained ankles than other drugs commonly used in hospital emergency departments, according to a new study.

In fact, a standard nonprescription dose of *ibuprofen* brought better relief—at least in the minds of patients—than a prescription dose of codeine, reports study head Dr. Eric Clark, an emergency medicine specialist at the University of Ottawa School of Medicine. Ibuprofen was also tested against *acetaminophen*, the active ingredient in Tylenol.

"No one had done comparison studies on the pain medications we use [on children]," says Clark. "Some of us were already using ibuprofen more than the others, and I think this [study] just confirms our clinical experience."

THE STUDY

His study tracked 300 children, ages 6 to 17, who were brought to the emergency department of the Children's Hospital of Eastern Ontario with a musculoskeletal injury to their extremities, neck or back. Each child was asked to rate their pain level, from "no pain" to "the worst pain they have ever felt."

Clark's team randomly assigned the children to one of the three treatment groups. The children, parents and research assistants who asked them about pain did not know which medication each child received. Each was given a standard dose orally, prescribed by the child's weight.

After the children took the medicine, they were asked to describe the pain every 30 minutes for two hours, using the same description as before.

"The primary outcome [we were looking at] was at one hour," Clark says. At the one-hour mark, the ibuprofen group had better pain relief. Those given ibuprofen were least likely to ask for more medicine for pain relief after an hour, he adds.

THE REACTION

Clark's results come as a surprise to some doctors. "I would have guessed codeine" would bring better relief, notes Dr. Dennis Woo, of Santa Monica-UCLA and Orthopaedic Hospital in California.

Indeed, codeine, a more powerful drug, has a reputation of being more effective against acute pain.

Still, Woo says that Clark's study is good news. He personally tries to avoid giving codeine for kids' pain management because "it spaces them out," he says.

Bottom line for parents: "When we send parents home with children with bumps, bruises and broken bones, we suggest parents use ibuprofen as well," says Clark. The same applies for treating musculoskeletal injuries not severe enough to seek medical care.

info The Nemours Foundation has more on children's pain relievers at *www.kids health.org.*

Funny Ways to Ease Kids' Pain—Watch Cartoons

Carlo Bellieni, MD, Neonatal Intensive Care Unit, Le Scatte Clinic, University of Siena, Siena, Italy.

Jess Shatkin, MD, MPH, director of education and training, and child and adolescent psychiatrist, New York University Child Study Center, New York City.

Brenda Bursch, PhD, clinical director, Pediatric Psychiatry Consultation Liaison, University of California, Los Angeles, David Geffen School of Medicine.

Archives of Disease in Childhood.

B ugs Bunny, Scooby-Doo and the Power Rangers might soon find a place in the doctor's office. Researchers in Italy say that watching cartoons helps distract children from the pain of minor medical procedures.

"We found that watching TV has an analgesic power, even greater than active distraction obtained by a mother's efforts," notes lead author Dr. Carlo Bellieni of the University of Siena.

THE STUDY

Bellieni reached this conclusion after studying the pain reaction of 69 children, ages 7 to 12, during a blood test. One group of kids watched a TV cartoon show during the procedure. In the second group, mothers tried to distract their children by talking, soothing or caressing them. The third group had no distraction as blood was drawn.

Those watching TV had pain levels three times less severe than those with no distraction,

say researchers. Children distracted by their mothers had less pain than those with no distraction, but significantly more pain than the TV watchers.

Explanation: "During a minor procedure, children experience fear, pain and stress that must be recognized and overcome," Bellieni says. "Caregivers should make efforts to provide distraction to children during painful events. Parents' presence must be encouraged, and television should be used as a routine tool, together with appropriate analgesic drugs, whose effectiveness it may increase."

THE REACTION

Experts are not surprised by the findings. In fact, more doctors are using TV specifically to distract kids as they undergo medical procedures.

"It's a good use of television as long as the kids are watching something that's approved," says Dr. Jess Shatkin, director of education and training at the New York University Child Study Center.

But the boob tube is not a replacement for parents. "It's important for parents to be in the room," Shatkin notes. Parents can also be coached on how to distract their child.

It may be that cartoons work best because they capture both the visual and auditory attention of the child, adds Brenda Bursch, clinical director of the Pediatric Psychiatry Consultation Liaison at UCLA's David Geffen School of Medicine.

By comparison, a parent's attention signals concern—something that can actually make the child more fearful.

"The mom's attempts to distract by talking, caressing or soothing might signal to the child that something bad is going to happen," she explains. "This is not to say that moms should not be present, but (this) study suggests that additional distractions may be more useful for pain reduction."

info For more on children and pain from the National Institutes of Health, visit *http:// painconsortium.nih.gov/genderandpain/chil dren.htm.*

Diet for a Pain-Free Life

Harris H. McIlwain, MD, a rheumatologist and pain specialist with Florida's largest rheumatology practice, and adjunct professor at University of South Florida College of Public Health, both in Tampa. He is coauthor, with Debra Fulghum Bruce, PhD, of *Diet for a Pain-Free Life*. Marlowe.

As many as 150 million Americans live with ongoing pain. This usually is caused by such problems as arthritis or injuries to the neck or back.

Being overweight and having a poor diet are crucial factors, too. Fatty tissue is an endocrine (hormone-producing) organ, just like other organs in the body. Studies show that patients who are overweight produce high levels of cytokines, C-reactive protein and other proinflammatory chemicals—substances that promote joint and tissue damage and increase pain.

Good news: Losing as little as 10 pounds can significantly reduce inflammation, pain and stiffness—regardless of the underlying cause of the discomfort. People who combine weight loss with a diet that includes anti-inflammatory foods (and excludes proinflammatory ones) can reduce pain by up to 90%. The effect rivals that of *ibuprofen* and similar painkillers—without gastrointestinal upset or other side effects.

PAIN-FREE DIET

The saturated fat in beef, pork, lamb and other meats is among the main causes of painful inflammation. People who eat a lot of meat (including poultry) consume *arachidonic acid*, an essential fatty acid that is converted into inflammatory chemicals in the body.

Although a vegetarian diet is ideal for reducing inflammation and promoting weight loss (no more than 6% of vegetarians are obese), few Americans are willing to give up meat altogether.

Recommended: A plant-based diet that includes little (or no) meat and poultry...at least two to four weekly servings of fish...and plenty of fiber and anti-inflammatory foods. Patients who follow this diet and limit daily calories to about 1,400 can lose 10 to 25 excess pounds within three months.

Helpful: It takes at least two to three weeks to establish new dietary habits. People who give up meat entirely usually find that they don't miss it after a few weeks—while those who continue to eat some meat may find the cravings harder to resist.

My favorite cookbooks: *Vegan with a Vengeance* by Isa Chandra Moskowitz (Marlowe) and *Pike Place Market Seafood Cookbook* by Braiden Rex-Johnson (Ten Speed).

Here are the best painkilling foods and beverages. *Include as many of these in your diet as possible...*

RED WINE

Red wine contains *resveratrol*, a chemical compound that blocks the activation of the COX-2 enzyme, one of the main substances responsible for pain and inflammation. Resveratrol may be more effective than aspirin at relieving pain from osteoarthritis and other inflammatory conditions.

Other beverages made from grapes, such as white wine and grape juice, contain some resveratrol, but not as much as red wine.

Servings: No more than two glasses daily for men, and no more than one glass for women.

Alternative source of antioxidants for nondrinkers: Two or more cups of tea daily. Both green and black teas contain *epigallocatechin-3 gallate* (EGCG), a chemical that blocks the COX-2 enzyme.

BERRIES

Virtually all fruits contain significant amounts of antioxidants, which prevent free radical molecules from damaging cell membranes and causing inflammation. Berries—particularly blueberries, cranberries and blackberries—are among the most powerful analgesic fruits because they're high in *anthocyanins*, some of the most effective antioxidants. One-half cup of blueberries, for example, has more antioxidant power than five servings of green peas or broccoli.

Servings: One-half cup of berries daily, fresh or frozen.

Bonus: Berries are very high in the antioxidant vitamin C, a nutrient that builds and protects joint cartilage.

PINEAPPLE

Fresh pineapple contains the enzyme *bromelain*, which is in the stem and fruit of the pineapple and inhibits the release of inflammatory chemicals. It has been shown in some studies to reduce arthritic pain. I advise patients with sports injuries to eat pineapple because of its healing powers.

Servings: At least two half-cup servings weekly, more if you're suffering from injuries or an arthritis flare-up. Bromelain also can be taken in supplement form—200 milligrams (mg) to 300 mg, three times daily before meals.

GINGER

Ginger contains potent anti-inflammatory substances and was found in one study to reduce knee pain in 63% of patients.

Servings: One teaspoon of ginger daily. Fresh and powdered ginger are equally effective and can be added to food.

FISH

I advise patients to substitute oily fish (such as salmon, tuna and sardines) for meat. Fish has little saturated fat (the main proinflammatory nutrient in the American diet) and is high in omega-3 fatty acids. Omega-3s increase the body's production of *inhibitory prostaglandins*, substances that lower levels of inflammatory chemicals and can reduce arthritis pain.

Servings: Two to four three-ounce servings of fish weekly or 1,000 to 2,000 mg of fish oil (available in capsule form) daily. If you don't like fish, omega-3s also are found in flaxseed, walnuts and soy foods.

WHOLE GRAINS AND BEANS

These are among the best sources of B vitamins —especially important for people who eat a lot of processed foods, which are usually deficient in these nutrients. Studies suggest that vitamins B-1 (*thiamin*), B-6 (*pyridoxine*) and B-12 (*cyanocobalamin*) may reduce inflammation.

Other B vitamins, such as B-3 (*niacin*), also reduce inflammation and may increase natural steroid levels and reduce the risk of osteoarthritis.

Servings: At least one-half cup of whole grains and/or beans daily.

Good choices: Brown rice, lentils, chickpeas, black beans and kidney beans.

Bonus: Grains and beans are high in fiber. High-fiber foods promote weight loss by increasing a sense of fullness and maintaining optimal blood sugar levels.

Soothe the Itch and Burn of Hemorrhoids

Deborah Nagle, MD, chief of colon and rectal surgery at Beth Israel Deaconess Medical Center, Boston. She is visiting assistant professor at Harvard Medical School, also in Boston, and chair of the Public Relations Committee of the American Society of Colon and Rectal Surgeons, based in Arlington Heights, IL.

Most people are embarrassed to talk about hemorrhoids. Yet hemorrhoids are among the most common conditions that doctors treat, affecting about half of all adults at some time in their lives.

Also known as piles, hemorrhoids are swollen veins in the anus and/or rectum. They can cause mild itching or discomfort and often bleeding. Less often, the blood inside a hemorrhoid forms a clot, or *thrombus*, causing a great deal of pain.

INTERNAL AND EXTERNAL

Two types of hemorrhoids…

•**External hemorrhoids,** which appear on the outer rim of the anus, are usually the most uncomfortable—partly due to abrasion (from sitting, rubbing against clothes, etc.). Also, this is where blood clots are most likely to form.

•**Internal hemorrhoids,** which usually cause no pain, are in deep portions of the anal canal and rectum, where there are few nerve endings. The presence of blood on toilet paper or in the bowl often is the only sign of internal hemorrhoids.

Exception: Internal hemorrhoids become visible, and much more sensitive, when they push out, or *prolapse*, through the anus. These may require treatment if they don't pop back inside on their own. It is safe to gently push a prolapsed hemorrhoid back in. Often, simply sitting down will do this.

Both types of hemorrhoids usually are due to excessive anal or rectal pressure. This pressure is often caused by straining to have a bowel movement…constipation and/or diarrhea…and prolonged sitting, particularly on the toilet. Hemorrhoids also are common during pregnancy because of increased pressure on the anal veins.

Important: Patients always should see a doctor if they see blood during a bowel movement.

Bright red blood is usually due to hemorrhoids—but it can also be a warning sign of colon cancer. Dark or black stools can indicate bleeding higher up in the colon, and may be a sign of colon cancer. Call your doctor immediately.

BEST AT-HOME TREATMENTS

Simple remedies…

•**Warm water.** Gently wash the area once or twice daily with a soft cloth moistened with warm water. Blot—don't rub—and don't use soap. It can increase anal irritation.

Also, sufferers can take a warm bath once or twice a day…or use a sitz bath, a basin that sits on top of the toilet seat and is filled with warm water.

•**Witch hazel,** the active ingredient in a number of hemorrhoid products, is an astringent that shrinks swollen tissue. It also acts as a topical anesthetic to reduce burning and itching.

•**Over-the-counter hydrocortisone.** Apply it to the hemorrhoid two to three times daily to reduce itching and inflammation. The cream is soothing and may reduce discomfort immediately. It is also available in suppository form.

Caution: Don't use hydrocortisone for more than a week without a doctor's recommendation—it causes thinning of the skin, which can cause bleeding or worsen anal irritation.

MEDICAL TREATMENT

External hemorrhoids: The most painful external hemorrhoids contain blood clots.

Self-test: Use a finger to feel the wall of the hemorrhoid. If there's a clot, you'll feel a hard "nugget" inside. The clot will break down and be reabsorbed by the body within seven to 10 days—but the pain may be so severe that the patient can't wait that long. For quicker relief, the hemorrhoid can be excised by a doctor. It is injected with an anesthetic, then a small incision is made to remove the clot.

Internal hemorrhoids: Banding is usually the first choice of medical treatment for a bleeding internal hemorrhoid. One or more small rubber bands are placed over the base of the hemorrhoid. This "strangles" the hemorrhoid by cutting off its blood supply. The hemorrhoid then disappears within a week. Banding can be done in a doctor's office and causes only mild discomfort. Patients should be up and about right away.

ADVANCED TREATMENT

Advanced treatment is most commonly required only for patients with Grade 3 or 4 hemorrhoids. Grade 3 is when a prolapsed hemorrhoid requires manual reduction (has to be pushed back in)…and Grade 4 is when a patient has hemorrhoids that are no longer reducible.

Two treatment choices…

•**Surgery:** The procedure, called *hemorrhoidectomy,* involves cutting out the matlike vein bundles that contain the hemorrhoids. The surgery requires a local anesthetic with sedation, a spinal anesthetic or a general anesthetic. It's almost always done as an outpatient procedure, but some patients stay overnight in the hospital. Postoperative pain can be intense and is optimally managed with several medications, including narcotics, nonsteroidal anti-inflammatory drugs (NSAIDs), such as *ibuprofen,* and topical agents.

•**Stapling** is a new procedure in which a circular device snips off a prolapsed hemorrhoid at the base and simultaneously staples the remaining tissue so that it stays in the proper position. This usually requires general anesthesia and is done as an outpatient procedure.

Stapling can be a good choice for patients with large internal (but not external) hemorrhoids. It causes less discomfort than traditional surgery, and patients recover more quickly. I tell most patients to plan to be off work for one week if they have traditional surgery and a long weekend for the stapling procedure. However, the results of stapling may not be as durable as those from surgery. In a recent study of 269 patients who underwent stapling, 23 had recurrences—compared with only four patients in a comparable group of surgical patients. It's a judgment call as to which procedure is better.

PREVENTION

Patients who are prone to hemorrhoids can reduce their symptoms by making lifestyle changes…

•**Eat 25 to 30 grams (g) of fiber daily.** High-fiber foods (fruits, vegetables, whole grains, etc.) cause stools to absorb water in the colon. This makes the stools softer and larger, which reduces straining and pressure on the anal veins. High-fiber breakfast cereals are a good choice for people who have trouble getting enough fiber. Look for a product that contains at least five grams of fiber per serving. Or try an over-the-counter high-fiber supplement.

•**Drink six to eight glasses of water daily** to keep the stools lubricated. This is especially important for patients who have increased their fiber intake.

•**Practice good "bowel habits."** Go to the bathroom as soon as you feel the urge (waiting can cause stools to harden)…don't sit on the toilet for more than five minutes (no reading!)…and avoid straining to have a bowel movement. If you don't feel the urge, get up and try again later.

Hangover Helpers

Christine Lay, MD, neurologist, The Headache Institute at St. Luke's-Roosevelt Hospital Center in New York City.
Khursheed Navder, PhD, RD, registered dietitian and associate professor of nutrition and food science program, Hunter College, The City University of New York, New York City.
US National Institutes of Health.
American Headache Society, Mt. Royal, NJ.

With all the breakthrough studies on the heart-helping impact of moderate drinking, you may wonder what's being uncovered about helping to offset the pain of a hangover.

The research is ever evolving, but scientists have some tips on how to reduce that morning-after misery.

BOOZE CLUES

What causes a hangover (besides the obvious —too much alcohol)? *According to Dr. Christine Lay, a neurologist at The Headache Institute at St. Luke's-Roosevelt Hospital Center, alcohol affects the body in these ways…*

•**Blood vessels dilate,** which may contribute to the throbbing headache.

•**The liver's ability to produce glucose is impaired,** which leaves you feeling weak and tired, clouds your thinking and makes you moody.

•**It "fragments" sleep.** Although alcohol is sedating and initially promotes sleep, it is often poor-quality sleep with frequent awakenings due to factors such as decreased rapid eye movement (REM) sleep.

•**The main byproduct of metabolized alcohol,** acetaldehyde, is a toxin that can make your heart race and lead to headache, sweatiness, flushed skin, nausea and vomiting.

•**It causes dehydration and electrolyte imbalance.** Alcohol promotes urination by inhibiting the release of the brain hormone that normally protects against dehydration. When dehydration is accompanied by sweating, vomiting or diarrhea, there is additional fluid and mineral loss leading to electrolyte imbalances. The result? Excessive thirst, lethargy, dizziness and light-headedness.

PREVENTING PROBLEMS

The first step in preventing problems caused by too much alcohol is to consume plenty of water—ideally, a full glass between each alcoholic drink. Dehydration is perhaps the most common cause of hangover symptoms.

"Those pounding headaches and everything else are related to the shriveling of the cells because they lose so much water," says Khursheed Navder, a registered dietitian and associate professor of nutrition and food science program at Hunter College.

So while you are drinking—and before going to bed—force yourself to drink water. "If you forget to drink water before going to bed, then do it first thing in the morning," she says. "The sooner you replenish your fluid loss, the quicker you'll bounce back."

Exercise can help with hangover symptoms by boosting blood flow to the brain and inducing sweating, which helps the body purge alcohol, she said. *Other tips…*

•**Eat soups to replace salt and potassium depleted by alcohol,** and fruits and vegetables can help replenish lost nutrients.

•**Take pain-relief medications** such as ibuprofen and naproxen sodium to reduce headache and muscle aches (as long as your stomach isn't upset). Antacids can help ease nausea and gastritis.

285

•**All things considered,** lighter-colored alcohol may reduce the severity of a hangover. That's because beverages such as vodka, gin and white wine have fewer congeners—a toxic byproduct of fermentation and aging—than darker-colored drinks such as whisky, brandy and red wine.

Price also matters: More expensive alcohol generally contains fewer congeners because it goes through a more rigorous distillation process that filters out more congeners.

info The Mayo Clinic Web site has more about hangover prevention and treatment at *www.mayoclinic.com/health/hangovers/ds00649.*

■ ■ ■ ■

Meat Eating Linked to Gout

In a study of more than 41,000 men, those who consumed the most meat (beef, poultry, pork and seafood) increased their risk for gout, a common form of inflammatory arthritis that often occurs in joints of the feet and ankles, by 41%.

Theory: Uric acid, which causes gout, is created in the body as meat is metabolized.

Self-defense: Limit your meat intake to four to five ounces daily.

Gary Curhan, MD, ScD, associate professor of medicine, Harvard Medical School, Boston.

Jolt of Java Eases Gout

Hyon K. Choi, MD, DrPH, Brigham and Women's Hospital, Boston.
Arthritis & Rheumatism.

Four or more cups of coffee a day may help keep the gout away, suggests a study published in *Arthritis & Rheumatism.* Gout, the most common form of inflammatory arthritis in adult males, is caused by having an excess of uric acid in the joints.

THE STUDY

American and Canadian researchers tracked almost 46,000 men for 12 years. They were aged 40 to 75 at the start of the study and had no history of gout. The researchers found that men who drank six or more cups of coffee a day were 59% less likely to develop gout than those who never drank coffee, while the risk was 40% lower for men who drank four to five cups a day. The findings were independent of all other risk factor for gout.

Decaffeinated coffee offered somewhat less protection against gout. Tea drinking and total caffeine consumption did not have an effect on the incidence of gout. This suggests that it's not caffeine but other components of coffee that are responsible for helping prevent gout, said researcher Dr. Hyon K. Choi of Brigham and Women's Hospital in Boston.

While he and his colleagues did not suggest that men should start drinking four or more cups of coffee a day, they said their findings may help men make an informed decision about coffee consumption.

13

Savvy Consumer

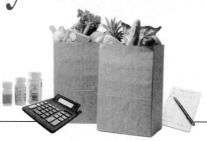

Better Prices, Great Care In Overseas Surgery

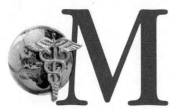 **M**ore and more Americans are traveling to Europe, the Far East and Mexico for medical treatment.

Key reason: Low prices on top-quality care.

In the past, this kind of medical tourism has been associated with elective plastic surgery and experimental treatments not available in the US. But two years ago, more than 55,000 Americans went abroad for necessary but non-emergency operations, such as angioplasty, knee replacement and cataract surgery.* Less expensive labor and administrative costs make foreign treatment 50% to 75% cheaper. That can be a bargain even with the additional costs of airfare and accommodations. *Costs of medical*

*US insurance companies currently do not pay for overseas surgery if it is not an emergency.

procedures vary widely, within the US and internationally, but here are a few examples...

- **Cataract surgery** in the US costs about $3,000 an eye...in Eastern Europe, it costs $1,200 an eye.

- **Repairing a herniated disk** in the US can range from $30,000 to $90,000...in Bangkok, Thailand, it starts at $3,500.

- **A total knee replacement** in the US is about $48,000...in India, $5,500.

- **Angioplasty** in the US, around $80,000... in Singapore, $15,000.

- **Root canal** in the US can range from $500 to $900...in Mexico, less than $300.

FINDING THE BEST

Flying thousands of miles from home for an operation is not for everyone, but it's worth exploring if you don't have adequate health insurance. Of course, you would want to use only

Rudy Rupak, founder of PlanetHospital, a foreign medical-treatment company based in Calabasas, CA, that arranges affordable surgeries overseas and offers free evaluations to those seeking surgery abroad. *www.planethospital.com.*

top-quality foreign hospitals and physicians. *Here's how to find them…*

•**Start by word of mouth.** Ask friends and associates who have had medical procedures overseas for recommendations. Also ask doctors who specialize in the type of surgery you need.

•**Check with Harvard Medical International (HMI).** This is a self-supporting, not-for-profit subsidiary of Harvard Medical School. Its role is to extend internationally the school's tradition of improving the quality of health care. HMI is affiliated with dozens of overseas medical institutions and hospitals. (617-535-6400, *www.hmi.hms.harvard.edu*).

•**Contact the Joint Commission International (JCI),** the global arm of the institution that accredits US hospitals. JCI hospitals have to meet rigorous standards of patient care, medication safety and infection control. (630-792-5000, *www.jointcommissioninternational.org*).

•**Choose a hospital with an international patient coordinator** on staff. He/she will help you coordinate doctor's appointments, diagnostics and treatment at the hospital, as well as arrange postoperative recuperation. He also can help with practical matters, such as airport pickup, currency exchange, hospital meal choices and interpreters if necessary.

•Ask the foreign doctor/hospital for references from Americans who have had the same type of treatment.

TOP FOREIGN HOSPITALS

These are foreign hospitals I would trust for myself and my family…

•**India**

•Apollo Hospitals has hospitals in Delhi, Chennai and Hyderabad that cater to foreigners and specialize in heart-related procedures.

•Wockhardt Hospitals Group has hospitals in Mumbai (formerly Bombay) and Bangalore that specialize in heart, eye, bone, brain and spinal surgery. Associated with HMI. *www.wockhardt hospitals.net.*

•The Max Hospital, New Delhi, offers state-of-the-art surgery for brain and pituitary tumors, aneurysms and vascular malformations. *www.max healthcare.in/corporate/index.asp.*

•**Thailand**

•Bumrungrad Hospital is Bangkok's leading health-care institution. Specialties include endocrinology, nephrology and neurology. *www.bum rungrad.com.*

•Samitivej Hospitals has branches in Bangkok and Chonburi. Specialties include cardiac and cancer surgery. *www.samitivej.co.th/index_en.aspx.*

•**Singapore**

•Parkway Group Healthcare. Three hospitals specializing in cardiac surgery and neurosurgery—East Shore, Gleneagles and Mount Elizabeth. *www.ipac.sg.*

•**Belgium**

•The De Smet Clinic, Ghent specializes in hip-related surgery. *www.hip-clinic.com/en/html/home_en.html.*

•**Mexico**

•Hospitales Angeles has six hospitals in cities such as Tijuana and Juarez. Specializes in neurosurgery and dental surgery. *www.mediks.com* (site is in Spanish only).

GETTING QUALITY CARE

•**Ask for a full diagnosis** from your own doctor first. Develop a treatment plan you both feel comfortable with. Your doctor should be willing to forward all diagnostic information and communicate with the foreign surgeon to discuss your condition. Once you arrive, the foreign doctor also will evaluate you prior to surgery.

•**Bring a family member or friend.** You need someone for emotional support and to serve as your advocate. That person should bring with him/her your health-care power of attorney, which will be honored by international hospitals. This document allows him to make health decisions for you if you are unable to communicate your own wishes.

While a second person doubles the cost of the airfare, most foreign hospitals will allow a companion to stay as a guest in your room for no extra charge.

•**Know the costs.** Most international hospitals and/or health-care providers expect 50% of their fee to book the surgery and the rest of the cost of treatment at the time of admission. If complications prevent you from returning home immediately, hospitals will accommodate you longer, but ask for the rates so that you can plan accordingly. Also, you should be able to change any airfare you book multiple times with minimal penalty.

Important: Check with your insurance company to make sure it will pay for the treatment of any complications once you arrive home.

•**Confirm that the hospital gives you the same rights** that you have in the US. Reputable hospitals and surgeons will guarantee these rights in writing before you travel overseas. *You should have the right to...*

•Receive complete and current information concerning your diagnosis, treatment and prognosis in terms that you can understand, including serious side effects or risks, problems related to recovery and the likelihood of success.

•Have access to all information contained in your medical records.

•Accept or refuse any treatment and be informed of the consequences of any such refusal.

•Request consultation with the hospital ethics/oversight committee regarding complaints and ethical issues involved in your care.

•Be transferred to another facility at your request or when it is medically appropriate.

•Examine your bill and receive an explanation of the charges.

•**Understand that your legal rights are limited** if medical malpractice is committed overseas. You cannot sue in American courts, and most foreign countries strictly limit malpractice damage awards.

Helpful: If your overseas doctor has a medical board certification in the US, you can complain to the board and seek sanctions.

■ ■ ■ ■

Flying Soon?

Avoid catching a cold or the flu by taking the dietary supplement lactoferrin. People who travel on planes often get colds within a week of travel. The supplement, which is made from whey, is identical to the lactoferrin protein that occurs naturally in the gut. This protein boosts the production of immunoglobulins, compounds that fight bacteria and viruses.

Helpful: Take 200 mg of lactoferrin twice daily two days before you fly, and continue taking it for three days afterward. It is available in health-food stores.

Erika T. Schwartz, MD, internist in private practice in New York City.

What You Must Know Before Having Surgery

Charles B. Inlander is a consumer advocate and health-care consultant based in Fogelsville, PA. He was the founding president of the nonprofit People's Medical Society, a consumer advocacy organization credited with key improvements in the quality of US health care in the 1980s and 1990s, and is the author of 20 books, including *Take This Book to the Hospital with You: A Consumer Guide to Surviving Your Hospital Stay.* St. Martin's.

Each year, more than 80 million Americans undergo some type of surgery. Over the last 35 years, I have advised thousands of surgical patients on the information they should give their doctors and the questions that must be asked to ensure the best possible odds for a successful operation and recovery. *Here are the areas that are most often overlooked or cause confusion among patients...*

•**Medications and/or supplements before surgery.** If you take a blood thinner, such as *warfarin* (Coumadin), you will likely need to stop taking it three or more days before any major surgery, such as a coronary bypass or a hysterectomy, to prevent excessive bleeding. You will probably need to modify your medication schedule even for less invasive surgery, such as knee surgery or removal of a growth.

Caution: Do not assume that your surgeon knows the drugs and/or supplements you are taking. In fact, he/she probably doesn't. Give him a list of all your prescription and nonprescription drugs, such as aspirin or antacids, as well as all vitamins and other supplements that you take.

Self-defense: When your surgery is scheduled, ask your surgeon to write down the specific drugs and/or supplements you should stop taking before surgery and exactly how many days prior to the operation you should discontinue them. Also, be sure to mention any chronic conditions you have, such as diabetes, heart disease or allergies, which may affect the outcome of your surgery.

•**New drugs before surgery.** It's not uncommon that the surgeon will ask you to take an antibiotic (to prevent infection) or an anticoagulant drug (to prevent blood clots) several days before surgery.

Self-defense: Don't wait for the surgeon to tell you this. As soon as your operation is planned, ask about presurgery medications. Get this in writing as well.

•**Fasting.** Many types of surgeries require that you fast or go on a liquid-only diet the day prior to the procedure. Among other reasons, fasting is necessary to prevent the patient from vomiting and possibly choking. You also may need to take a laxative to empty your bowels before the operation.

Self-defense: When surgery is scheduled, ask your surgeon for a written schedule of when you should stop eating solid foods…when you should take a laxative (if necessary)…and when you must stop ingesting anything, including liquids.

•**Medical tests.** Presurgical tests may be required a few days before the operation to rule out any reasons to delay, alter or cancel the surgery. However, often, those same tests were performed only a week or two earlier to diagnose your condition.

Self-defense: Ask the surgeon or his staff to check whether you need to repeat a recently performed test. You have enough to do prior to surgery without going for unnecessary tests.

•**Conflicting instructions.** Your surgeon may tell you that it's okay to take a certain drug prior to surgery while one of your other doctors says to stop it.

Self-defense: When your surgeon gives you instructions that differ from what one of your other doctors has told you, ask that the doctors speak with each other and give you their joint recommendation.

One Dose of Antibiotics Prevents Post-Surgery Infection

Philip Tierno, MD, PhD, director of clinical microbiology and immunology, New York University Medical Center, and author, *The Secret Life of Germs* (Atria) and *Protect Yourself Against Bioterrorism* (Simon & Schuster). *Archives of Surgery.*

If you're facing surgery, ask your doctor about getting an antibiotic before your procedure. New research shows a single pre-operative dose of antibiotic seems to prevent surgical site infections just as well as multiple doses given afterwards for 24 hours.

This finding, made by Brazilian researchers, could lower your hospital bill without affecting your recovery.

THE STUDY

In their study, researchers compared infection rates and costs for more than 12,300 patients who underwent surgery.

They found no difference in infection rates between those getting one-dose pre-surgery therapy and those getting multiple doses of antibiotic following it and it appears to save money as well.

Infection after surgery is a common complication, and antibiotics are often used to reduce the chance a patient will develop an infection at the surgical site.

THE REACTION

"I think that the paper is a step in the right direction," says Dr. Philip Tierno, the director of clinical microbiology and immunology at New York University Medical Center and author of *The Secret Life of Germs* and *Protect Yourself Against Bioterrorism.*

Tierno is also a member of the Infection Control Committee at the medical center.

"However, I think that there are some surgeries that are inherently more at risk for development of infection like heart, bone, GI and colon, such that some institutions may elect to exclude those surgical procedures from the one-dose protocol," Tierno says.

How to Save Money On Organic Food

Ronnie Cummins is national director of the Organic Consumers Association, a nonprofit organization that promotes food safety, children's health and environmental sustainability, Finland, MN. *www.organicconsumers. org*. He is author of *Genetically Engineered Food: A Self-Defense Guide for Consumers*. Marlowe & Company.

M any people who would like to eat organic fruits, vegetables, dairy, meat and poultry are put off by the high prices. Organic foods can cost 25% to 100% more than regular foods—but if you're willing to do a bit of sleuthing and look beyond traditional grocery stores, you can find organic products for much less.

My organization's Web site, *www.organic consumers.org,* has links to most of the resources suggested below...

•**Compare prices of conventional and organic foods** when shopping at regular grocery stores. Occasionally, the price gap narrows dramatically, or organic foods may even be cheaper.

•**Shop at a farmers' market.** You can find bargains if you prowl around the stalls of your local farmers' market. You'll save even more if you haggle. Farmers may be especially willing to negotiate prices if produce is misshapen or closing time is approaching.

Sample savings: Organic apples at a farmers' market often are 25% to 50% cheaper than organic apples at grocery or natural-food stores.

•**Consider purchasing a share in a community-supported agriculture program (CSA).** There are more than 1,000 of these programs around the US. Through a CSA, you purchase produce from an organic farmer in a region near you. You'll receive a weekly basket that contains produce, flowers and perhaps even eggs and milk. A share in a CSA typically costs several hundred dollars for one growing season, which could last half a year (prices vary dramatically depending on location). In mild regions, such as California, you can receive just-picked produce year-round. Each week, it's fun to discover what goodies are in the basket.

Sample savings: In rural Minnesota, where I live, I pay $450 for the season and split my weekly harvest with another family. This is at least 50% cheaper than store prices.

Helpful: Most CSAs deliver produce orders to a central location. You may be able to reduce the price of your weekly delivery if you allow your front porch to serve as a delivery spot for your neighborhood.

CSAs can be found at the Web site of Local Harvest (*www.localharvest.org*), as well as on my Web site.

•**Join a food co-op.** Co-ops typically offer high-quality organic food and produce at a discount for members. You may be required to volunteer your time for a certain number of hours each month. For a list of co-ops, see my organization's Web site.

•**Buy in bulk.** This is a great way to save money on long-lasting and nonperishable organic food, such as dried beans, lentils, pasta, rice, cereals, trail mix, nuts and even peanut butter. Health-food stores, Whole Foods, and even some supermarkets sell bulk items.

Cheaper still: Join a wholesale buying club (regular yearly membership fee is between $35 and $50). The minimum order for the club I belong to is $1,000 every three months, so I share a membership with several families in my area.

Typical savings: 30% to 50% off retail.

There is no national directory of buying clubs. Ask your local natural-food store for the names of its organic-food suppliers and contact them.

•**Eat seasonally.** You're sure to overpay if you buy organic fruits and vegetables off-season. That's when you want to buy frozen or canned. When produce is bountiful and cheap, you may want to can, freeze or dry it for the coming months.

■ ■ ■ ■

Steps to Safer Produce

S everal deaths as a result of *Escherichia coli*–contaminated spinach have left many people wary of fresh produce. In the case of the contaminated spinach, even washing the leaves doesn't seem to have eliminated the risk. That's why the government must ensure safe growing conditions and handling by the food industry. *Meanwhile, consumers should follow these food-handling guidelines from the not-for-profit Partnership for Food Safety Education...*

•**Check that fresh-cut fruits and vegetables,** such as packaged salads and precut melons, are refrigerated by the store.

•**Wash hands with warm water and soap** for at least 20 seconds before and after handling produce.

•**Wash surfaces and utensils with hot water and soap** before and after preparation of produce.

•**Rub firm-skin produce under running tap water or scrub with a vegetable brush while rinsing.** With leafy produce, such as spinach, rinse until the water comes through the food clear. Dry with a clean cloth towel or paper towel. Never use detergent or bleach to wash produce.

•**Throw away any produce that won't be cooked** if it has touched raw meat, poultry or seafood.

info For more information on food safety, visit *www.fightbac.org/images/pdfs/produce bro-bw.pdf.*

■ ■ ■ ■

Enjoy Fruit and Veggies Without Pesticides

For good health, most of us have been told that we should significantly increase our intake of fruits and vegetables. At the same time, we have been warned about the potential health hazards of pesticides, and little research is available to determine the long-term health effects of regularly eating foods with low levels of pesticide residues. *What to do...*

•**Wash and scrub fruits and vegetables.** Soaking in water can loosen debris, and scrubbing with a soft brush helps remove contaminants in crevices. Running water is an effective way to rinse off residue—commercial produce rinses are only slightly more effective.

•**Choose organic.** This is especially important for foods known to have the most pesticide

residue, such as nectarines, peaches, apples, spinach and celery. Large natural-food stores often have the widest selection and most competitive prices.

•**Buy conventional produce selectively.** If you can't always buy organic, choose fruits and vegetables that have the lowest amounts of pesticide residue—asparagus, avocados, bananas, broccoli, cauliflower, sweet corn, kiwi, mangos, onions and papaya.

info For more information, contact the Environmental Working Group at 202-667-6982, or download their Shopper's Guide to Pesticides in Produce at *www.foodnews.org/walletguide.*

Suzanne Havala Hobbs, DrPH, RD, clinical assistant professor, School of Public Health, University of North Carolina at Chapel Hill. She is the author of *Being Vegetarian for Dummies* and *Vegetarian Cooking for Dummies* (both from Hungry Minds).

■ ■ ■ ■

Super Juices That Fight Alzheimer's, Cancer, More

Gulp for gulp, purple grape, cranberry and cloudy apple juices contain the most health-benefiting antioxidant nutrients found in morning beverages.

So say a team of Glasgow University scientists who compared various fruit juices believed to help prevent diseases such as Alzheimer's, heart disease and certain cancers.

A REALLY-FULL GLASS

What makes those the best beverages? They contain the highest concentrations of the very strongest antioxidants to fight free radicals, renegade cells that damage healthy ones and precipitate many harmful conditions.

Juice made with Concord grapes has the best range of polyphenols with the highest antioxidant capacity.

Advice: "Supplementing a healthy diet with a regular intake of a variety of fruit juices such as purple grape juice, grapefruit juice, cloudy apple juice and cranberry juice will, without major dietary changes, increase the consumer's intake of phenolic antioxidants," notes study author and researcher Alan Crozier, professor of plant biochemistry and human nutrition at Glasgow University.

Alan Crozier, professor of plant biochemistry and human nutrition, Glasgow University, Scotland.
Journal of Agriculture and Food Chemistry.

The Best Honey For Your Money

Rosa Ana Perez, MS, PhD, main researcher, Department of Food and Agriculture Research, Instituto Madrileno de Investigacion y Desarrollo Rural, Agrario y Alimentario, Madrid, Spain.
Journal of the Science of Food and Agriculture.

If you're looking for the healthiest honey, consider darker-colored "honeydew" varieties from bees that collect the sugary "dew" secretions that insects leave on plants.

According to a new study of Spanish varieties, honeydew varieties have higher levels of disease-fighting antioxidants than honey that bees make from nectar.

"Besides its value as a great sweetening agent, honey has proved that it also has effective antioxidant and antibacterial activities," says study coauthor Rosa Ana Perez, a researcher with the Instituto Madrileno de Investigacion y Desarrollo Rural, Agrario y Alimentario in Madrid.

THE BUZZ ON HEALTH

In recent years, honey has gained a reputation as a health food, especially in light of research suggesting that it has germ-fighting powers and is high in antioxidants, which block certain types of cell damage caused by molecules called free radicals.

"There is increasing evidence that free radicals contribute to the development of diseases, such as neurodegenerative disease, chronic inflammatory disease, cancer, cardiovascular disease and aging," notes Perez.

In past research, scientists noted that antioxidant levels increased in people who ate between four and 10 tablespoons of honey per day, depending on their weight. It wasn't clear, however, which varieties of honey might harbor the most antioxidants.

THE STUDY

In this new research, Perez's team looked at 36 varieties of Spanish honey in two groups— clover honey made by bees from the nectar of flower blossoms, and honeydew honey, made by bees from a sweet, sticky substance secreted by insects such as aphids that live off plants.

Honeydew types, which are darker and more acidic, consistently proved to have the highest antioxidant content. This variety is relatively rare in the US.

But be warned: With the high nutrient content comes a price—honey is about 80% sugar, so it can pack on the pounds.

info To find out more about honey's healthful properties, visit *www.whfoods.org,* the Web site of the World's Healthiest Foods.

■ ■ ■ ■

How to Use Honey as a Natural Antibiotic

Honey's natural acidity creates an inhospitable environment for germs…and it contains a small amount of germ-killing hydrogen peroxide.

Important: Heat can destroy honey's beneficial properties, so buy the raw and unpasteurized kind. Honey can be used on most wounds. If you have a puncture wound, consult your doctor.

What to do: Work one tablespoon of warmed honey into a four-inch by four-inch gauze pad, then place it on the wound. Change the dressing at least twice daily until the wound heals.

Caution: Do not use on children under one year of age. (They should not ingest honey.)

Peter Molan, PhD, professor of biological sciences, University of Waikato, Hamilton, New Zealand.

More Americans Paying Medical Bills with Credit Cards

Mark Rukavina, executive director, The Access Project, Boston.

Cindy Zeldin, federal affairs coordinator, Economic Opportunity Program, Demos.

More Americans are using credit cards to pay their medical bill—whether or not they have health insurance.

But it's not out of convenience, say experts. It's because they don't have the cash.

"People are using high-interest credit cards to pay for their health care," notes Mark Rukavina, coauthor of a new report, *Borrowing to Stay Healthy: How Credit Card Debt Is Related to Medical Expenses.*

Health-care costs have been rising for decades, and the cost of health insurance continues to outstrip wages and inflation.

As a result, employers are looking for ways to reduce their insurance costs—often leaving workers to take on more of the financial burden.

HARDSHIPS EN MASSE

"Nearly 60 million adults in the US are at risk of incurring medical bills they will not be able to afford," says Rukavina. "Many people are just an illness away from becoming medical debtors, and medical debt can have a detrimental effect on health-care access."

Past research indicates that half of all declared nonbusiness bankruptcies in the US result from medical costs.

To assess how US households are dealing with medical debt, The Access Project, along with the consumer advocacy group Demos, commissioned a national survey of 1,150 low- and middle-income households. To be included in the survey, participants had to have credit-card debt of three months or longer at the time of the survey.

Nearly one in three participants reported that medical expenses contributed to their credit card balances. Within that group, the overwhelming majority reported a large medical expense in the past three years.

Among the report's other findings...

• **Households with medical debt had higher levels of credit card debt than households without medical debt**—on average, 46% more.

• **Those with medical debt were nearly twice as likely to carry credit card balances over $10,000.**

• **Households that were medically indebted were more likely to be called by bill collectors** than nonmedically indebted households, 62% versus 38%.

• **Credit card debt was high for both insured and uninsured medically indebted households**—$10,973 and $14,512, respectively. "This indicates that even those who do have health insurance aren't always protected," notes Cindy Zeldin, a report coauthor and federal affairs coordinator with Demos' Economic Opportunity Program.

 Read the full report at *www.accessproject. org/adobe/borrowing_to_stay_healthy.pdf.*

How to Get Great Care At Walk-In Clinics

The American Geriatrics Society.

The number of walk-in medical clinics in retail malls in the US doubled last year, indicating a new trend in the way people seek healing. How can you make the most of these no-appointment-necessary facilities?

DO

• **Clearly explain to the walk-in medical clinic's health care professional *all* of your medical problems** and any allergies or problems you have with medications.

• **Bring a complete list of your current medications**—including over-the-counter products—and ask the clinic health-care provider to check the list to be certain that the drugs on the list agree with any new medications the clinic doctor may prescribe.

• **Get a report from the clinic with your diagnosis and follow-up instructions.** Take that report with you the next time you see your doctor.

DON'T

• **Go to a walk-in medical clinic in a retail mall if you have major new symptoms,** such as chest pain, shortness of breath, leg swelling, or a cough that lasts more than three weeks. These symptoms require immediate attention by your doctor.

• **Visit a walk-in medical clinic in a retail mall if you notice a change with a medical problem** that you've had for a long time and is already being treated by your doctor. See your own doctor.

• **Use a walk-in medical clinic in a retail mall for the majority of your health care.** These clinics provide only basic treatments and tests.

Secrets for Staying Safe In the Hospital

David J. Sherer, MD, a board-certified anesthesiologist in clinical practice at Falls Church Ambulatory Surgery Center in Falls Church, VA, affiliated with Mid-Atlantic Permanente Medical Group. He is author of *Dr. David Sherer's Hospital Survival Guide: 100+ Ways to Make Your Hospital Stay Safe and Comfortable.* Claren.

As many as 195,000 patients die each year in US hospitals because of medical errors, according to a recent study by HealthGrades, a leading health-care rating company. Here's how to stay safe next time you're in the hospital. If you're too incapacitated by your illness or injury to do these things for yourself, a family member can do many of them for you.

1. Keep a list of prescribed medications with dosages. You can get this list from the attending physician (the doctor in charge of your case), an intern, resident or nurse. Receiving the wrong medication is one of the most common—and dangerous—hospital errors. When a hospital staff member hands you a pill or starts to hook an intravenous (IV) bag to your arm, ask what you're being given. *If the drug isn't on the list of medications you have been prescribed…*

• Ask "What does this treat?" If the answer isn't a condition that you think you have, double-check that the drug provider knows your name and birthday, to confirm you're the patient he/she thinks you are.

• Make sure it's not a drug with a similar name. If you've been prescribed Zantac and someone's trying to give you Xanax, someone may have misheard the instructions and provided the wrong medication.

• Also, if it is a drug you've been prescribed but you previously received a different dosage, make sure the change was intentional.

2. Label yourself. If you're in the hospital for an operation on a limb, a lung or anything else that you have more than one of on or in your body, use a marker or ballpoint pen to write "this arm," "this leg" or just "yes" on the side that should go under the knife, so there is no confusion in the operating room. (At some hospitals, your surgeon will sign his initials to the body part in advance of your operation.) Don't use an "X" to mark the spot, because an "X" is ambiguous—it could be misinterpreted as "not here."

• If you're allergic to any medications, make a sign to this effect and post it over your hospital bed.

Example: "Allergic to Penicillin."

3. Schedule your hospital stay wisely. New interns, residents and medical school students begin assignments at teaching hospitals in early July. If possible, postpone elective procedures until a different time, when young medical professionals have more experience.

• If you can't avoid a July stay in a teaching hospital, be wary about what you let interns and medical students do. If one wants to draw blood, insert a catheter or perform another common hospital task, ask how many times he/she has done it before. If the answer doesn't fill you with confidence, insist that a nurse or resident take over.

• Also, at any time of the year, try to schedule your surgery for early in the day. By the end of a long day, even the most skilled surgeons aren't at the top of their game. Also, because patients aren't allowed to eat or drink before surgery, a late operation means extra hours of hunger, thirst and worry.

4. Get to know the staff. A wide range of doctors, nurses, physician's assistants, interns, residents, orderlies and others might be involved in your care. Whenever a new face arrives, politely ask his name and what his role is, unless his name tag makes this obvious, then engage in some friendly conversation.

•If you make a personal connection with everyone involved in your care, it reduces the odds that you'll be mistaken for a different patient with potentially dangerous results. It also increases the odds that you'll get prompt care. Because most hospital patients are preoccupied with their health problems, the few who remain composed, personable and interested in the hospital staff often are treated more favorably.

5. Know who should do what. Find out when you can expect your attending physician to visit your bedside, and save any questions you have until then. Answers you receive from anyone else might not be definitive.

•Don't let a UAP (also known as unlicensed assistive personnel or nurse assistant) insert an IV or catheter, change a sterile dressing, give you a shot or feed you through a tube. Such tasks should be handled by trained medical staff, such as a registered nurse. Check the person's name tag. If there's no designation, such as RN, ask what his training is.

6. Select the right surgeon. Unless it is an emergency, you shouldn't necessarily settle for the first surgeon you're sent to. *When you meet with a surgeon for a consultation, ask...*

•Are you board-certified in this specialty? Or check this on the Web site of the American Board of Medical Specialties (*www.abms.org*). You will have to register, but it is free.

•How many times have you performed this exact procedure? You want someone who has done it hundreds or even thousands of times. If the procedure is rare, you at least want a surgeon who performs it dozens of times per year.

7. Find the right hospital. If your surgeon has privileges at more than one hospital in your area, the annual "America's Best Hospital Guide" of *US News and World Report* (*www.us news.com* and click on "Best Hospitals") can help you decide which facility is best for a given procedure. Be aware that your health insurance might limit you to a particular hospital or restrict your choice of surgeons.

8. Plan for the unexpected before you wind up in a hospital. Ask your doctor now which emergency room in your region he considers the best, assuming that there's more than one. (Of course, in situations where every second counts, the closest ER is almost always the best choice.)

9. Speak up. Make no effort to conceal your pain in a crowded emergency room—the ER staff might equate a quiet patient with a low-priority medical problem and treat others ahead of you. If you must wait, let the staff know if the pain gets worse...you have trouble breathing ...feel increasingly light-headed...or lose feeling in, or control over, part of your body.

10. Encourage bedside visitors. Visitors don't just keep you company in the hospital. They can keep an eye on the quality of your care when you're unable to do so yourself. And because hospital employees know that family members keep an eye on what's going on, more visitors tend to mean more attention from the staff.

11. Warn your anesthesiologist of any loose teeth. A loose tooth could be knocked out during intubation (when a breathing tube is placed in your windpipe), causing a potentially serious infection if the tooth reaches your lungs. Also, ask your doctor about removing any dentures or artificial teeth before you're taken to the operating room.

Vitamins—Are They More Harm Than Good?

Robert M. Russell, MD, director and senior scientist at Jean Mayer USDA Human Nutrition Research Center on Aging at Tufts University, Boston, and former chairman of the Institute of Medicine's Food and Nutrition Board.

At least half of American adults take vitamins and other supplements regularly, spending more than $23 billion a year on these nutritional aids in the belief that supplements can help prevent disease and improve health. However, evidence suggests that many supplements may be ineffective—and, in large doses, some may even do more harm than good.

Here's what you need to know now...

MULTIVITAMINS

According to a recent report by a panel of advisers at the National Institutes of Health, there is not enough evidence to recommend the use of multivitamin and mineral supplements to prevent chronic disease. And most people taking multivitamins don't really need them.

Reason: These individuals tend to be health conscious anyway, getting important nutrients from the food they eat.

There are, however, some people who do need supplements...

•**Anyone who eats fewer than 1,500 calories per day** should take a daily multivitamin that contains 100% of the Recommended Dietary Allowance (RDA) of all key nutrients.

•**Women who are trying to conceive** and those who are in the first trimester of pregnancy should take a daily prenatal multivitamin—which has 400 micrograms (mcg) of folic acid. Folic acid has been shown to reduce the risk of birth defects.

•**People over age 50** should take a B-12 supplement or a multivitamin containing at least the RDA of 2.4 mcg of B-12 if they don't get that amount in fortified foods, such as cereals. That's because as people age, the stomach produces less acid to digest food, making it difficult to absorb B-12 from food.

•**Those over age 70** have trouble getting enough calcium and vitamin D from food.

Example: To get the recommended amount of calcium, they would have to drink a quart of milk a day. People in this age group should have at least 600 international units (IUs) of vitamin D (15 mcg) and 1,200 milligrams (mg) of calcium a day.

MEGADOSES

The real concern is with the millions of Americans who consume nutrient-specific supplements in dosages that far exceed the RDAs.

Examples: Many people take vitamin C pills in hopes of boosting immunity and preventing colds...vitamins B and E to protect their hearts...beta-carotene and other antioxidants to help fight cancer.

Below are common supplements and the possible health problems that may result from taking high doses...

•**Vitamin E.** Although this antioxidant has been touted to improve heart health, recent "gold-standard" studies—randomized trials in which participants who are not aware of whether or not they are taking a supplement or a placebo are carefully tracked—show the opposite may be true. One meta-analysis, led by researchers from the Johns Hopkins School of Medicine, analyzed 19 previous trials involving almost 136,000 people and found that vitamin E supplements—especially in the often-sold daily dosage of 400 IUs—caused a slight increase in death from heart attack. In another study of 9,500 people, those who took vitamin E had a 13% higher risk of heart failure.

Another danger: Vitamin E supplements could interfere with chemotherapy or radiotherapy by suppressing free-radical production, which is necessary to kill cancer cells.

•**B vitamins.** Until recently, the belief was that vitamins B-6, B-12 and folic acid reduced the risk of heart attack and stroke by lowering the level of homocysteine in the blood, a well-documented risk factor for coronary artery disease. However, one recent study published in *The New England Journal of Medicine,* which followed people who had had a heart attack, found that the risk of a second attack increased after taking B-vitamin supplements.

Another danger: In animal studies, high doses of B vitamins seemed to stimulate cancer growth. There is no proof of this effect in humans, but there is a theoretical risk.

•**Vitamin C.** Contrary to popular wisdom, there's no credible evidence that vitamin C supplements help prevent colds, although they may shorten the duration by a day or so. For people who eat healthfully, supplementing with vitamin C does not seem to boost immunity.

Dangers: Vitamin C supplements raise the risk of kidney stones. As with vitamin E, vitamin C supplements should be avoided by cancer patients who are undergoing chemotherapy or radiotherapy.

•**Vitamin A and beta-carotene.** Vitamin A comes in two forms—as preformed vitamin A or as one of several carotenoids, of which beta-carotene is the best-known. Both forms of vitamin A supplements have proved risky.

Beta-carotene supplements have been found to speed the risk of death from lung cancer and heart disease in people who smoke. More recently, a study of 75,000 people found that supplements of preformed vitamin A—as well as diets rich in vitamin A—increased the risk of hip fractures by 48%. This was observed with dosages just slightly above the RDAs of 900 mcg for men and 700 mcg for women.

Other dangers: Unless you are deficient in vitamin A—rare in the US—taking supplements containing more than 3,000 mcg (10,000 IUs) can cause liver damage. In pregnant women, high-dose vitamin A supplements may cause birth defects.

•**Glucosamine and chondroitin sulfate.** In a recent federally sponsored clinical trial, the often-used combination of glucosamine and chondroitin sulfate, once believed to reduce osteoarthritis knee pain by rebuilding cartilage, proved no more effective than a placebo for most of the 1,583 participants. Only a small group of patients with severe arthritis experienced slight relief.

Dangers: Mild gastrointestinal upset is a possible side effect. Theoretically, people with seafood allergies may be allergic to glucosamine, which is derived from shellfish.

•**Saw palmetto.** Although taken by millions of men with an enlarged prostate, the herb saw palmetto didn't relieve symptoms any better than a placebo in a recent well-respected randomized trial published in *The New England Journal of Medicine.*

Dangers: Saw palmetto should not be taken with blood thinners, such as aspirin or *warfarin* (Coumadin). Possible side effects of saw palmetto include stomach pain, nausea, diarrhea and impotence.

•**Zinc.** Another antioxidant nutrient, zinc was once believed to help boost immunity and prevent colds. However, in most studies, supplements seem to benefit only those with zinc deficiency, which is rare among Americans eating a balanced diet.

Danger: Zinc supplements lower the body's copper levels, which in turn may increase the risk of cardiac arrhythmia.

•**Copper.** In adequate amounts—the RDA of 0.9 mg—copper helps in the formation of red blood cells, nerve fibers and collagen for healthy skin and bones. It also acts as an antioxidant. However, in higher amounts, copper may work as a pro-oxidant, promoting free-radical damage that could contribute to Alzheimer's disease—especially in people who eat a high-fat diet.

In a six-year study of 3,718 people whose average age was 75, recently published in *Archives of Neurology,* the rate of memory loss and other cognitive decline was equivalent to 19 years of aging in those who consumed 2.75 mg of copper per day—levels found in some multivitamins—and ate a diet rich in saturated and trans fats. However, copper intake wasn't associated with mental decline in people who ate low-fat diets.

Another danger: The risk of liver damage occurs with dosages above 10 mg a day.

THE BOTTOM LINE

Although high levels of certain nutrients help prevent disease and improve health, the benefit typically comes from diets rich in those vitamins and minerals. Foods also contain health-protecting *phytochemicals*—some of which have not yet been identified—and these substances are not in supplements.

The old advice still is best—eat a healthful, well-balanced diet to meet the RDAs of necessary nutrients.

Hidden Dangers of Acetaminophen You Need To Know Now

Janice Stumpf, clinical associate professor of pharmacy, University of Michigan, Ann Arbor.
Journal of the American Pharmacists Association.

One of the most common causes of sudden liver failure in the US is acetaminophen overdose—the popular pain reliever found in over-the-counter drugs such as Tylenol and in various prescription drugs.

Researchers say that excessive use of this medication—whether over time or from a single large dose—can cause severe liver damage or even death.

Yet, new research finds that most Americans are completely unaware of the dangers associated with this commonly consumed medication, found in many pain and cold medications, as well as prescription drugs such as Vicodin, Darvocet, Tylox, Percocet and Lorcet.

SHORTAGE OF KNOWLEDGE

To test how little is known about the dangers of this drug, University of Michigan researchers surveyed 104 patients visiting a general internal medicine clinic. *What they found...*

•**Most of those surveyed say they use acetaminophen,** but none could identify the maximum dose of either regular or extra-strength preparations of the drug.

•**More than 60% of those surveyed** say they had never received or weren't sure they had received information about the possible dangers of high doses of acetaminophen.

•**The majority also couldn't say what problems** might arise as a result of acetaminophen overdosing.

•**Most couldn't identify** which drugs contain acetaminophen.

Study author Janice Stumpf says she hopes these findings prompt pharmacists to provide better education on the safe use of acetaminophen.

Until that happens, it's essential that you read nonprescription drug labels carefully and be aware of the potential hazards of overdosing on a medication.

Bar Codes Mean Fewer Medicine Mistakes

Using bar coding in hospital pharmacies may help prevent dangerous prescription errors, according to a new study. Researchers at Brigham and Women's Hospital in Boston compared the rates of medication dispensing errors before and after bar coding technology were implemented at the hospital pharmacy.

HOW IT WORKS

With the new technology, every dose of medication was affixed with a bar code, and these codes were scanned in as an additional step to ensure that the right medications were being dispensed. Without the bar coding, the pharmacists relied on visual inspections alone to make sure they were dispensing the right medication.

After implementing the bar coding technology, the rate of dispensing errors fell by 85%, and the rate of dispensing errors with the potential to harm patients fell by 63%.

The bar coding technology was most effective when it required the pharmacy staff to scan *all* doses of medications.

"Overall, the use of bar code scanning technology appears to have a significant impact on the rate of dispensing errors that were serious enough to potentially harm patients," said lead author Eric Poon, an associate physician in the hospital's department of general medicine, in a prepared statement.

info For more on medication safety, go to the Institute for Safe Medication Web site at *www.ismp.org.*

8 Great Ways to Get More Accurate Lab Tests

Marjory Abrams, publisher, *Bottom Line Personal.*

Last fall, we held a health fair at our office. One employee who had recently had her annual physical decided to have her cholesterol levels measured again at the fair. To her surprise—and dismay—the reading on the second cholesterol test was almost 20% higher than the first. Which results should she believe?

I recounted this incident to Kandice Kottke-Marchant, MD, PhD, clinical pathologist at the renowned Cleveland Clinic. She told me that many factors can influence test results. These include diet, medications, differences between laboratories, even season (cholesterol counts tend to increase in winter). Patients can't control all of these factors—but there are ways to increase lab test accuracy. *Steps to take in advance…*

•**Make sure the lab is accredited.** The physician and the insurance carrier dictate where a test is performed. Labs are typically accredited by reputable organizations, but it is a good idea to check that the lab has accreditation.

•**Use the same lab every time,** if possible, since there can be significant testing differences between laboratories. In my colleague's case, only the first test actually involved lab work. The health-fair test was the "instant" kind—so disparate results were more likely.

•**Follow all instructions**—for example, eating a meal exactly two hours before a two-hour postprandial blood sugar test or abstaining from sexual intercourse for two days prior to a prostate-specific antigen (PSA) test.

•**Review your medications, dietary supplements and herbal remedies** with your doctor. These can affect lab test results. For example, high levels of vitamin C interfere with certain tests…birth control pills can increase blood sugar…some antidepressants and blood pressure medications can decrease blood sugar. Generally, these factors can be taken into account when interpreting the test results, but your doctor may advise a change in your regimen prior to the test.

•**If you have experienced significant stress recently** or exercised strenuously, tell your doctor. Those factors can increase blood levels of *C-reactive protein* (CRP), an inflammation indicator associated with heart disease.

•**To avoid bacterial contamination,** clean yourself with soap and water before giving a urine sample, or particularly for women, use the special wipes available at testing facilities.

Dr. Kottke-Marchant warns that patients should keep a watchful eye during a test, too. *For example…*

•**If blood flows too slowly as it is drawn,** clots may form, invalidating the results for some tests, especially hematology and coagulation tests (drawn in tubes with purple or light blue tops). A simple tilt of the tube back and forth may detect a clotted sample.

•**Check that the sample is labeled accurately.** Confirm your name, type of test, date drawn and, if at a hospital, patient ID number.

Treatment decisions generally should not be made on the basis of a single out-of-range reading, says Dr. Kottke-Marchant. A second test, drawn from a new sample, helps to confirm whether an out-of-range result is in line with prior results.

Sometimes trends can be more important than absolute numbers. A Johns Hopkins University study, for example, suggests that the annual rate of increase in PSA may be more significant than simply looking at whether the numbers are within the normal range.

As for my colleague—after her elevated cholesterol readings, her physician decided to change her cholesterol-lowering medication. Her total cholesterol count is now lower, and she expects it to continue to drop. She is delighted —and so am I!

Pill Splitting Cuts Drug Costs for Patients, Health Plans

Hae Mi Choe, PharmD, assistant clinical professor, pharmacy, University of Michigan School of Pharmacy.
Eric Michael, PharmD, pharmacist and principal, Mercer Human Resource Consulting, Minneapolis.
Greg Scandlen, president, Consumers for Health Care Choices, Hagerstown, MD.
American Journal of Managed Care.

A practice patients often use to cut down on drug costs, called "pill splitting," can also save money for insurance companies and employers, a study of the University of Michigan's own health benefit plan shows.

In pill splitting, patients cut larger-dose tablets in half to equal a smaller-dose prescription —for example, dividing 40-milligram tablets to create twice as many 20-milligram doses for the same price. And since drug companies and pharmacies don't usually double the price of medications as the dose doubles, that can mean lower overall per-pill drug costs and fewer drug store copays for consumers.

THE STUDY

The pill-splitting study involved more than 100 university health plan members who take cholesterol-reducing drugs, such as statins. Statins tend to be good candidates for splitting, the researchers noted, because they linger in the body for a long time, and any impact splitting might have on their action wouldn't greatly alter their effects.

The authors cautioned, however, that not all pills can be safely split. For example, drugs that pass through the body quickly, or have special time-release coatings, are not good candidates for splitting.

RESULTS

After the six-month randomized trial, 89% of participants said they'd be willing to continue splitting their cholesterol medications in exchange for a 50% reduction in their prescription copays, the study found.

In 2006, the university's health benefit plan (which covers 80,000 employees) offered the pill-splitting program for three cholesterol-lowering statin drugs. The program saved 500 employees who chose that option a total of $25,000 in copay reductions. In turn, the university saved $195,000 in drug costs, reported Hae Mi Choe, assistant clinical professor of pharmacy at the University of Michigan.

Splitting copays might not be quite enough of a financial incentive to get large numbers of patients to take the extra trouble to split pills, according to Greg Scandlen, president of the nonprofit Consumers for Health Care Choices, based in Maryland. If insurance carriers or employers "shared savings 50–50 with the patient, that would be a real incentive," he added.

And with an increased use of health savings accounts—from which consumers pay 100% of drug costs—"you'd have a substantial incentive," added Scandlen, whose group supports private health insurance.

Already, some managed-care plans require pill splitting without financial incentive for appropriate medications, explained pharmacist Eric Michael, of Mercer Human Resource Consulting in Minneapolis.

SPLITTING PILLS SAFELY

According to Choe, participants in the University of Michigan study used pill-splitter devices to avoid problems with pills crumbling or being too hard to cut.

Michael said he favors having pharmacists, not patients, split the pills, and some states—but not all—already authorize pharmacists to do this for customers. For one thing, certain patient groups, such as the elderly, might not be appropriate for pill splitting because of problems with dexterity, he said.

Choe agreed that those kinds of concerns should be considered when deciding what pills to include in a splitting program. "If doubling the dose will lead to detrimental consequences, I wouldn't recommend splitting," she said.

info For more on safe medication use, go to the Web site of the National Council on Patient Information and Education at *http://www.talkaboutrx.org/*.

The Disability Insurance Trap

Frank N. Darras, managing partner in the law firm of Shernoff Bidart & Darras LLP, Ontario, CA, the largest disability insurance and long-term-care law practice in the US. He has recovered more than $500 million in wrongfully denied benefits.

One out of every four Americans will miss at least 90 consecutive days of work because of an injury or illness between the ages of 35 and 65. Disability insurance can prevent these medical disasters from becoming financial disasters.

However, most disability insurance is obtained through deeply flawed group policies offered by employers. Employees with such group coverage often aren't adequately protected.

In representing clients, I have seen what can go wrong with employer-sponsored disability policies. *Here's what to watch out for and how to get the best coverage...*

PROBLEMS WITH EMPLOYER PLANS

Employer-sponsored disability policies—in which all or part of the premiums are paid by the employer—typically claim to replace 60% or 70% of an employee's income when he/she is disabled beyond the typical 90- or 180-day elimination (waiting) period. However, these promises are empty and deceptive. Insurers are allowed to reduce the benefits they pay dollar for dollar for any benefits the disabled employee receives from his state worker's compensation program…Social Security disability program…the state's disability program…and even cash settlements received for pain and suffering if the employee was injured in an accident that caused his disability.

Even worse: Any money these insurers pay out to group disability policyholders is taxed.* Beneficiaries end up with only a small fraction of what they thought they were insured for.

Other drawbacks…

•**An employer might eliminate** its disability plan at any time.

•**An employee may not be able to take this disability policy** with him if he quits or is fired.

•**If a claim is ultimately denied,** an employee in the group plan must appeal the denial in a timely manner, then sue in federal court to recover only his past-due benefits, some interest and attorney fees if the court allows. The horror of group disability litigation is that there is no trial by jury, no recovery for emotional distress and no opportunity to seek punitive damages under the Employee Retirement Income Security Act (ERISA). The carrier is required to pay only what it owed—in my opinion, this is like robbing a bank and returning the money years later without any penalty or jail time.

ADVANTAGES OF INDIVIDUAL COVERAGE

It's best to purchase your own individual disability coverage through an insurance agent, whether or not you are covered through an employer's group plan. You will receive the maximum benefit you're owed—tax free—even if you get other forms of compensation for your injury…you, not your employer, have control over the coverage…and if necessary, you can take the insurer to court, get a trial by jury and seek not only the benefits owed but also punitive damages if your state allows.

The downside is cost. A 55-year-old man in good health might spend $280 per month for a well-designed disability policy that replaces

*There are some employer plans that allow workers to pay all or part of the premiums with after-tax dollars so that payouts aren't taxed.

60% of wages up to $4,000 a month after a 90-day waiting period. A 55-year-old woman might spend around $325 (women are more likely to become disabled, so their coverage costs more). For a 45-year-old man, the cost might be $199 a month. For a woman, it might be $281 a month.

Two ways to cut the cost of your coverage…

•**Increase your waiting period** from 90 to 180 days. This should reduce premiums by about 20% compared with a 90-day wait—but this strategy makes sense only if you can afford to live half a year without income. With a six-month waiting period, you begin to accrue payable benefits in the seventh month and would get a check at the 225th-day (seven-and-a-half-month) mark.

•**Women should ask their insurance agents** to check whether unisex policies are available. These might cost 10% to 20% less.

MUST-HAVE FEATURES

Expect insurers to offer coverage for up to two-thirds of your current wages, not to exceed $15,000 per month.

Three provisions that you also should insist on…

•**"Own occupation" protection.** Without this provision, your insurer could reduce benefits by the amount you're capable of earning—even in a line of work that doesn't appeal to you.

Example: A stroke makes it impossible for a woman to continue her career as a surgeon. Without "own occupation" protection, her disability insurer might argue that she still could work as a janitor and then reduce her benefits by the $2,000 a month she could earn in that job. With "own occupation" protection, the woman receives her full benefit for as long as she can't perform surgery.

•**Noncancelable and guaranteed renewable to age 65.** With this clause in the contract, your insurance company can't terminate your coverage until you turn 65, even if your health deteriorates. Guaranteed renewable policies also have fixed premiums.

•**Total disability and partial disability coverage.** Some individual policies provide for both total and partial disability benefits.

Example: A woman has a heart attack but still can work 20 hours a week. If her policy covers only total disability, her insurer won't owe her a dime. With total and partial coverage, she will be compensated based on the percentage of her income that she has lost.

RECOMMENDED FEATURES

•**Cost-of-living adjustment.** This feature increases your monthly benefits after disability strikes to keep pace with inflation. It's highly recommended for those younger than 40 but not vital for those over 50—inflation won't have as much time to deplete the value of their benefits. Expect a policy that provides an annual 3% to 6% increase in benefits to cost 8% to 12% more than one that does not provide such an increase.

•**Future increase option.** It makes sense to add more disability coverage over the course of your career to keep pace with your rising wages. A future increase option gives you the right to buy more coverage at the initial contract rate, even if your health declines. This provision typically isn't available past age 50.

WHAT TO AVOID

•**"Except fraud" provision.** If an "except fraud" clause is written into your contract, your insurance company can attempt to take away your policy at any time by claiming that you materially misstated your medical, financial or occupational status when you applied for coverage. Insurance companies sometimes use this clause to deny benefits to honest policyholders when they find the slightest hint of an error on the application.

Better: Ask for a "two-year contestability policy" instead. After your contract has been in force for two years, the insurance company cannot contest any statements in your application.

BUYING DISABILITY COVERAGE

Ask trusted financial professionals or friends to recommend disability insurance agents…or call the top insurers to find agents in your area. Make sure an agent is licensed by your state.

There are four major individual disability insurance companies in the US…

•**Guardian** (866-425-4542, *www.guardian life.com*).

•**Mass Mutual** (800-272-2216, *www.mass mutual.com*).

•**Northwestern Mutual** (414-271-1444, *www. nmfn.com*).

•**UNUM** (877-322-7222, *www.unum.com*).

Helpful: If the agent you speak with can't get you a quote from each of these insurers, call other agents until you can compare quotes from all four companies. There's nothing wrong with checking the rates offered by smaller insurers as well, but the best deals usually come from the big four.

Protect Your Legal Rights If You Become Ill

Barbara Ullman Schwerin, Esq., adjunct professor of law at Loyola Law School, deputy director of community programs at the Disability Rights Legal Center and the founding director of the Cancer Legal Resource Center (CLRC), all in Los Angeles. The CLRC, *www.disabilityrights legalcenter.org*, a joint program of Loyola Law School and the Disability Rights Legal Center, provides information about relevant laws and resources.

If you or someone you love is diagnosed with a serious ailment, such as cancer, heart failure or some other chronic or life-threatening disease, it's easy to become so consumed with the reality of the medical condition that you overlook important legal issues that may arise.

Most people know the importance of a will or trust, which provides for someone's estate after death, and an "advance directive" that appoints a person to make medical decisions on a patient's behalf in case the patient becomes unable to do so.

However, there are other important legal concerns for ill people—and often they are shrouded in myths that create unnecessary worry and confusion. *The most common legal myths facing patients—and the facts you need to know…*

Myth: You will lose your health insurance if you change employers while you have a serious illness.

Fact: The federal Health Insurance Portability and Accountability Act (HIPAA) allows you to move from one health plan to another without being excluded due to a preexisting medical condition, such as cancer, heart disease, etc.

Medicare, which covers Americans age 65 and older (as well as people of any age who meet Social Security disability requirements), cannot be revoked because of a serious illness. People have the option of enrolling in traditional Medicare or a Medicare Advantage plan, which is basically a medical HMO.

The same applies to people who are covered by Medicaid, the federal-state program for low-income Americans. For more information, contact the Centers for Medicare and Medicaid Services, 800-633-4227, *www.cms.gov*.

Another little-known fact: Some employers will request that a representative from your health insurance provider come to your workplace to explain coverage. This usually happens if an employer offers more than one health insurance plan—or as a part of the open enrollment period when employees can change from one plan to another. In other cases, your company's human resources department may provide guidance.

Myth: If you are unable to work because of a serious illness, you will lose your job.

Fact: The Americans with Disabilities Act (ADA) is a federal law that applies to employers with 15 or more employees. A person is protected by ADA if he/she has a physical or mental impairment that substantially limits a major life function. To qualify, a person must be able to perform the essential functions of the job—with reasonable accommodation, if necessary (which must be provided by the employer as long as it does not create undue hardship for the employer).

Examples: Extended periods of leave time, job restructuring and part-time work schedules.

Important: It is your choice whether to disclose your medical condition to your employer. If you do not require some type of accommodation, you are not obligated to disclose your illness. Some employees are concerned that if they tell their employers they have cancer, they will be treated differently and will face discrimination. However, you cannot claim discrimination if your employer was never told about your medical condition.

Another little-known fact: The Family and Medical Leave Act is a federal law that allows an employee to take up to 12 weeks of unpaid medical leave during any 12-month period without losing his job or health insurance coverage. It applies to employers with 50 or more employees, and the employee must have worked at the company for at least one year (and at least 1,250 hours in that year).

This type of leave can be tailored to the needs of your treatment.

Example: You can take all 12 weeks at once...or mornings off for radiation...or Fridays off for chemo. This leave can be used for an employee's own serious illness or that of a parent, child or spouse.

When on leave, people are usually looking for ways to cover their monthly expenses. Some states have a state disability insurance program that provides a portion of one's salary, usually for a maximum of one year.

Another option is payments under short- or long-term disability insurance. Not every employer offers this type of insurance.

Suggestion: If your employer does not offer disability insurance, you may want to purchase it privately.

Caution: Once you are diagnosed, it may be difficult to purchase private disability insurance. Contact an insurance agent who can explore options that might be available.

Myth: If you don't have health insurance when you're diagnosed with a serious illness, no insurer will cover you.

Fact: Many states have a high-risk pool that covers people who can't qualify for individual insurance and don't have access to group insurance, Medicare or Medicaid. These offerings vary from state to state, and premiums may be high. Also, depending on the state where you live, there may be other options available.

Another little-known fact: Some states have additional protections. The Breast and Cervical Cancer Treatment Program, administered by the states, pays for the treatment of uninsured women with breast or cervical cancer if they meet certain requirements. Some states may have coverage for men with prostate cancer.

The specific details of coverage vary from state to state. Check with the Department of Insurance in your state about all of the above.

Myth: If you lose income because of a serious illness, you won't be able to pay your bills.

Fact: The short-term disability insurance offered by some states can help. Social Security benefits may be available if you can demonstrate that you are disabled by a physical or mental impairment that is expected to last 12 months or longer.

Social Security Disability Insurance is based on a person's work history. Supplemental Security Income is based on a person's assets and resources. For more information, contact the Social Security Administration, 800-772-1213, *www.socialsecurity.gov.*

Important: There is a six-month waiting period before you are eligible to receive Social Security benefits. Apply for benefits as soon as it is determined that you are going to be disabled for at least 12 months.

Another little-known fact: Many people know that it's often possible to save on health insurance by electing coverage under a spouse's health insurance plan. However, many people don't know that HIPAA protection also applies to this situation, so a preexisting medical condition cannot legally preclude you from starting coverage under your spouse's employer-provided plan.

Also, some people may be eligible for lower utility and telephone bills, because their income has decreased.

Affordable Treatments Bring Better Vision For Patients

Donald Schwartz, MD, associate clinical professor of ophthalmology, University of California, Irvine, and the University of Southern California's Doheny Eye Institute, Los Angeles.

James Salz, MD, clinical professor of ophthalmology, University of Southern California, attending ophthalmic surgeon at Cedars-Sinai Medical Center, Los Angeles.

National Eye Institute.

Prevent Blindness America.

D ue to changes to Medicare guidelines, more folks than ever can take advantage of the latest technologies to sharpen their eyesight, ophthalmologists say.

More than 20 million Americans are afflicted with cataracts, a clouding of the lens that diminishes vision, and the elderly are particularly vulnerable.

"The new rules allow patients to make a decision whether they want to pay for these advances," says Dr. Donald Schwartz, associate clinical professor of ophthalmology at the University of California, Irvine, and the University of Southern California's Doheny Eye Institute.

AN EYE ON ADVANCES

Two new types of synthetic replacement lenses are available that can restore a cataract patient's vision better than ever. These "multifocal" lenses allow people to focus both far and near; older replacement lenses provided clear vision only at one specific distance.

One type of lens, called an accommodating lens (brand name Crystalens), acts much like a normal human lens when focusing, said Dr. James Salz, attending ophthalmic surgeon at Cedars-Sinai Medical Center in Los Angeles, and spokesman for the American Academy of Ophthalmologists.

"It replicates what the eye does when you go from far to near," Salz says. "The lens changes its shape, actually becoming thicker in your eye and focusing."

The other type of lens, marketed under the brand names ReZoom and ReSTOR, replicate normal vision through a "bull's-eye" design. Formed with concentric circles resembling a practice target, the lens allows a patient to shift his or her focus through slight eye movements.

NEW RULES, NEW OPTIONS

Until recently, these new lenses were financially out of reach for many senior citizens—who are most likely to develop cataracts—because Medicare would only pay for the old-style basic lens replacement.

But recent changes allow applying up to $2,000 toward the more expensive lenses that provide close-to-normal sight. That's the amount long allocated for a basic lens replacement.

"When patients get these new lenses, over 90% say they never wear glasses again," Salz says. "But they have to pay for it, up to a couple thousands of dollars per eye."

On the downside, the multifocal lenses can cause some problems with night vision, with patients suffering from halo effects and glare. "If I have somebody that does a lot of night driving, I don't think it's necessarily a good idea to

305

put one of these lenses in because it will bug them," he adds.

FOCUS ON THE FUTURE

The number of Americans with cataracts is expected to balloon to 30.1 million by 2020, according to Prevent Blindness America, an eye health and safety advocacy group.

By age 80, more than half of all Americans either have a cataract or have had cataract surgery, according to the National Eye Institute, part of the National Institutes of Health.

Cataracts form in one of two ways: Clumps of protein can adhere to the lens, reducing the sharpness of the image reaching the retina. Or the clear lens can slowly change to a yellowish/brownish color, adding a brownish tint to vision. Cataracts are usually painless.

See your eye doctor if you experience any of following...

• **Blurred vision,** double vision, ghost images, or the sense of a "film" over the eyes.

• **Lights that used to be sufficient that now seem either too dim for reading or close-up work,** or are now too strong and "dazzle" eyes.

• **Needing to change eyeglass prescriptions often,** without experiencing improvement.

• **Finding that a milky or yellowish spot has appeared in the pupil,** which is normally black.

Surprising! Antibiotics Useless for Most Cases of Bronchitis

Richard P. Wenzel, MD, chairman of internal medicine, Virginia Commonwealth University School of Medicine, Richmond.

Jeffrey Chapman, MD, director of interstitial lung disease, Cleveland Clinic.

New England Journal of Medicine.

M ost people who go to a doctor with bronchitis get an antibiotic. Most of them shouldn't, according to a new report reviewing most previous medical studies, clinical trials and other research related to bronchitis treatment.

"Physicians should be encouraged to avoid antibiotics in most cases," says Dr. Richard P. Wenzel, chairman of the department of internal medicine at Virginia Commonwealth and author of the new report.

Reason: Only a small percentage of bronchitis cases are caused by bacteria that doctors can treat with antibiotics, such as whooping cough. Most are caused by other agents, such as viruses, that do not respond to prescription medications, says Wenzel.

Yet about 70% to 80% of patients with bronchitis—an inflammation of the tiny airways of the lungs—are prescribed a course of antibiotics lasting five to 10 days.

SAVE MONEY, PREVENT PROBLEMS

Besides saving money, foregoing antibiotics for most cases of bronchitis makes good health sense. "All antibiotics have side effects, such as rash, diarrhea and abdominal pain," Wenzel says. Such side effects are acceptable only when a medication helps.

Another reason: Unnecessary use of antibiotics may make organisms more resistant to the drugs when you need them.

WHO'S TO BLAME?

So why are antibiotics routinely prescribed for the one in 20 Americans who develop bronchitis each year?

One reason is convenience, Wenzel says. "Think of all the patients we have to move through the office," he says. "I could take 15 minutes to explain why an antibiotic is not needed or write a prescription in 30 seconds."

Patient demand is another reason, notes Dr. Jeffrey Chapman, director of interstitial lung disease at the Cleveland Clinic. Many have long believed they need an antibiotic to feel better.

"But patients are getting more savvy," he says. "They understand that a lot of infections are viral and that giving them an antibiotic places them at risk."

To treat bronchitis, the American Academy of Family Physicians recommends getting lots of rest, drinking lots of noncaffeinated fluids, keeping the indoor humidity high and waiting for the condition to go away "after a few days or a week." If coughing and other symptoms persist, see your doctor; it could be a more serious condition, such as asthma or pneumonia.

Some Dialysis Centers Overmedicating Patients

Mae Thamer, PhD, senior associate, Medical Technology and Practice Patterns Institute, Bethesda, MD.

Daniel Coyne, MD, professor of medicine, Washington University School of Medicine, St. Louis.

Journal of the American Medical Association.

Large for-profit dialysis centers may be overtreating patients for anemia (a shortage of red blood cells), a common complication in people with kidney disease—and possibly putting their health at risk, finds new research.

Researchers say that the typical hospital-based dialysis center administers an average dose of 16,188 units per week of *epoetin*, a drug that helps correct anemia. But at for-profit chain facilities, an average of 20,838 units a week is given —an increase of some 3,300 units per week.

The problem: There's an increased risk of death from getting too much epoetin, says researcher Mae Thamer of the Medical Technology and Practice Patterns Institute in Bethesda, Maryland.

LIKELY EXPLANATION

Why would for-profit centers overuse the medication? Possibly because it's more profitable.

Epoetin is one of the few treatments for end-stage kidney disease that's readily reimbursed by Medicare, says Thamer. In fact, epoetin comprise 11% of all Medicare costs for end-stage kidney disease, with almost $2 billion in payouts for the drug each year.

And some experts say up to 25% of a dialysis center's profits may come from epoetin, a synthetic version of a hormone normally produced by the kidneys called erythropoietin.

This hormone stimulates the bone marrow to produce red blood cells, which carry oxygen to all of the other cells in the body. People with kidney disease don't always produce enough erythropoietin, and the result can be anemia.

There's still some debate about what the optimal levels of treatment should be.

THE STUDY

In her study, Thamer and her colleagues compared the treatment received at nonprofit and for-profit dialysis centers for nearly 160,000 dialysis patients over a two-month period.

They found vast differences in the way anemia was treated, depending on the type of center where someone received dialysis. But overall, for-profit facilities administered roughly one-third more units of epoetin per week.

Although each individual patient needs a varying dose of epoetin to combat anemia, reimbursement for (each patient) "would be based from a population standpoint," which averages the reimbursement to account for individual variations.

"Reimbursement needs to be tied to providing dialysis," notes Daniel Coyne, MD, of Washington University School of Medicine, who was not involved in the study. "Right now, we offer perverse incentives where wasting epoetin is beneficial even at the risk to the patient's health."

info Get more information on how anemia develops in people on dialysis from the National Institute of Diabetes and Digestive and Kidney Diseases at *http://kidney.niddk. nih.gov/kudiseases/pubs/anemia/.*

New Kind of Doctors Bring Better Hospital Care

Navneet Kathuria, MD, senior faculty, medicine/general medicine, and Brian A. Markoff, MD, assistant professor, medicine, both at Mount Sinai Medical Center in New York City.

Inpatient physicians, one of the fastest growing medical specialties, can now be found in American hospitals. These doctors only provide in-hospital care and are known as "hospitalists."

Upon admittance to a hospital, a patient is introduced to a hospitalist who will supervise his or her care for the duration of the hospital stay. (Attending physicians are often, but not always, hospitalists.) Not only does this physician treat the condition that caused the patient to be hospitalized, but he or she will also supervise care of any other medical conditions.

Two leaders in the field, Navneet Kathuria, MD, and Brian A. Markoff, MD, oversee the adult inpatient care at the Mount Sinai Medical Center in New York City. They described some of the benefits of this specialty.

Primary-care doctors spend many hours seeing patients in their offices and have a limited amount of time to make hospital rounds. Knowing that there is a doctor on site supervising care, reviewing all tests and evaluating the patient's progress throughout the day reduces the burden on the primary-care physician and reassures the doctor and the patient. In the past, the doctors were also supervising from their offices via telephone calls with the nurses and residents. Now, there is often 24-hour-a-day coverage with hospitalists.

WHO THE HOSPITALISTS ARE

The majority of hospitalists specialize in general internal medicine, although some are specialists in pulmonary and critical care medicine, cardiology or other subspecialties. A number of nurse practitioners and physician assistants also specialize in providing inpatient care. Additionally, there are pediatricians who work with hospitalized children.

At Dr. Kathuria's hospital, a hospitalist will supervise approximately 15 patients at a time who are almost always medical—not surgical—patients. However, in some hospitals, this too has begun to evolve—particularly in orthopedic surgery patients. With joint replacement on the rise for older people, more patients with other conditions that require monitoring are admitted. With a team approach, the orthopedist performs the surgery and the hospitalist monitors the medical aspects of the patient's needs in order to prevent complications—including chronic conditions, such as diabetes. With diabetes, for example, it is critical to keep blood sugar levels under control for the patient's health, and it's also very important for proper healing after surgery.

Effective communication is the cornerstone of hospitalists' work, whether with the patient, the primary-care physician or the other doctors involved in the patient's care. The hospitalists who are assigned patients at the time of admission gather background information from the primary-care doctor upon admittance to the hospital and keep the primary-care physician apprised of the patient's condition on a regular basis. While care may vary from hospital to hospital, you can expect your hospitalist to see you every day, and sometimes twice a day—often with an in-depth visit every morning and another visit late in the day.

The hospitalist also stops by any time there are tests to review or complications to deal with. (Generally, primary-care doctors can see the patient who has been hospitalized as well, but this can't replace the on-site, moment-to-moment care that hospitalists are able to provide.) The hospitalist also works closely with the patient at discharge.

The hospitalist gives the primary-care physician a written or verbal summary covering not only what happened during the hospitalization but also what the patient needs to do to continue care at home, including prescriptions and medical follow-up. The patients often get a copy of this discharge summary.

WHAT PATIENTS SHOULD DO

Dr. Kathuria and Dr. Markoff believe that there are several ways in which patients can maximize their experience with a hospitalist, stressing the vital importance of communication. They suggest having a general conversation with your primary-care doctor to learn who would be involved in your care if hospitalized. Will it be just your own doctor or will a hospitalist be assigned to you? While it's always good to be under your own doctor's care, the hospitalist is far more available to you while in the hospital. Depending on your potential needs, you may want to select a hospital specifically because it has hospitalists on staff and then work with your doctor to learn who would be assigned to your case.

Find out from your own doctor how you can best stay in touch with him/her during this time and how your doctor will be communicating with the hospitalist to ensure the hospitalist has all your pertinent background information... and that your primary-care physician will have all information once you are released. When in the hospital, it is absolutely key to get the name of the hospitalist(s) who supervised your care and all contact information for reaching this person later if necessary.

Having a designated hospitalist work on your case in the hospital is one way to potentially reduce the risks and help improve quality and continuity of care. And, in general, hospitalists reduce costs by providing efficient care and reducing the length of stay in the hospital.

 For more information, go to *www.hospital medicine.org.*

Choose the Right Mental Health Professional

Charles B. Inlander is a consumer advocate and health-care consultant based in Fogelsville, PA. He was the founding president of the nonprofit People's Medical Society, a consumer advocacy organization credited with key improvements in the quality of US health care in the 1980s and 1990s, and is the author of 20 books, including *Take This Book to the Hospital with You: A Consumer Guide to Surviving Your Hospital Stay.* St. Martin's.

Choosing the right counselor, psychiatrist or other mental health professional can be confusing. But when you face a mental health issue, it is important to get appropriate care, because primary-care doctors are not trained in diagnosing and treating these problems.

•**Psychiatrist.** A psychiatrist is a medical doctor (MD) or doctor of osteopathy (DO)—two degrees with virtually the same training (four years of medical school, followed by four additional years of training in psychiatry)—who specializes in the prevention, diagnosis and treatment of mental and emotional disorders. Psychiatrists use both medication and counseling. Because of their medical training, they are the only mental health professionals allowed to write drug prescriptions. Before choosing a psychiatrist, check to see if he/she is board-certified by the American Board of Psychiatry and Neurology. Go to the American Board of Medical Specialties Web site at *www.abms.org* and enter the practitioner's name, or call 866-275-2267.

Strengths: Good medical and psychological diagnosticians who can discover or rule out medical conditions that could be affecting your mental health.

•**Psychologist.** These professionals perform psychological testing and practice psychotherapy. Most psychologists hold an advanced degree, such as a doctor of philosophy (PhD) in psychology, a doctor of psychology (PsyD) or doctor of education (EdD) in psychology, all of which require the same minimum amount of schooling. Psychologists are licensed in the state where they practice. Some states also license psychologists holding master's degrees, but a certain level of work experience is required before a license can be granted. To determine if a psychologist is licensed, contact your state's health department.

Strengths: Best trained in a wide range of diagnosed mental health problems that require counseling.

•**Mental health social worker.** Social service agencies, hospitals and crisis centers employ mental health social workers, who usually hold a master's degree in social work with an emphasis in psychology. Licensing requirements for social workers vary widely from state to state. Contact your state's health department to find out if a specific practitioner is licensed.

Strengths: Skilled at helping people adjust to a new problem, such as a cancer diagnosis, and find resources and services.

•**Family, marriage or pastoral counselor.** These are general terms that are used by psychologists, social workers or even members of the clergy who specialize in particular areas of counseling. Some states require licensing for anyone calling himself/herself a "counselor," although no states require clergy to be licensed in order to offer counseling.

Strengths: Good general counselors for less serious mental health problems.

•**Psychiatric nurse.** Registered nurses with advanced training in psychiatry are called psychiatric nurses. They are found in general hospitals, psychiatric facilities and some nursing homes. They often administer and monitor medications and facilitate patient therapy sessions.

14

Stroke Prevention

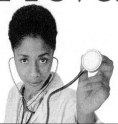

Are You Headed For a Stroke?

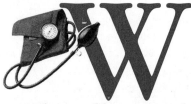

What would you do if you knew in advance that you were at risk for a stroke? You might assume that an alert would cause people to seek medical attention, so that you/your doctor could take measures to prevent a stroke. Usually, that's not the case with many people.

Each year, an estimated quarter-million Americans receive a warning in the form of a transient ischemic attack (TIA), commonly known as a "ministroke." Unfortunately, the majority of patients who experience a TIA don't recognize its importance—and fail to get prompt medical care that likely could prevent a full-blown stroke. About 11% to 20% of patients who experience a TIA go on to suffer a stroke within three months.

Good news: Patients who experience a TIA and then take preventive steps can greatly reduce their risk for further problems.

Important: A TIA is an emergency, and everyone should know the symptoms. If you experience one of the symptoms described below for at least five minutes, see a doctor the same day —go to the emergency room, if necessary.

BE ON THE ALERT FOR THESE SYMPTOMS

Like the majority of strokes, a TIA is usually caused by a blood clot and/or material that breaks free from artery walls and temporarily blocks blood flow to parts of the brain. The blockage of the artery lasts long enough to stop blood flow and cause stroke-like symptoms, but not long enough to kill brain cells.

What to watch for...

James F. Toole, MD, Walter C. Teagle Professor of Neurology and director of the Stroke Research Center at Wake Forest University Baptist Medical Center in Winston-Salem, NC. He is immediate past president of the International Stroke Society, *www.internationalstroke.org*.

•**A dizzy spell that occurs for no obvious reason,** such as standing too quickly...or dizziness from a middle-ear disease.

•**Weakness and/or numbness on one side of the body**—usually in the face or an arm or leg.

•**The sensation that there's something in the eye,** causing blurriness, double vision or even temporary blindness.

•**Difficulty speaking or difficulty understanding what others are saying.**

People should not panic if they experience one or more of these symptoms—they aren't always caused by a TIA. Dizzy spells can be caused by something as simple as a plug of earwax. The only way to know for sure whether you've suffered a TIA is to see a doctor.

DIAGNOSING TIAS

Researchers are in the process of identifying brain enzymes that are released during a TIA. Blood tests that diagnose TIAs based on the presence of these enzymes are being developed.

In the meantime, doctors diagnose most TIAs by taking a medical history of the event—what the patient felt, how long the symptoms lasted and whether the person has stroke risk factors, such as high blood pressure, family history, diabetes or smoking.

Physical findings: Atherosclerosis (hardening of the arteries) is the underlying cause of most TIAs (and the majority of strokes). Patients who have atherosclerosis elsewhere in the body, such as in the arteries leading to the legs, kidneys, heart, etc., are very likely to also have damaged carotid arteries—blood vessels in the neck that carry blood to the brain.

In some cases, a doctor can detect problems in the carotid artery by listening carefully with a stethoscope. There are characteristic sounds (bruits) that indicate atherosclerosis.

In other cases, additional tests are required...

•**Carotid ultrasonography** uses sound waves to detect blood-vessel narrowing and/or clots in the carotid arteries. This is a good screening test for people with stroke risk factors or a family history of strokes or TIAs.

•**Magnetic resonance imaging (MRI)** also measures blockages in the carotid arteries.

If atherosclerotic blockages of 50% to 70% are found from either test, further evaluation and treatment is necessary.

TREATMENT APPROACHES

Patients with carotid artery blockages of 50% or more are usually advised to take strict steps, including the use of medication, to reduce risk. *If their disease progresses to 70% blockage, surgery is typically recommended...*

•**Carotid endarterectomy** is an inpatient procedure in which an incision is made to expose the carotid artery, and plaques are removed from the artery. When performed by a skilled surgeon, the risk for stroke or death is less than 1%, and the patient recovers within a week.

•**Stenting** is an inpatient procedure in which an expandable metal net is threaded into the carotid artery. The net presses against the artery walls...dilates the opening for better circulation...and helps prevent the artery from "shedding" more clots.

Stenting, however, has not been performed long enough for its long-term effectiveness and durability to be known. One possible risk is that a dislodged blood clot could get carried in the bloodstream to the brain.

TIA patients who don't require surgery are almost always treated with drugs to prevent blood from clotting. *Main drug therapies...*

•**Aspirin is most often used.** Taking a regular aspirin (three times weekly) or baby aspirin (daily), depending on the patient, can reduce stroke risk by up to 20%.

•**Aspirin plus an anticlotting drug.** Adding other active ingredients to aspirin can reduce stroke risk by an additional 3% to 5%.

Example: Aspirin plus *dipyridamole* (Aggrenox).

•**Aspirin alternatives,** such as *clopidogrel* (Plavix) and *ticlopidine* (Ticlid), can prevent excessively sticky platelets from clumping together and forming clots. These drugs are a good choice for patients who are allergic to aspirin or who have an ulcer or acid reflux disease, which can be aggravated by aspirin.

■ **More from Dr. Toole...**

How to Prevent a Stroke

Most stroke risk factors can be reduced with lifestyle modifications. *Most important...*

- •**Not smoking.**
- •**Limiting dietary fat.**
- •**Eating fruits and vegetables.**
- •**Exercising regularly.**

Patients who maintain healthy blood pressure readings (less than 120/80) and total cholesterol levels (less than 200)...avoid (or reverse) obesity...and control underlying diseases, such as diabetes, are far less likely to develop hardening of the arteries, thereby reducing their risk for TIAs and stroke.

Stroke Incidence Is Declining

Philip A. Wolf, professor of neurology, Boston University School of Medicine.

Virginia Howard, MSPH, assistant professor of epidemiology, University of Alabama, Birmingham.

Journal of the American Medical Association.

The incidence of stroke has dropped over the last 50 years and yet stroke still remains a major problem for older Americans.

An estimated 700,000 Americans suffer a new or recurring stroke every year. Nearly 157,000 people die each year from stroke, making it the No. 3 cause of death after heart disease and cancer.

THE STUDY

The following findings, from the Framingham Heart Study, are based on an unusual, half-century follow-up of more than 9,000 residents of this Massachusetts town who were first recruited in 1948. Since then, the risk of stroke by age 90 has decreased from 19.5% to 14.5% in men 65 and older, and from 18% to 16.1% for women.

Still, one in every six men and one in every five women who remain in the study will suffer a stroke in their lifetime, said Dr. Philip A. Wolf, professor of neurology at Boston University, and a member of the research team. "The risk exists because everyone in Framingham is living longer," he said.

FINDINGS

The study shows that there clearly has been a good deal of progress in fighting the risk factors for stroke, such as high blood pressure, smoking, obesity and diabetes.

The study offers a snapshot in time on how we are doing concerning stroke. "The information from Framingham gives us that opportunity because of its very detailed surveillance. It gives us a handle on what's happening," Wolf said.

The research also helps fill in a blank in statistics about stroke, said Virginia Howard, assistant professor of epidemiology at the University of Alabama, Birmingham, and chairwoman of the American Stroke Association's stroke statistics committee.

"It is very exciting because a lot of what we know about stroke at this point is based on studies of risk factors," she said. "There are not a lot of studies about incidence."

Howard did see one limitation of the study—the fact that the participants are predominately of European origin, educated and middle class. Other studies have shown an increased risk of stroke in minority groups such as blacks.

"But the message is, 'yes,' we are making good progress in the education and treatment of risk factors, but there is still a way to go," she said. "We have to continue our education effort and also continue to support studies like this one that give us evidence on the success of that effort."

However, the study also contained some troubling news. The severity of strokes that do occur has not lessened, and the 30-day mortality rate has decreased significantly only for men, "perhaps due to an older age at onset of stroke and more severe strokes in women," the report said.

These sobering trends emphasize that while improved control of risk factors has lowered incidence of stroke, there is a need for greater prevention efforts.

info To learn more about the risk factors for stroke and what can be done about them, visit the American Stroke Association, *www. americanstrokeassociation.org.*

New Drug Could Help Fight Bleeding Strokes

Dr. Joseph Broderick, chairman of the guideline writing committee and professor and chairman in the neurology department at the University of Cincinnati.

American Heart Association.

The first proven treatments for often fatal intracerebral hemorrhage (bleeding strokes) are on the horizon, including a new drug called *recombinant activated factor VII* (rFVIIa) that slows bleeding and limits brain damage, according to updated guidelines from the American Heart Association (AHA). The new drug is approved in the US to treat hemophilia patients.

NEW GUIDELINES

The new AHA guidelines suggest that using the drug on intracerebral hemorrhage (ICH) patients within four hours of ICH onset may limit the amount of bleeding, reduce the risk of death, and improve survivors' functional outcome at 90 days.

ICH occurs when an artery in the brain bursts and floods the surrounding tissue with blood. Of the more than 60,000 people who have an ICH each year in the US, 35% to 52% die within a month and only 20% are expected to be functionally independent six months after the ICH.

The best way to prevent ICH is to avoid high blood pressure.

"We don't recommend routine surgical treatment of ICH, but people who have larger blood clots close to the surface of the brain may be an exception," said Dr. Joseph Broderick, chairman of the guideline writing committee and professor and chairman in the neurology department at the University of Cincinnati.

The guidelines do recommend surgery for patients with a larger ICH in the cerebellum that presses on the brain stem.

Broderick and colleagues also made recommendations about the use of medical imaging technology to diagnose ICH.

Newer Form of Heparin Lowers Risk of Clots Up to 43%

David G. Sherman, MD, professor, medicine and neurology, University of Texas Health Science Center at San Antonio.

Richard M. Weinberg, MD, chief quality officer, Stamford Health System, Stamford, CT.

The Lancet.

A newly engineered form of the blood-thinning drug *heparin* has proven more effective at preventing life-threatening clots in people who suffer strokes than the older version of the drug.

NEW FINDING

The incidence of clots in the lungs and legs of stroke patients who got the engineered form, *enoxaparin,* was 43% lower than in those who received ordinary heparin.

The finding is potentially applicable to more than 700,000 people who suffer strokes in the US each year, said lead researcher Dr. David G. Sherman, a professor of medicine and neurology at the University of Texas Health Science Center in San Antonio. These patients are at high risk of clotting because of their forced inactivity. In fact, the 1,762 stroke patients in the study received anticoagulant treatment only if they were unable to walk.

THE STUDY

Half of the patients were given an injection of enoxaparin, while the other half received heparin. They were then studied for the presence of blood clots in the legs and lungs.

The study included only patients who suffered ischemic stroke, the most common kind. In this type of attack a blood clot blocks a brain artery. However, Sherman said there are indications that the results also apply to people who have hemorrhagic strokes, in which a blood vessel bursts.

IMPLICATIONS

Cost remains a potential issue, however, because enoxaparin is much more expensive than ordinary heparin. Sherman's group is working on an analysis determining the economic impact of a shift to using enoxaparin on the total cost of treating stroke.

One prior study has indicated that introducing the drug might actually lead to cost reductions, said Dr. Richard M. Weinberg, chief quality officer of the Stamford Health System in Connecticut. His team tracked costs across 33 hospitals.

"There are several possible explanations for the lower overall cost," Weinberg said. "Most patients getting Lovenox *(enoxaparin)* can be managed without the frequent tests needed for heparin. In addition to reduced laboratory testing, a reduction in the length of stay and less time spent in the ICU [intensive care unit] are possible explanations."

"This is the first big trial in which the two treatments have gone head to head," said Sherman. "Enoxaparin pretty convincingly appears to work better."

info To learn more about stroke treatment, visit *www.medicinenet.com/stroke/article. htm.*

Lowering Cholesterol Reduces Risk For Stroke

Eric E. Smith, MD, assistant neurologist, Massachusetts General Hospital Stroke Service, Boston.
American Academy of Neurology.

Many American stroke patients have cholesterol levels higher than the national guidelines. A number of these patients may not have had a stroke if their cholesterol had been properly managed by following the guidelines.

THE STUDY

Researchers found that 27% of 1,040 people hospitalized for stroke or transient ischemic attack (TIA, a short-term reduction in blood flow to the brain resulting in temporary symptoms like numbness, weakness and inability to talk) had cholesterol levels higher than the national guidelines.

"If this high cholesterol had been recognized and the guidelines followed, then 93% of these people would have been treated with cholesterol-lowering drugs," said Dr. Eric E. Smith, of the Massachusetts General Hospital Stroke Service in Boston.

"Studies have shown that these drugs reduce the risk of stroke, so it's probable that, if the guidelines had been followed, at least some of these strokes and TIAs would have never happened," Smith said.

The study also found that 30% of the stroke/TIA patients previously diagnosed with high cholesterol, and 19% of those taking cholesterol-lowering drugs, did not have ideal cholesterol levels, which are based on a person's risk of stroke or heart disease.

RECOMMENDATIONS

"Unfortunately, we found that the people who were at the greatest risk for a stroke or heart attack were also the least likely to be at the guideline-recommended cholesterol levels," Smith said.

He said the study findings suggest that all people hospitalized with stroke or TIA should have their cholesterol levels checked, and those with high levels should be treated to lower their cholesterol.

info The US National Institute of Neurological Disorders and Stroke has more information about stroke prevention, *www.ninds.nih.gov.*

A Quick Test That May Help Predict Major Stroke Risk

S. Claiborne Johnston, MD, associate professor, neurology, University of California, San Francisco.
Brett L. Cucchiara, MD, assistant professor, neurology, University of Pennsylvania, Pittsburgh.
The Lancet.

Neurologists say they've developed a quick test to assess the risk if someone who suffers a transient ischemic attack (TIA) or "ministroke," will have a major stroke in the following 48 hours.

"It's important to assess the immediate danger, because half of those strokes will occur within the first two days after a TIA," said lead author Dr. S. Claiborne Johnston, associate professor of neurology at the University of California, San Francisco. About 240,000 TIAs are diagnosed in the US each year, and up to 20% of them are followed by a major stroke.

THE NEW TEST

The test combines elements of two earlier predictive assessments. Those tests were designed to determine the risk of a stroke within seven and 90 days, respectively.

The new test can be administered in a few minutes. It measures blood pressure, speech impairment, weakness on one side of the body, diabetes and age.

Using the tests on a large number of people who had TIAs showed that 21% were at high risk, meaning they had a 1-in-12 chance of having a stroke in the following 48 hours. Another 45% were classified as being at moderate risk, with a 1-in-25 chance of a stroke.

"This is the first large-scale study to validate these scores," Johnston said. "We are at a new level where we feel confident that the scores are useful in clinical practice in the Western world."

ACTION PLANS

The test can help determine which patients should be hospitalized and which can safely be sent home. "We are hoping that neurologists, emergency physicians and primary-care doctors will hear about this score and start using it widely," Johnston said. "Currently, it doesn't seem that physicians are making decisions based on risk. They are hospitalizing people whether they are at high risk or not."

Dr. Brett L. Cucchiara, assistant professor of neurology at the University of Pennsylvania, said he currently hospitalizes every patient who suffers a TIA. The reason, he said, is the real doubt about the value of all risk-assessment tests.

Cucchiara's view of the new report is that it is "very interesting and suggests that this strategy may be useful. But we really need to see these kinds of findings replicated by an independent group before they are ready for prime time."

Rural Patients Benefit from 'On-Call' Stroke Therapy

American Academy of Neurology.

Stroke patients in rural hospitals can receive safe, effective treatment with a clot-busting drug when an expert from a larger hospital guides the therapy over the telephone.

"Expert guidance of this treatment over the telephone appears to be safe, practical and effective," according to study author Dr. Anand Vaishnav, of the University of Kentucky Medical Center in Lexington.

THE STUDY

The study included 121 ischemic stroke patients treated with the clot-busting drug *tissue plasminogen activator* (tPA) at a rural community hospital. Treatment was guided via phone by a stroke neurologist from a larger center.

To be effective, tPA must be given within three hours of a stroke. On average, the patients in this study started receiving tPA therapy within 132 minutes of stroke onset.

"This is less time than the average 144 minutes it took from stroke onset to tPA treatment in the National Institute of Neurological Disorders and Stroke (NINDS) tPA study, which was a large national study in 1995. We also had lower rates of bleeding in the brain and death than the original NINDS study," Vaishnav said.

BACKGROUND STUDY

In the original NINDS study, 6.4% of patients had symptomatic bleeding in the brain, compared with 2.5% of the rural patients in this study. The patient death rate in the NINDS study was 17%, compared with 7.5% in this new study.

 The American Academy of Neurology has more about tPA at *www.aan.com*.

Beauty Shops Spread the Word on Strokes

American Stroke Association.

Beauty shops may be an ideal place to educate minority women about the key warning signs of a stroke, according to a new study.

THE STUDY

Researchers gave lessons on stroke prevention and warning signs to beauticians in African-American–run beauty shops in Cincinnati and Atlanta. The beauticians then discussed stroke-related issues with their clients, who also received a packet that included heart-healthy cookbooks, wallet cards listing stroke warning signs and other stroke-related materials.

The beauty shop clients were also given stroke knowledge surveys at the start of the study and again five weeks and five months later. Nearly 400 women completed the baseline survey, and 318 women completed the five-month survey.

FINDINGS

At the start of the study, 40.7% of the women surveyed knew three stroke-warning signs, compared with 50.6% after five months. The study also found an 8% increase (to a total of 93%) in the women who knew to call 911 immediately in the event of a stroke, and a 7% increase (to a total of 92%) in the women who recognized stroke when they were given a clinical scenario.

CONCLUSION

Overall, the findings demonstrate that these kinds of community-based programs are an effective method of educating minority groups about stroke risk, said study lead author Dr. Dawn Kleindorfer, a stroke neurologist and associate professor at the University of Cincinnati College of Medicine in Ohio.

"We know that this program works. Two women had a stroke during the study in the beauty salon, and the beauticians called 911 and got them to the hospital within 45 minutes. The beauticians said they would not have known what to do before our project," Kleindorfer said.

Weekends Worst Time For Stroke

Gustavo Saposnik, MD, assistant professor, medicine, University of Toronto, Canada.

Larry B. Goldstein, professor, medicine, Duke University, Durham, NC, and chairman, American Heart Association's Stroke Council.

Stroke.

Canadian researchers report that strokes treated on weekends are 14% more deadly than those treated on weekdays.

"And while the study included only Canadians, the best guess is that the difference in outcome might be even worse in the United States," said lead author Dr. Gustavo Saposnik, assistant professor of medicine at the University of Toronto.

"We don't have information on what's going on in the United States," Saposnik said. "But here, we have universal health insurance with no copayment. With all the different plans in the United States, it might be a little worse."

THE STUDY

Saposnik and his colleagues had information on almost 26,700 people admitted to 606 Canadian hospitals for ischemic stroke. Ischemic strokes occur when a clot blocks a brain artery. More than 80% of strokes are ischemic; the rest are hemorrhagic, occurring when an artery bursts.

About a quarter of those people came to the hospitals on Saturdays or Sundays. After adjusting for age, gender and other complicating factors, the researchers found that people admitted on a weekend had a 14% higher risk of dying within seven days than those who came in on weekdays. They were also less likely to survive and go home.

IMPLICATIONS

This "weekend effect" was greater for people admitted to rural rather than urban hospitals, and if the physician in charge was a general practitioner rather than a specialist.

The reasons for the difference are not clear, Saposnik said. "There may be some differences in resources in different hospitals on weekends. We are doing another study trying to address the underlying mechanism for our findings."

Whatever the reason, the experts' advice to people who suspect someone may be having a stroke remains the same no matter what day of the week it is, no matter what time of day," Saposnik said.

"In a rural or an urban area, they should seek medical attention right away," he said. "Call 911 and get to the nearest emergency room."

RECOMMENDATIONS

Quick action is needed because, in a stroke, "time means brain." Faster treatment means fewer brain cells will die.

This rule was stressed by Dr. Larry B. Goldstein, professor of medicine and director of the stroke center at Duke University, and chairman of the American Heart Association's Stroke Council.

He offered the following suggestion for those who believe a loved one might be experiencing a stroke: "Don't put a person in a car. It could be something other than a stroke. Just call 911, and hopefully the system will make sure that the patient gets to the appropriate facility."

Stroke symptoms include abrupt difficulty in speaking or understanding, weakness or numbness of an arm or leg and unexpected difficulty walking.

Appropriate help should be available "24/7," Goldstein said. There is a national system for accrediting round-the-clock stroke centers, and states including New York, Florida and Massachusetts have their own accrediting mechanisms, he said.

"The difference in weekend admissions found in this study may be real, but the potential benefits of early treatment well outweigh the risk of waiting," Goldstein said.

Stroke Risk Almost Double for Siblings of Stroke Victims

American Academy of Neurology.

If you have a sibling who's suffered a stroke, you might be nearly twice as likely to have one yourself, says a new study.

THE STUDY

Researchers assessed stroke risk in 807 siblings of 181 people, aged 45 to 65, who had strokes in Nueces County, Texas. Nearly 60% of the stroke patients were Mexican-American, while the rest were non-Hispanic whites.

The stroke patients suffered either an ischemic stroke (where blood flow to the brain is blocked) or a transient ischemic attack, a mini-stroke.

The study found that brothers and sisters of people who had a stroke were almost twice as likely as the average American to have a stroke. The risk was even higher among Mexican-Americans.

CONCLUSION

"The findings show there may be a genetic link to ischemic strokes in this ethnic group," said study author Lynda D. Lisabeth, of the stroke program and department of epidemiology at the University of Michigan in Ann Arbor.

"Other possible explanations could include shared environmental factors such as diet, physical activity and smoking habits. Medical conditions like high blood pressure and diabetes, which cluster in families, may also play a role," Lisabeth stated.

Deadly Dangers of Combining Heart and Stroke-Prevention Surgeries

Richard M. Dubinsky, MD, associate professor of neurology, University of Kansas Medical Center, Kansas City.

Ethan Halm, MD, associate professor of medicine and health policy, Mount Sinai School of Medicine, New York City.

Neurology.

Combining heart-bypass surgery with a common stroke-prevention surgery appears to increase the risk that a patient will die or suffer a postoperative stroke.

BACKGROUND

Heart-bypass surgery reroutes blood flow around clogged arteries, while carotid endarterectomy, the most commonly used stroke-prevention surgery, removes plaque in the carotid arteries, which supply blood to the brain.

The idea behind combining the procedures is to protect the carotid artery from becoming blocked during the heart-bypass surgery, and to reduce the overall risk by having just one surgery. But while the frequency of combined surgery has increased, evidence of any real benefit is unclear.

THE STUDIES

For the first study, the researchers reviewed hospital discharge data on almost 658,000 patients from the Nationwide Inpatient Sample, all of whom were admitted to US hospitals for carotid endarterectomy or coronary bypass artery surgery from 1993 to 2002.

Patients who combined the two procedures had a 38% greater chance of death or postoperative stroke than patients who underwent coronary artery bypass surgery alone, the study found.

However, one problem with the study is that the authors weren't able to compensate for disease severity. "The excess of mortality may just be that they're sicker," said first study lead author Dr. Richard M. Dubinsky, associate professor of neurology at the University of Kansas Medical Center in Kansas City. Women had a lower risk of postoperative death or stroke than men. This is the first study to show this, the researchers noted.

"This means that the benefit of combining the two-in-one operation on one hospital stay hasn't been proven," Dubinsky said. "This is something that would be worthy of a randomized controlled trial."

A second study found that fewer elderly people are undergoing carotid endarterectomy for the wrong reasons. This is the result of the publication of randomized controlled trials that concluded that about one-third of these surgeries were unnecessary.

"Fewer patients are undergoing stroke prevention surgery for the wrong reasons, and this can be viewed as a success of evidence-based medicine and public investment in rigorous evaluation of surgical procedures," said Dr. Ethan Halm, lead author of this study and associate professor of medicine and health policy at the Mount Sinai School of Medicine in New York City.

Only 8.6% of procedures were deemed unnecessary, the study found. That's still a large number, however—11,500 in the US annually.

Still, more patients without symptoms are undergoing the operation. "That's a concern because asymptomatic patients have less to gain from the surgery," Halm said.

■ ■ ■ ■

Stroke Danger

Among 10,405 adults ages 49 to 73, people with early-stage age-related macular degeneration (AMD), an eye disorder that gradually destroys central vision, were 87% more likely to suffer a stroke over a 10-year period than those without AMD.

Theory: AMD risk factors, such as hypertension and smoking, also increase stroke risk.

If you're diagnosed with AMD: Ask your doctor whether you should be monitored for stroke risk factors, including hypertension and diabetes.

Tien Yin Wong, MD, PhD, MPH, professor of ophthalmology, University of Melbourne, East Melbourne, Australia.

■ ■ ■ ■

Improved Stroke Detection

Researchers studied 356 people who received magnetic resonance imaging (MRI) or computed tomography (CT) scans after suffering stroke-like symptoms, such as slurred speech or weakness on one side of the body.

Conclusion: Doctors accurately diagnosed strokes 83% of the time when patients received MRI scans, compared with 26% of the time when CT scans were given.

Reason: MRI scans detect changes within minutes after the onset of a stroke...a CT scan may not be accurate until hours later.

Julio A. Chalela, MD, medical director, Neuroscience Intensive Care Unit, Medical University of South Carolina, Charleston.

Deadly Blood Clots

Geno J. Merli, MD, a leading vascular expert, director of the Jefferson Center for Vascular Diseases at Thomas Jefferson University Hospital, and Ludwig A. Kind Professor of Medicine at Jefferson Medical College, both in Philadelphia.

Blood clots that form in the coronary arteries cause heart attacks. However, many people don't realize that clots also can form in other parts of the vascular system—particularly in the deep veins of the legs, causing *deep vein thrombosis* (DVT). These clots can be even more dangerous than clots in the coronary arteries because they are more likely to go undiagnosed.

Of the 200,000 Americans who die each year from clots due to DVT, about 80% of them experience no symptoms. The worst danger of DVT is *pulmonary embolism*, in which one or more clots travel from the legs to the lungs. One in five people who experience a pulmonary embolism dies from it.

Clots that form in veins near the surface of the skin (superficial thrombosis) are rarely serious. But those that form in the deep veins in the legs—particularly in the *femoral* (thigh), *iliac* (groin) or *popliteal* (behind the knee) veins—are often life-threatening. They rarely dissolve on their own. If anything, they're likely to keep growing—and eventually break free and travel to the lungs.

Even for patients who survive a pulmonary embolism, the risk for complications is high. About 4% to 5% will go on to develop pulmonary hypertension (high blood pressure in the lungs). Others are at risk for *venous insufficiency*, in which the leg veins are damaged, resulting in chronic leg swelling, skin thickening and skin ulceration.

MAJOR RISK FACTORS

About 10% of patients with DVT have a genetic tendency to form blood clots. *Other risk factors...*

•**Prolonged periods of inactivity** can allow dangerous blood clots to form. This can occur during lengthy (more than five hours) plane flights or car trips. Long-distance air or car travelers who have other risk factors, such as congestive heart failure, previous heart attack, obesity or a history of previous blood clots, are at even greater risk than healthy people of developing DVT.

Orthopedic surgery, particularly hip or knee replacement, causes immobilization, often for days to weeks. Anticlotting drugs are given to prevent clots from forming.

•**Lung, pancreatic or ovarian cancer.** Patients with these cancers have increased levels of procoagulants, substances in the blood that promote clotting.

•**Pregnancy and childbirth.** Pulmonary embolism is a cause of death in women during childbirth. Many women who die from pulmonary embolism during or soon after childbirth may have an underlying genetic disorder that increases the risk for clots.

Women who take the breast cancer drug *tamoxifen* (Nolvadex) or supplemental estrogen in birth control pills or hormone therapy also are at increased risk for DVT and pulmonary embolism.

DIAGNOSIS AND TREATMENT

Although patients with DVT frequently do not have symptoms, when clots completely block a vein, persistent symptoms of leg swelling, redness, increased warmth and pain develop.

Red flag: A pulmonary embolism from DVT typically causes sudden shortness of breath, chest pain or a cough that produces blood-tinged mucus. If you experience these symptoms, get to an emergency room *immediately.* About 10% of patients with pulmonary embolism die within one hour.

DVT usually can be diagnosed with ultrasound, a painless, 30-minute test that uses high-frequency sound waves to view the veins.

If your doctor suspects that you have a pulmonary embolism, he/she may recommend a pulmonary computed tomography (CT) scan, in which a dye is injected into an arm vein and computerized images are taken as the dye passes through the blood vessels in the lungs.

Most patients require medication to prevent the clot from growing—and to prevent additional clots from forming.

Typical treatment approaches...

•**DVT patients with a pulmonary embolism who are hemodynamically stable—that** is, their blood pressure and level of oxygen in the blood are close to normal—are hospitalized for five to seven days and treated with intravenous heparin, an anticoagulant medication.

Recent development: A new formulation known as low-molecular-weight heparin, which is better absorbed and lasts longer than intravenous heparin, can be given as a subcutaneous shot at home for five to seven days.

After one of these initial treatments, *warfarin* (Coumadin) is given for three to six months.

•**DVT patients with a pulmonary embolism who are hemodynamically unstable** are at the greatest risk for death—they have low blood pressure and poor oxygen saturation. These patients are typically given tissue *plasminogen activator* (tPA), an intravenous, clot-dissolving drug that is often used to treat stroke patients. This therapy is followed by intravenous or subcutaneous heparin for five to seven days. Warfarin is then given for three to six months to prevent recurrent clots.

In rare cases, when a patient cannot receive anticoagulant therapy because of bleeding, recent surgery or an allergy to the medication, doctors may use a vein filter, a small metal trap that's inserted into the *inferior vena cava* (the large vein that carries blood from the lower part of the body to the heart). The filter prevents pulmonary embolism by catching clots before they can be carried to the lungs.

PREVENTING DVT

Patients at risk for DVT who are hospitalized and bedridden are usually treated with subcutaneous heparin.

If they cannot take heparin, they may be fitted with graduated compression stockings or external pneumatic compression sleeves (which inflate and deflate every 30 seconds by air compression). Both exert varying amounts of pressure along the legs to keep blood from pooling in the legs and forming clots.

Other ways to prevent DVT...

•**Rotate your ankles and flex your toes** at least every 20 minutes when traveling by plane or car. On airplanes, periodically stand and rise up on your tip-toes repeatedly. These exercises flex the calf muscles, which pushes blood out of the legs and helps prevent DVT.

•**Walk daily.** Walking, like other forms of leg exercise, keeps blood moving upward out of the leg veins. The more that blood moves, the less likely it is to form unwanted clots. It's particularly important for hospitalized patients to attempt to walk with appropriate supervision or at least move their legs while they're in bed.

Recent studies indicate that about 15% of hospitalized patients get DVT. Bedridden patients also should flex their feet, ankles and calves every 20 to 30 minutes when awake for clot prevention.

•**Drink water.** Airplane and car travelers on trips of five hours or more should drink two to four eight-ounce glasses of water during the flight or car ride. This increases blood volume, which may help prevent blood clotting.

■ **More from Dr. Merli...**

What Is Deep Vein Thrombosis?

Deep vein thrombosis (DVT) occurs when blood clots form in the deep veins—far from the surface of the skin, most often in the legs. Each year, approximately 1 million Americans are diagnosed with DVT, using imaging tests. Millions of other Americans are believed to have the condition. DVT can be life-threatening if a blood clot breaks loose and travels to the lungs.

15

Women's Health

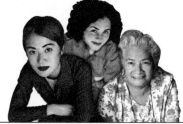

High Trans Fat Intake Triples Heart Disease Risk

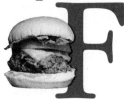

Food rich in unhealthy trans fats, like that found in fast-food restaurants, are even more dangerous to women than previously believed, according to new research.

That study finds that women who regularly consume these heart-hurting fats have three times the risk of heart disease as those with the lowest intake.

"This study just reinforces the idea that trans fat is bad—worse than saturated fat—and we need to make a concerted effort to reduce trans fats," says Dr. Frank Hu, senior author of the study and an associate professor of nutrition and epidemiology at the Harvard School of Public Health in Boston.

THE IMPACT

Trans fats, also called hydrogenated fats, are man-made compounds made from processed liquid oils. These harmful fats will raise bad cholesterol and could lower a person's good cholesterol levels. Because these fats are so thick and stiff, they can also clog up arteries and blood vessels, which can lead to heart attack or stroke.

These fats are commonly found in processed foods such as potato chips, cookies, doughnuts, cakes and many fast foods.

Previous research had already implicated dietary trans fat as a major player in the development of heart disease. However, past research had been done using self-reported dietary information.

Frank Hu, MD, PhD, associate professor of nutrition and epidemiology, Harvard School of Public Health, Boston.

Nieca Goldberg MD, cardiologist, author of the award winning book *Women Are Not Small Men: Lifesaving Strategies for Preventing and Healing Heart Disease*, recently started her own practice "Total Heart Care" in Manhattan. She is the former chief of the Cardiac Rehabilitation and Prevention Center at Lenox Hill Hospital and a national spokesperson for the American Heart Association. During her time at Lenox Hill, Dr. Goldberg founded the "Women's Heart Program," the only cardiac rehabilitation and prevention program for women in New York City.

Circulation, American Heart Association.

THE STUDY

Hu's new study includes an objective measure of trans fat intake—levels found in red blood cells. He notes that because red blood cells live for six months or more, trans fat levels in those cells are a good indicator of average trans fat intake.

His Harvard team examined blood samples collected from almost 33,000 women participating in the ongoing Nurse's Health Study. During the six-year study period, 166 women developed heart disease. The researchers then pulled information on 327 healthy women to serve as controls. Men were not studied.

The women were grouped into four different quartiles based on the levels of trans fats in their blood.

Results: Those with the highest trans fat levels had three times the risk of heart disease when compared with women with the lowest levels. Women in the second and third quartiles had a 60% greater risk of heart disease than those eating the least amount of trans fat.

WHAT IS TOO MUCH?

Hu and his colleagues also estimated the average daily trans fat intake from the trans fat blood levels. Women in the lowest quartile were estimated to consume an average daily trans fat intake of 2.5 grams, while women in the highest quartile were estimated to take in 3.6 grams per day of trans fats.

These are rough estimates, but the US Food and Drug Administration (FDA) estimates that the average American diet contains about 5.8 grams of trans fat daily. The American Heart Association advises that trans fat should make up no more than 1% of your daily caloric intake.

TRIMMING THE TRANS

"Trans fats are a dangerous and unnecessary component of our diet. When you look at data like this, it's scary," says Dr. Nieca Goldberg, medical director of the Women's Health Program at New York University Medical Center and author of *The Women's Healthy Heart Program: Lifesaving Strategies for Preventing and Healing Heart Disease in Women.* "Just a small change gives you a great increase in risk."

In January 2006, the FDA required labeling changes to list trans fat content. This makes it easier for people to know what's in packaged foods, but it's still difficult to know what's in restaurant or fast foods.

When buying packaged goods, look for foods that have no trans fat. However, under current rules, products with 0.5 grams or less trans fat can label their products as having zero grams of trans fat. That means if you have four foods with 0.5 grams of trans fat each, you've unwittingly eaten 2 grams.

Given that this study found that averaging just one extra gram daily can significantly increase your heart disease risk, Hu says the labeling is probably "something we should consider."

In the meantime, if a product is labeled zero grams of trans fat, but the ingredient list includes "partially hydrogenated vegetable oil," the food *does* contain some trans fat, he notes.

Small Steps Lead to Heart Health for Women

Nieca Goldberg MD, cardiologist, author of the award winning book *Women Are Not Small Men: Lifesaving Strategies for Preventing and Healing Heart Disease*, recently started her own practice "Total Heart Care" in Manhattan. She is the former chief of the Cardiac Rehabilitation and Prevention Center at Lenox Hill Hospital and a national spokesperson for the American Heart Association. During her time at Lenox Hill, Dr. Goldberg founded the "Women's Heart Program," the only cardiac rehabilitation and prevention program for women in New York City.

Jennifer Mieres, MD, director of nuclear cardiology, and associate professor of clinical medicine, New York University School of Medicine, New York City, and a national spokeswoman, American Heart Association.

For years, doctors have been fighting the perception that heart disease is a mainly male affliction.

In fact, cardiovascular disease is the number one killer of women: Two of every five women in the US die from heart disease or stroke—more than from all types of cancer combined.

But because heart disease affects women differently than men, it is harder to detect and treat. So health officials are now rethinking how to educate women about their risks—and what they can do to prevent problems.

TRANSLATE KNOWLEDGE INTO ACTION

One problem: Getting information is one thing; applying it is another.

"The problem I see is that women are much more knowledgeable, but they aren't translating that knowledge into action," says Dr. Jennifer Mieres, director of nuclear cardiology and associate professor of clinical medicine at New York University School of Medicine, and a national spokeswoman for the American Heart Association. "That's where the disconnect is."

So the AHA has launched its "Go Red for Women" campaign, which includes an on-line self-survey to evaluate an individual woman's specific risk factors.

"That way, women can increase their thought process about their risk factors," says Dr. Nieca Goldberg, a cardiologist and associate professor of medicine at New York University, and medical director of the university's Women's Heart Program. "We still have to get women to take the plunge to personalize it. If you ask the average woman on the street, she will not say, 'It's going to affect me.'"

A big part of the problem is that women often don't experience a heart attack the same way men do.

WOMEN'S SYMPTOMS DIFFERENT FROM MEN'S

"Women's symptoms can be more subtle," Goldberg says. "It can be shortness of breath without any chest pain. Some suddenly feel very exhausted with minimal activity. Pain often is felt lower in the chest and mistaken for a stomach problem."

Because the symptoms are less obvious, women often wait too long to get treatment.

"If you look at statistics of women who've died suddenly of heart attack, two-thirds died before they could reach the hospital," notes Goldberg.

THE GENDER GAP

Heart disease also often takes place in women differently than it does in men.

In men, plaque forms on the walls of blood vessels in specific places, eventually causing a "kink" in the vessel that stops blood flow. To treat it, doctors will often implant a stent—an artery-opening mesh tube—at the point of blockage to reopen the blood vessel.

But as many as 30% of women suffer from microvascular coronary disease, Goldberg says. The plaque distributes more evenly throughout the blood vessels, slowing blood flow without creating a flow-stopping kink.

In those cases, arteries have difficulty dilating during exercise or exertion, causing extreme fatigue in women.

"When women go to have an angiogram, there have been situations where doctors don't see any blockages, even though the patient has symptoms and a bad stress test," she adds.

Since there's no specific blockage, treating microvascular coronary disease is much harder.

"When doctors go in to look, there are no kinks, so they can't be stented," Goldberg says. "Women are given drugs to thin the blood and take care of symptoms, as well as reduce cholesterol levels."

PREVENTION IS THE KEY

Since heart disease is often harder to detect and harder to treat in women, prevention is the key to saving most women's lives, say experts. Women need to take a hard look at their risk factors.

"If they can't recite their cholesterol levels or blood pressure, they need to schedule a visit with their doctor because that shows those probably haven't been checked in a while," says Goldberg.

Women also should consider whether or not a relative has had heart disease. There is a genetic risk involved, and family members often share the same lifestyle risks, such as drinking, smoking or eating unhealthy foods.

Once that risk is known, women can take steps to improve their health, adds Mieres.

She recommends taking small steps that lead to bigger ones—walking 10 minutes a day and increasing that to 30 minutes, or eating an apple for a snack instead of a candy bar.

"Everyone thinks it's so overwhelming in terms of making lifestyle changes," Mieres says. "Doctors want women to realize that simple steps can make a world of difference in terms of your heart health."

info For more information on the "Go Red for Women" campaign, visit *www.gored forwomen.org.*

Hot Flashes in Women Tied to Higher Blood Pressure

Linda Gerber, MD, professor of public health and medicine, and director of the biostatistics and research methodology core at Weill Cornell Medical College, New York City.
Menopause.

Hot flashes in women are linked with high blood pressure, suggests a new study that may be the first to discover the connection.

In the study of 154 women, women who experienced hot flashes had an age-adjusted systolic blood pressure of 141 while awake, and an average "top-number" reading of 129. However, those who were not experiencing hot flashes had readings of 132 and 119.

The women in the study were between 18 and 65; the mean age was 46.

"One-third of the women we studied reported having hot flashes within the past two weeks. Among these women, systolic blood pressure was significantly higher—even after adjusting for whether they were premenopausal, menopausal or postmenopausal," notes study lead Dr. Linda Gerber, professor of public health and medicine, and director of the biostatistics and research methodology core at Weill Cornell Medical College in New York City.

That's significant, since high blood pressure is a major risk factor for heart disease, which accounts for half of all deaths among American women age 50 and older. And during and following menopause, the risk of heart disease increases.

Previous research has linked menopause—but not hot flashes, per se—to high blood pressure.

■ ■ ■ ■

Better Hot Flash Therapy

Nearly 500 postmenopausal women applied an estrogen gel (Bio-E-Gel) or a placebo gel to their upper arms once a day for 12 weeks.

Result: Hot flashes were reduced in the low- (0.87 g daily), mid- (1.7 g daily) and high-dose (2.6 g daily) gel groups by 71%, 80% and 85%, respectively, compared with 45% in the placebo group. Bio-E-Gel increases estrogen concentrations to help reduce hot flashes, but at a dose lower than FDA-approved products.

Theory: Lower-dose estrogen may lead to fewer side effects and less long-term risk for breast cancer. The gel is currently undergoing FDA review.

James A. Simon, MD, clinical professor of obstetrics and gynecology, George Washington University, Washington, DC.

■ ■ ■ ■

Warning for Women

Postmenopausal women are more prone to vaginal infections, irritation and pain during intercourse. That's because the labia—the folds of tissue that surround and protect the vagina—loses plumpness when estrogen levels drop after menopause.

Self-defense: Ask your doctor about local estrogen therapy—creams, suppositories, rings or tablets inserted into the vagina—that can deliver small amounts of estrogen to help keep tissues plump.

Irwin Goldstein, MD, editor-in-chief, *The Journal of Sexual Medicine*, 715 Albany St., Boston 02118.

A Woman's Brain Hit Harder by Alcohol Abuse

Barbara Flannery, PhD, senior scientist, RTI International, Baltimore.
Matthew Torrington, MD, clinical research fellow, Integrated Substance Abuse Programs, University of California, Los Angeles, and medical director, PROMETA Center, Santa Monica, CA.
Alcoholism: Clinical and Experimental Research.

Alcohol causes damage faster in the brains of women compared with men—even with fewer drinks, according to new research.

New research shows that women suffer a faster rate of intelligence loss, as well as problems with memory, spatial planning, problem-solving and cognitive flexibility, says study Barbara

Flannery, a senior scientist at the research institute RTI International in Baltimore.

These effects were gathered after comparing test results from male and female alcoholics and nonalcoholics from Russia.

THE STUDY

Overall, as you may expect, the tests reveal that nonalcoholics trumped the alcoholics—who had been abstinent for three weeks—in a series of computerized tasks. The tasks evaluated the ability to match patterns in shapes, remember the locations of certain items, and name colors when confronted with contradictory information.

Female drinkers fared significantly worse in most instances than their male counterparts, a finding that prompted Flannery to call for a "gender-sensitive public awareness campaign that highlights these cognitive deficits."

On average, female alcoholics in the study had used alcohol for 10.6 years, compared with 14.8 years for the males.

The study corroborated previous research that finds female alcoholics score lower than their male counterparts in tests that assess working memory, visual skills and the ability to process information.

In past studies, female drinkers have been found to experience accelerated damage to the liver, heart and muscles, compared with males.

QUESTIONS CONTINUE

It's not known to what degree and at what period of sobriety alcoholics can recover from this brain damage.

But research on adolescent rats subjected to binge doses of alcohol at Duke University suggests the brain of the alcoholic teen is more adversely affected by memory loss than adult alcoholics. This indicates that teen girls who abuse alcohol may be most vulnerable to long-term cognitive loss.

"The higher percentage of body fat in females means alcohol is twice as toxic," says Dr. Matthew Torrington, a substance abuse specialist at UCLA and medical director of an addiction-treatment center in Santa Monica.

According to the World Health Organization, at-risk females are those who consume at least seven drinks a week, whereas at-risk males are those who consume at least 14 drinks.

Hormone Therapy— Best Time to Start

Sam Gandy, MD, PhD, chairman, medical and scientific advisory council, Alzheimer's Association, and director, Farber Institute for Neurosciences, Thomas Jefferson University, Philadelphia.
American Academy of Neurology.

Women who start hormone therapy before age 65 could cut their risk of developing Alzheimer's or another dementia, a new study suggests.

This new finding stands in contrast to previous research showing that starting HRT appears to increase dementia risk.

"The magnifying glass has moved slightly earlier, and it looks like, if women started taking HRT early, they did show a decreased risk of Alzheimer's," notes Dr. Sam Gandy, chairman of the Alzheimer's Association's medical and scientific advisory council, and director of the Farber Institute for Neurosciences at Thomas Jefferson University in Philadelphia.

THE STUDY

In this study, 7,153 women aged 65 to 79 without dementia provided information on past hormone therapy exposure.

Women who reported using any form of estrogen HRT before they turned 65 were nearly 50% less likely to develop Alzheimer's disease or another dementia than women who did not use such therapy by that age.

However, starting HRT *after* age 65 doubles their risk of Alzheimer's. The risk was nearly double among women using combined (estrogen plus progestin) therapy.

Gandy has a possible biological explanation for differences observed in younger and older postmenopausal women.

"If you give HRT early, you prevent menopause from ever happening. The brain never sees menopause," he explains. "But if you allow menopause to happen, the brain goes from 30 years of a hormone-rich environment to a hormone-deficient environment, then a reintroduction of hormones after menopause. I think the brain reacts to those two scenarios very differently."

GUIDELINES

Official guidelines recommend that women take HRT for relief of menopausal symptoms only and then at the lowest dose possible for the shortest possible time. Extended use of hormone therapy has been linked to a variety of significant health problems, including breast cancer, heart attack and stroke.

Hormone therapy in older women seems to increase the risk for different dementias. But, in younger postmenopausal women, the relationship between hormone therapy and Alzheimer's disease is less clear.

Previous research had suggested that low levels of estrogen in the brain may raise the risk for developing Alzheimer's, which could be an argument for using HRT.

■ ■ ■ ■

Women on Hormone Replacement Therapy May Suffer Hearing Loss

A recent finding shows that women who are taking *progestin*—the most common form of hormone replacement therapy (HRT)—have 10% to 30% higher risk of hearing loss than women taking estrogen alone or not using HRT at all.

If you are taking progestin: Have your hearing checked every six months.

Robert D. Frisina, PhD, University of Rochester Medical Center, Rochester, NY, and senior author of a study of 124 women, published in *The Proceedings of the National Academy of Sciences.*

Hormone Therapy's Benefits May Outweigh the Risks

A recent study found that the rate of the most common form of breast cancer dropped by 15% between August 2002 and December 2003

—possibly because millions of women halted hormone treatment after a 2002 study showed that it increased breast cancer risk slightly.

How it helps: Hormone therapy can improve quality of life if frequent hot flashes or night sweats make a woman unable to go about her daily activities or get a good night's sleep.

To minimize risk: Take the lowest dose possible for the shortest amount of time necessary. Women who have been on hormone therapy for several years should ask their physicians about weaning themselves off the drugs. Women just starting out should see whether they can get by on half the standard dose.

JoAnn Manson, MD, DrPH, chief of preventive medicine, Brigham and Women's Hospital, and professor of medicine, Harvard Medical School, both in Boston. She is author of *Hot Flashes, Hormones, & Your Health.* McGraw-Hill.

Speedy Recovery from Fibroid Surgery

Jonathan Moss, MB, interventional radiologist, Gartnavel Hospital, Glasgow, Scotland.

New England Journal of Medicine.

A new, minimally invasive procedure called embolization to treat uterine fibroids allows for quicker recovery—allowing women to get back on their feet faster than other methods.

Embolization involves blocking the arteries that supply blood to the fibroids. The procedure uses angiographic techniques similar to those used in heart catheterization, in which a catheter is placed into the uterine arteries. Small particles are injected into the arteries to block blood. This technique is essentially the same as that used to control bleeding that occurs after birth or pelvic fracture.

In a new study, Scottish researchers report that hospital stays for embolization average just a day, compared with about five days for more traditional surgery procedures to remove fibroids, such as hysterectomy.

THE STUDY

The scientists randomly assigned 157 women with uterine fibroids to undergo either embolization or surgery. Of those, 106 had embolization, 43 had hysterectomies in which the uterus is removed; and eight had myomectomies, in which each individual fibroid is removed.

The purpose was to track hospital stays and recovery rates. Researchers found that the average hospital stay was one day for embolization, compared with five days for surgery. Those who underwent embolization also got back to their daily activities faster than women in the surgical group.

Women in the embolization group were able to drive a car after an average of eight days, compared with 34 days for the surgical group. And they returned to work, on average, 20 days after the procedure, versus 62 days for the surgery group. Embolized women were able to resume sexual activity within 21 days, compared with 53 days for those who had surgery.

"The biggest problem of surgery, whether myomectomy or hysterectomy, is the time to recover from the operation. This was much faster following embolization," notes lead author Dr. Jonathan Moss, a consultant interventional radiologist at Gartnavel Hospital in Glasgow.

"The other problem with hysterectomy is not every woman is happy with that option," he adds. With embolization, "you keep your uterus."

NEW OPTION

Embolization is a relatively new technique—introduced in 1995—to treat fibroids, which are noncancerous growths that develop in the uterus. As many as one in five women of childbearing age develop fibroids.

Most fibroids don't require treatment, but some cause excessive bleeding and may cause pain. When they do, they are treated with hormone therapy, surgery and now another option, uterine-artery embolization.

DRAWBACK

The biggest problem with embolization is that it doesn't always work. As many as 20% of patients will ultimately need it repeated or have to undergo hysterectomy. It is typically recommended for women who know they don't want to have additional children.

Shot That Keeps Women's Bones Strong

Paul Brandt, PhD, assistant professor of neuroscience and experimental therapeutics, Texas A&M Health Science Center College of Medicine, College Station.

Nanette Santoro, MD, director of reproductive endocrinology, Montefiore Medical Center, New York City.

Steven R. Goldstein, MD, professor of obstetrics and gynecology, New York University School of Medicine.

New England Journal of Medicine.

A once-a-year injection of a common osteoporosis drug may provide an easy way to protect women against the risk for bone fractures—and might even replace bone-building pills, say researchers. The findings could open the door to the US Food and Drug Administration's approval of once-a-year *zoledronic acid.*

"Here we've got something we can give to patients when they're in the clinic with a 15-minute IV, and it lasts for a whole year," says Paul Brandt, an assistant professor of neuroscience and experimental therapeutics at Texas A&M Health Science Center College of Medicine in College Station.

Brandt was not involved in a new study that shows great promise in this quarter-hour treatment. "The FDA hasn't approved it for a single-year injection, but I hope it will. It sure is going to be a good kick in the right direction."

THE STUDY

The research examined the efficacy of annual injections over three years.

Almost 4,000 postmenopausal women were randomly assigned to receive either a single 15-minute infusion of zoledronic acid, or a placebo, at the study's start, and then again 12 months and 24 months later. Participants were followed out to the three-year point.

Those treated with zoledronic acid injections had a 70% lower risk of vertebral fractures and were 41% less likely to suffer hip fractures.

They also experienced significant improvement in bone mineral density and bone metabolism markers.

The downside to the injections: They have a higher incidence of an irregular heart rhythm called atrial fibrillation. Other side effects were similar in both groups, say researchers.

A BETTER OPTION?

Experts say these results are encouraging—especially when they consider that many women in the study were already take bone-preserving pills called oral bisphosphonates.

These pills are not for everyone, says Dr. Nanette Santoro, director of the division of reproductive endocrinology in the department of obstetrics and gynecology and women's health at Montefiore Medical Center in New York City.

"For now, women who do not tolerate oral bisphosphonates well but who are good candidates will be able to take the medication in a relatively convenient form," she says.

The pills work by slowing the body's natural resorption of bone. But one common problem with bisphosphonates is that patients don't take the drugs as they should.

"The big concern has been in patient compliance," says Brandt. "The monthly pills run into problems where women start to forget. It's also a pain to take these drugs. You have to sit upright and there's a risk of acid reflux, esophageal damage."

Women also have to take the pills with a full glass of water while fasting.

Another expert, Dr. Steven R. Goldstein, a professor of obstetrics and gynecology at New York University School of Medicine and author of *The Estrogen Alternative* and *Could It Be Menopause...*, believes the new study to be "a very nice alternative."

He calls the injection "an attractive alternative for a significant number of people who cannot or will not take traditional antiresorbtive medication."

info The National Osteoporosis Foundation has more on osteoporosis at *www.nof.org*.

■ ■ ■ ■

Women, Watch Your Knees!

Women have wider hips than men, which puts more stress on the knees, according to a new report. Women also have more estrogen, which makes ligaments flexible but also reduces their ability to absorb shocks.

Harvard Health Publications.

Bone-Building Drug Backfires

Salvatore Ruggiero, DMD, MD, chief of oral and maxillofacial surgery at Long Island Jewish Medical Center, New Hyde Park, NY.

The drug *alendronate* (Fosamax), one of the bisphosphonates developed to help prevent bone loss and treat it, is often prescribed as a long-term remedy for women in postmenopause. It's been deemed as safe for the life of the patient. A recent study has cast long shadows on that assumption.

DETERIORATING JAWBONES

Salvatore Ruggiero, DMD, MD, chief of oral and maxillofacial surgery at Long Island Jewish Medical Center in New Hyde Park, New York, was astonished to see a rare condition develop with the jawbone in a set of female patients. The condition, *osteonecrosis of the jaw* (ONJ), tends to occur after dental work that causes trauma to the jaw. Doctors often detect it when the jawbone becomes exposed and sometimes an infection has set in.

ONJ had been associated with bisphosphonates before Fosamax, but previously, patients had been administered bisphosphonates as IV treatment for cancer. What Dr. Ruggiero observed was ONJ had also developed in another group of patients who had undergone oral surgery at his hospital over a three-year period. These women were taking bisphosphonates orally for the treatment of osteoporosis. (Besides Fosamax, other bisphosphonates for osteoporosis include Boniva and Actonel.)

FDA RULES

Dr. Ruggiero stresses that while the Food and Drug Administration (FDA) now requires that drug manufacturers add labeling stating that ONJ is a potential side effect of bisphosphonates, the condition as associated with osteoporosis is extremely rare. Of the 159 ONJ patients from his medical center, just 25 had taken the medication orally and the overall percentage of women on oral bisphosphonates who develop ONJ is much smaller than that—well under 1% of all patients, he says.

Some doctors think that ONJ is just the first sign of a broader bone deterioration problem.

Prior to the FDA disclosure, the main reported side effects of bisphosphonates were gastrointestinal problems. As long as women's "tummies didn't rumble" they saw no reason to suspend use of the medication. Besides, *ibandronate* (Boniva), a newer bisphosphonate drug that requires taking just once a month rather than daily or weekly, as with Fosamax, seemed to help with GI side effects.

Dr. Ruggiero feels it is time to rethink the length of time osteoporosis patients are allowed to stay on any drugs. He anticipates that the next step may be to have "drug holidays" in which women go off the medication for several years at a time, and return to it for the same period before suspending its use once again. Women would need to be monitored in this period for any bone deterioration with bone-density scans…and they must also be careful to continue vigilance about protecting their bone strength in more traditional ways, such as taking their calcium and Vitamin D, exercising regularly, limiting alcohol and not smoking.

DENTAL CARE

Dr. Ruggiero is concerned about overreaction among patients who are avoiding routine dental care and even among dentists who are reluctant to treat this group of patients. He stresses that routine dental care is not likely to open the gates to ONJ—it is bone that was once traumatized that fails to heal properly that causes the problem…for example, work that involves trauma to the jaw including extractions and implants.

Furthermore, he says it is critical for all women on bisphosphonates to get regular careful dental care. That is how they can be sure their teeth will stay strong so they will not end up needing extractions or implants. He says for those women who do have to have dental work that will involve jawbone healing, current information shows that there is nothing to worry about if they have been on oral bisphosphonates for up to five years.

The exception: For those patients taking steroids and a bisphosphonate, the time window is much less, or as little as two years. For those who have taken them longer, Dr. Ruggiero suggests going off the medication for at least a few months before elective dental work. Even though these drugs stay in the bones for an extremely long time, he says that a year off them does seem to make ONJ more manageable—assuming that normal bone cell function can be restored and metabolically supported, based on the ebb and flow of bone cell formation and resorption.

TELLTALE SIGNS OF ONJ

Symptoms of ONJ are pain and/or numbness in the jaw, swelling, loosened teeth, gum infections and exposure of bone within the oral cavity. Women who experience any of these signs should see their doctor right away.

Dr. Ruggiero says not to be alarmed about the possibility that problems like this could develop in other bones in the body, from bisphosphonates. To date, there have been no reports of this complication occurring anywhere other than the jaw, he added.

info For more on ONJ, including symptoms, treatment options and the bisphosphonate connection, visit *www.onj-net.org* or *www.bonehealthcouncil.org*.

■ ■ ■ ■

Ginkgo Biloba May Cut Ovarian Cancer Risk by 60%

In a study of 668 women with ovarian cancer and 721 healthy women, those who took the herbal supplement ginkgo biloba for at least six months (for any reason) were 60% less likely to develop ovarian cancer.

Theory: Ginkgo inhibits *platelet activating factor*, which can stimulate cancer cell growth.

Self-defense: Women at elevated risk for ovarian cancer (due to family history, for example) may want to ask their doctors about taking ginkgo biloba.

Caution: Do not use ginkgo if you take a blood thinner.

Daniel W. Cramer, MD, ScD, professor of obstetrics, gynecology and reproductive biology, Brigham and Women's Hospital, Boston.

■ ■ ■ ■

Pap Tests Still Needed After Some Hysterectomies

Women who had partial hysterectomies, in which the uterus was removed but not the cervix, and women who had total hysterectomies to treat invasive cervical cancer or a precancerous condition should continue to get annual Pap tests because they still are at risk for cancer. Women who had total hysterectomies for noncancer-related reasons, such as endometriosis or fibroids, do not need Pap tests—but they still should have yearly pelvic exams to check their ovaries.

Mary Jane Minkin, MD, clinical professor of obstetrics and gynecology, Yale University School of Medicine, New Haven, CT.

■ ■ ■ ■

Better Cervical Cancer Screening

In a study including 1,305 women ages 40 to 50, researchers analyzed the results of Pap smears and testing for human papillomavirus (HPV), a common cause of cervical cancer.

Result: Twenty-one percent of the women who tested positive for HPV at the beginning of the study developed cervical cancer or precancerous cervical lesions within a 10-year period, even though the results of their Pap smears, which also had been performed at the beginning of the study, were negative. If you are over age 40, ask your gynecologist about receiving an HPV test with your PAP smear.

Susanne Krüger Kjær, MD, DMSc, professor, Danish Cancer Society, Copenhagen.

■ ■ ■ ■

Are You Taking This Potent Anticancer Vitamin?

Vitamin D can drive down mortality rates from 16 types of cancer, including breast and ovarian, by up to 70%. As a possible cancer preventive, be sure to get at least 1,000 IU of vitamin D-3 (*cholecalciferol*—not D-2, *ergocalciferol*, which is less effective) in summer and 2,000 IU in winter. For most people, it is best to take 1,500 IU daily in supplement form.

William B. Grant, PhD, founding director, Sunlight, Nutrition and Health Research Center, *www.sunarc.org.*

■ ■ ■ ■

Trans Fats May Increase Infertility Risk

In a recent finding, women who obtain as little as 2% of total calories from trans fats instead of monounsaturated fats are twice as likely to have ovulation-related fertility problems. Each 2% increase in trans fat consumption raises ovulation-related infertility by 73%. Trans fats are found mainly in commercially baked and fried products.

Self-defense: Be extra vigilant about avoiding trans fats if you are childbearing age and are planning to have children.

Jorge E. Chavarro, MD, ScD, research fellow, Harvard School of Public Health, Boston, and leader of a study of trans fats and infertility, published in *The American Journal of Clinical Nutrition.*

Air Pollution Raises Heart Risk in Postmenopausal Women

Joel D. Kaufman, MD, professor of environmental and occupational medicine and epidemiology, University of Washington, Seattle.

Len Horovitz, MD, pulmonary specialist, Lenox Hill Hospital, New York City.

New England Journal of Medicine.

Postmenopausal women who live in areas with higher air pollution levels have a greater risk of developing cardiovascular disease and dying from it, says new research. The study was the first to look at new cases of cardiovascular disease, not just death, and to look at air pollution levels within cities.

"The risk of having a cardiovascular event, that is, a heart attack, stroke or needing bypass surgery, or of dying of a cardiovascular cause, was increased," said study senior author Dr. Joel Kaufman, professor of environmental and occupational medicine and epidemiology at the University of Washington.

THE STUDY

For the study, Kaufman and his colleagues looked at 65,893 postmenopausal women in 36 US metropolitan regions who were part of the Women's Health Initiative, a large, government-funded study designed to look at heart health, cancer and osteoporosis in women. All participants were free of cardiovascular disease at the start of the study in 1994.

Each small increase of fine particulate matter per cubic meter was associated with a 24% increase in the risk of a cardiovascular event and a 76% increase in the risk of death from cardiovascular disease.

"It's an important study," said Dr. Len Horovitz, a pulmonary specialist at Lenox Hill Hospital in New York City. "They showed that very small particulate matter can penetrate into the lungs and cause damage over time."

Fine particulate matter is comprised of tiny particles of soot or dust carried in the air. "They mostly come from combustion of fossil fuels, although vegetative burning has an impact in some cities," Kaufman said. "In the United States as a whole, we're mostly talking about power plants, coal burning and motor vehicle exhaust, especially diesel exhaust."

Women having a higher long-term average exposure had a higher risk. Also different health risks within cities were often larger than those between cities.

IMPLICATIONS

Scientists aren't sure how fine particulate air pollution increases these health risks, although it's possible that inhaling the particles may be speeding the development of atherosclerosis or hardening of the arteries.

"The EPA [US Environmental Protection Agency] did tighten 24-hour standards but failed to listen to its scientific advisers on long-term standards. They could be tightened," Horovitz said.

Kaufman added, "This is not a study that necessarily spells individual-level health decisions. It's not like we can say people should move. We really need to work harder to lower these levels, and we need to think about pollution as a risk factor, like smoking and diabetes and cholesterol. We need to think of pollution as a cause of health effects now and not just a nuisance factor and something that causes haze on the horizon."

Cardiovascular disease is the leading cause of death in the United States, accounting for one in three deaths. Reducing fine particulate air pollution could result in less cardiovascular disease and fewer deaths, the study authors stated.

info Daily pollution readings for more than 150 cities can be found on the EPA's Web site, *www.epa.gov.*

Fight Osteoporosis The Natural Way

Dr. Mark Stengler is a licensed naturopathic medical doctor and a leading authority on the practice of alternative and integrated medicine. An associate clinical professor at the National College of Naturopathic Medicine in Portland, OR, Dr. Stengler has served on a medical advisory committee for the Yale University Complementary Medicine Outcomes Research Project and is the author or coauthor of 16 books, including two best sellers—*The Natural Physician's Healing Therapies* and *Prescription for Natural Cures.* Dr. Stengler is the founder and director of the La Jolla Whole Health Clinic in La Jolla, CA. *www.DrStengler.com.*

Misconceptions abound when it comes to osteoporosis, a dreaded disease marked by porous, brittle bones and hunched backs. Most people think of osteoporosis as a women's disease, but it's more than that. While 8 million American women have been diagnosed with osteoporosis, more than 2 million men also are affected by it.

OSTEOPOROSIS: A SILENT PROBLEM

Osteoporosis can develop because, starting at about age 35, our bone cells do not make new bone as fast as it is broken down. Our bones become more frail and fracture more easily. Fractures, especially of the hip, spine and wrist, are more likely to occur, even without trauma. Osteoporosis has no symptoms until a bone is fractured. Many people go for decades without a diagnosis of osteoporosis—until they fall and an X-ray reveals porous bones.

Bone density can be measured with a dual-energy X-ray absorptiometry (DEXA) scan, but many people don't get this test. I recommend a baseline DEXA scan by age 50, and if results are normal, follow-ups every three to five years.

The most worrisome risk for a person with osteoporosis is a hip fracture. According to the National Osteoporosis Foundation (*www.nof.org*), an average of 24% of hip-fracture patients age 50 or older die in the year following their fractures, often as a result of long-term immobilization that leads to blood clots or infection. Six months after a hip fracture, only 15% of patients can walk unaided across a room.

Virtually every person with osteoporosis who has come to my clinic is confused about the best way to promote bone health. Conventional doctors typically prescribe osteoporosis medication, such as *alendronate* (Fosamax) and *ibandronate* (Boniva). However, these drugs can cause side effects, such as digestive upset and blood clots, and they don't address the underlying nutritional deficiencies that promote bone loss.

The natural protocol I recommend includes a healthful diet (rich in vegetables, fruit and fish and low in refined-sugar products and red meat) …weight-bearing exercise (such as walking and stair-climbing)…and good hormone balance (deficiencies of some hormones, such as testosterone, accelerate bone loss). I also suggest certain bone-protecting supplements.

Caution: People with kidney disease should not take supplements without consulting a doctor. With kidney disease, the kidneys cannot process high doses of nutrients.

My recommendations for women and men: To help prevent osteoporosis, take the first three supplements listed below. *If you have osteoporosis or osteopenia (mild bone loss that can be diagnosed with a DEXA scan), take the first three supplements listed and as many of the others as you're willing to try, in the dosages recommended…*

SUPER TRIO PREVENTS AND TREATS OSTEOPOROSIS

•**Calcium** is the most prevalent mineral in bone tissue. Taking supplements helps prevent a deficiency. Most studies have found that calcium slows bone loss but does not increase bone density when used alone. Women with osteoporosis should take 500 mg of calcium twice daily with meals. It should be a well-absorbed form, such as citrate, citrate-malate, amino acid chelate or hydroxyapatite. To boost absorption, take no more than 500 mg per dose. Calcium carbonate, which is widely used, is not well-absorbed. For osteoporosis prevention, men and women, as well as boys and girls starting at age 13, should take 500 mg daily.

Calcium supplementation for men with osteoporosis is more complicated. Some recent research has identified a link between high calcium intake (from dairy products) and increased prostate cancer risk. A meta-analysis in the *Journal of the National Cancer Institute* that reviewed 12 studies on this association concluded, "High intake of dairy products and calcium may be associated with an increased risk for prostate cancer, although the increase appears to be small." A recent study found that calcium intake exceeding 1,500 mg a day (from food and supplements) may be associated with a higher risk of advanced, and potentially fatal, prostate cancer. The saturated fat in dairy products may raise prostate cancer risk.

Until there is more definitive information, I recommend that men who have osteoporosis, regardless of whether they have eliminated calcium-rich foods from their diets, take no more than a 500-mg calcium supplement daily. Men with prostate cancer should consult their doctors before using calcium supplements.

•**Vitamin D** promotes absorption of calcium. Deficiencies of this vitamin are more common in Americans over age 50 than in younger adults. Sun exposure prompts the body to produce vitamin D, and the kidneys help convert it to its active form. As we age, our skin cannot synthesize vitamin D as effectively from sunlight, and our kidneys become less efficient. People with darker skin, those with digestive problems (due to malabsorption conditions, such as Crohn's disease) and those with limited exposure to sunlight are also at greater risk for vitamin D deficiency. Preliminary studies indicate that an inadequate intake of vitamin D is associated with an increased risk of fractures.

For the prevention of osteoporosis, I recommend 600 IU to 800 IU of vitamin D daily. People with osteoporosis should take 800 IU to 1,200 IU daily. Vitamin D is fat soluble, meaning it is better absorbed when taken with meals (containing small amounts of fat).

For many patients with low vitamin D levels, I recommend 2,000 IU of vitamin D daily. To ensure that vitamin D levels are optimal, I monitor blood levels once or twice a year. Overdosing can lead to heart arrhythmia, anorexia, nausea and other ill effects.

•**Magnesium,** an important constituent of bone crystals, is crucial for the proper metabolism of calcium. A deficiency of magnesium impairs bone-building cells known as *osteoblasts*. Like calcium, magnesium requires vitamin D for absorption.

Researchers at Tel Aviv University in Israel looked at the effect of magnesium supplementation on bone density in 31 postmenopausal women with osteoporosis. This two-year, open, controlled trial (both the researchers and patients knew who was receiving the placebo or the supplement) involved giving the participants 250 mg to 750 mg of magnesium daily for six months and 250 mg for another 18 months. Twenty-two patients (71%) experienced a 1% to 8% increase in bone density. The mean bone density of all treated patients increased significantly after one year and remained at that level after two years. Among an additional 23 postmenopausal women not receiving magnesium, mean bone density decreased significantly.

For osteoporosis prevention, take 400 mg to 500 mg of magnesium daily...for osteoporosis, take 500 mg to 750 mg daily. In both cases, take in divided doses.

Are Flexible Joints The Key to Chronic Fatigue Syndrome?

Peter Rowe, MD, professor of pediatrics, Johns Hopkins Children's Center, Baltimore.

Leonard Jason, PhD, professor of psychology and director, Center for Community Research, DePaul University, Chicago.

Journal of Pediatrics.

Researchers believe that extreme joint flexibility may increase the risk of developing chronic fatigue syndrome, a painful and fatiguing condition usually affecting women—often, with no reasonable explanation.

The link was first discovered accidentally at Johns Hopkins Children's Center, where a young girl was being treated for chronic fatigue syndrome for three years before it was noticed that she could bend and twist her joints much more than normal.

"I was chagrined that my physical examination had not included that. So, we decided to look into it," notes pediatrician Dr. Peter Rowe.

THE DISCOVERY

Rowe soon learned that most of the 60 children and teens who had been treated at his center for CFS had hypermobility in at least four joints. That means they could move their joints well beyond the normal range of motion, such as being able to bend a pinkie 90 degrees backward, touch the thumb to the forearm, or bend at the waist and rest both hands flat on the ground.

"Some of the kids would be able to put their leg behind their head in a seated position," says Rowe. "Others could do the splits. Once we saw this over and over, we thought it was something that needed more study."

That's significant, considering that no more than two in 10 people in the general population have a single hyperflexible joint.

Although this link doesn't mean that hypermobility will result in CFS, it offers new clues into how the painful and fatiguing syndrome develops—and possibly, a new way to identify at-risk patients.

REMOVING STIGMA

In the past, some doctors regarded the syndrome as a psychosomatic byproduct of depression. And those who saw it as a legitimate illness could find few physiological signs of it. CFS often generates ambiguous complaints about pain in the joints and a general malaise.

At the very least, Rowe's connection may remove some stigma associated with CFS, which strikes about four per 1,000 adults. Children are less affected.

"In the past, you had a tremendous amount of skepticism about [CFS], which created a certain amount of stigma for people who have it," says Leonard Jason, a professor of psychology and director of the Center for Community Research at DePaul University in Chicago.

DIAGNOSING CHRONIC FATIGUE SYNDROME

Now, a CFS diagnosis is made if a patient has a sudden onset of fatigue that lasts at least six months and at least four of the following eight symptoms: impaired memory, sore throat, tender neck or tender lymph nodes in the armpit, muscle pain, joint pain, new headaches, troubled sleep and a feeling of malaise after exertion.

THE EXPLANATION

How could joint hypermobility be connected with CFS? That's currently under study, but there are some theories...

Rowe says that flexible joints may stress the peripheral nerves in the arms and legs, thereby fatiguing the entire nervous system, or the excessive range of motion may indirectly cause the syndrome.

"For example, if you're prone to injury because of your joints, you might decrease your activity, which studies have shown can lead to [the syndrome]," he notes.

info Get more on CFS from the Web site of CFIDS Association of America (chronic fatigue and immune dysfunction syndrome) at *www.cfids.org*.

Experts Help Women Predict Heart Disease Risk

Paul Ridker, MD, MPH, cardiologist and director, Center for Cardiovascular Disease Prevention, Brigham and Women's Hospital, and professor, medicine, Harvard Medical School, Boston.

Nieca Goldberg MD, cardiologist, author of the award winning book *Women Are Not Small Men: Lifesaving Strategies for Preventing and Healing Heart Disease*, recently started her own practice "Total Heart Care" in Manhattan. She is the former chief of the Cardiac Rehabilitation and Prevention Center at Lenox Hill Hospital and a national spokesperson for the American Heart Association. During her time at Lenox Hill, Dr. Goldberg founded the "Women's Heart Program," the only cardiac rehabilitation and prevention program for women in New York City.

Journal of the American Medical Association.

Women may soon have a better idea of what their actual cardiovascular disease risk is for the next 10 years and beyond. Researchers from Brigham and Women's Hospital in Boston have developed a new cardiovascular disease assessment tool specifically for women.

NEW ASSESSMENT TOOL

The new risk model, called the Reynolds Risk Score, includes age, systolic blood pressure (the top number in a blood pressure reading), total and HDL ("good") cholesterol levels, smoking status, levels of high sensitivity C-reactive protein (CRP, a marker of increased systemic inflammation), and family history of cardiovascular trouble (whether or not a parent had a heart attack before the age of 60).

"The Reynolds Risk Score provides a very easy way for women and physicians to truly understand what the cardiovascular risk is, not only for 10 years, but for 20 and 30 years," explained the study's lead author, Dr. Paul Ridker, director of the Center for Cardiovascular Disease Prevention at Brigham and Women's Hospital in Boston. "Of the approximately 10 million American women who have an intermediate risk of heart disease based on current guidelines, about 50% would be classified into higher or lower categories (based on the Reynolds Risk Score)."

BACKGROUND

Heart disease remains the leading killer of American women. "Women need to understand that their risk of suffering a heart attack, stroke or other cardiovascular disease is the same as it is for men, but it happens about 10 years later," Ridker says.

But, the current guidelines, originally designed in the 1950s and 1960s, don't fully capture a woman's heart disease risk. In fact, as many as 20% of all women who have had heart attacks don't have any of the known major risk factors, and, according to Ridker, about half of all heart attacks occur in women who have normal cholesterol levels.

THE STUDY

To develop a better model of female risk, Ridker and colleagues assessed 35 different risk factors in nearly 25,000 women taking part in the Women's Health Study. All of the women were over 45 years old and heart disease–free at the start of the study. Additionally, none of the women included in the risk-score study had diabetes, because being diabetic automatically puts a woman in the high-risk category for heart disease.

The average follow-up time was 10.2 years. The researchers used information from two-thirds of the group to design the new risk model and the other third to validate the Reynolds Risk Score.

According to the study, about 40% to 50% of women classified as having an intermediate risk actually had a higher or a lower risk, based on the Reynolds Risk Score.

IMPLICATIONS

"By adding CRP and family history, we can do a much better job on assessing risk," said Ridker. "This will have an enormous impact on prevention. We can get aspirin and statins to women who truly need them, without exposing those who don't. It's cost-effective as well as being good medicine."

"This is great news that we're starting to look at and fine-tune the risk of heart disease in women," said Dr. Nieca Goldberg, medical director of the Women's Heart Program at New York University Medical Center and author of *Women Aren't Small Men: Lifesaving Strategies for Preventing and Healing Heart Disease in Women*.

"But, not every woman needs to have her CRP levels measured, and there are some limitations to using CRP levels. While diet and exercise can lower CRP levels, there's currently no evidence that lowering CRP can lower heart disease risk," she said.

The new scoring tool will be useful as part of a global assessment of all of a woman's risk factors, including lifestyle factors, such as diet and exercise habits.

"This is just one tool, not the sole measure of a woman's risk of heart disease," Goldberg added.

The most important risk factor for heart disease is still smoking, but this study found that family history and CRP are also key. Ridker recommended that women let their doctors know if their parents had heart disease before they were 60.

info The new risk assessment tool for cardiovascular risk can be found on-line at *www.reynoldsriskscore.org*.

Migraines During Pregnancy Linked to Heart Disease, Stroke

Cheryl Bushnell, MD, assistant professor, medicine (neurology), Duke Center for Cerebrovascular Disease, Duke University Medical Center, Durham, NC.

Richard Lipton, MD, director, Montefiore Headache Center, and professor, neurology and epidemiology, Albert Einstein College of Medicine, New York City.

American Academy of Neurology.

Women who experience migraines while they're pregnant are significantly more likely to suffer a stroke, heart attack or other vascular problems. Although many questions remain, there are steps women can take to protect themselves, said the authors of a new study.

GOOD ADVICE

"Clearly this is not proving a cause and effect. It's an association that we've found and it has to be looked at in more studies," said study author Dr. Cheryl Bushnell, an assistant professor of medicine (neurology) at the Duke Center for Cerebrovascular Disease at Duke University Medical Center.

"But I think that we can assume that women who have migraines also seem to have vascular disease, and women who have migraines and vascular risk factors should be trying their best to modify or control those risk factors while they're pregnant. That's a common-sense approach," Bushnell added.

Dr. Richard Lipton, director of the Montefiore Headache Center and professor of neurology and epidemiology at Albert Einstein College of Medicine in New York City, said, "People with migraine should view migraine the same way they would view diabetes or high cholesterol, as a medical problem that should be managed to make life better today and prevent complications tomorrow. Rather than being alarmed, people with migraine should get the migraines treated and make sure they modify risk factors for heart disease and stroke by maintaining a normal body weight and treating high blood pressure."

Previous research by the study authors had shown that migraines were a risk factor for having a stroke during pregnancy. Migraines had also shown up as a predictor of heart disease during pregnancy.

Migraines have also been associated with stroke and heart disease in nonpregnant women. "Migraine, particularly migraine with aura, is known to be a risk factor for heart disease and stroke, and there's lots of evidence for that," Lipton confirmed.

THE STUDY

For the new study, the authors looked at pregnancy discharge data from the years 2000 to 2003 for almost 17 million women nationwide. Almost 34,000 women had been treated for migraines.

Women who were treated for migraines during pregnancy were 19 times more likely to suffer a stroke, five times more likely to have a heart attack and more than twice as likely to have heart disease, blood clots and other vascular problems.

Women who were 35 or older when they delivered their baby were also more likely to have migraines while pregnant. The findings make sense on a biological level, Bushnell said, as migraine is a vascular headache.

One lingering problem is identifying those people with migraines who are truly at risk for other problems.

"The underlying mechanism is certainly real," Bushnell said. "However, how do we know, of these hundreds of thousands of people with migraine, who is going to be at risk? We don't have a good marker for that.

"In the meantime, women might consider the information in the study as a window of opportunity," she added. "Especially women who delay pregnancy and who have already developed other risk factors such as diabetes, hypertension and obesity."

info Visit the American Pregnancy Association at *www.americanpregnancy.org* for more on migraines during pregnancy.

Index

Hip fractures, 332
Homeopathy, for constipation, 224–225
Honey, benefits of, 293
Hormone replacement therapy (HRT)
    and Alzheimer's disease, 325–326
    and breast cancer, 58–60
    and hearing loss, 326
Hormone therapy, for prostate cancer,
    80–81
Hospitalists, 307–309
Hospitals
    inpatient doctors for, 307–309
    and MRSA-related pneumonia, 152–154
    safety, while in, 295–296
    and stroke care, 316–317
    top foreign, 288
Hot flashes, 324, 326
HRT. *See* Hormone replacement therapy
Human papillomavirus (HPV)
    and cancer screening, 83, 330
    vaccine for, 74–76
Humidifiers, and sinus health, 29
Hydration
    to prevent hemorrhoids, 285
    and sexual function, 134
Hydrogenated fats. *See* Trans fats
Hypertension. *See* Blood pressure, high
Hypnosis, for breast cancer biopsy
    pain, 48
Hypoglycemia, and memory problems,
    90–91
Hysterectomies, and Pap tests, 329

I

Ibuprofen, for children, 280–281
Immune boosters
    during cancer therapies, 72–73
    eating less, 258–259
    T'ai Chi, 22–23
Implantable cardioverter defibrillators
    (ICDs), 182
Infants
    car seats, risks of, 167
    and cough and cold medications,
    162–163
    SIDS, 164–165
Infections
    and adrenal fatigue, 144
    misdiagnosis of, 150
    prevention of, before surgery, 290
    protection against, 155–156
Infertility, risk of, and trans fats, 330
Inflammation, reduction of, 241,
    282–283. *See also* Omega-3 fatty acids
Influenza
    drugs to prevent the spread of, 154–155
    herbal teas for, 212
    and pneumonia prevention, 154
    shots, blocking of, by NSAIDs, 17
Insomnia
    and chronic pain, 279
    herbal teas for, 212
    relief for, from music, 142
Insulin, inhaled form, 101
Insulin levels, to diagnose diabetes, 93
Insulin resistance
    and cancer prevention, 64
    saturated fat and diabetes risk, 99
Insurance
    disability, 301–303

health, 294
    medical, during serious illness,
    303–304
Intensity modulated radiation treatment
    (IMRT), for breast cancer, 55
Intercourse, pain during, 324
Iron, depletion of, by reflux drugs, 107
Iron supplementation, for hair growth,
    216
Irritable bowel syndrome
    functional medicine approach to,
    240–241
    herbal teas for, 212
Itching, relief of, from hemorrhoids,
    283–285

J

Jet lag, treatment with Viagra, 121
Joint flexibility, and chronic fatigue
    syndrome, 333–334
Juices
    best to prevent Alzheimer's disease,
    292–293
    for health, 260

K

Kidney disease
    and anemia treatments, 112
    dialysis, and epoetin, 307
    and supplements, 332
Kidney stones, treatments for, 159
Knees, problems in women, 328

L

Lab tests, accuracy of, 299–300
Larynx cancer, 217–218
Left ventricular assist devices (LVADs),
    198–199
Leg length, uneven, and arthritis risk, 16
Leg pain, and peripheral arterial
    disease, 13
Legal rights, during serious illness,
    303–305
Legs, cramping of, 2
Lemonade
    to fight kidney stones, 159
Leptin, and breast cancer risk, 60
Libido
    low, herbal teas for, 212
    natural help for increasing, 133–134
Lice, head, 169–170
Licorice, and drug interactions, 226
Lidocaine, topical, 269–270
Lifestyle changes
    for adrenal fatigue, 143–144
    for bipolar disorder, 127–128
    and heart disease, 187–188
    for prediabetes, 86–87
Light/dark therapies, for bipolar
    disorder, 128
Liver cancer, risk of, 258
Liver disease, coffee as protection,
    213–214
Liver failure, 298–299
Longevity, 19–22
Low-fat diets, and breast cancer
    recurrence, 49–50
Lung cancer, and genetic testing, 82–83

Lung Centers, top US, 38–40
Lung health, and hostility, 230–231
Lutein, 220–221

M

Macular degeneration, 11, 12
Magnesium supplements
    for asthma, 36
    for constipation, 224
    and headaches, 232
    for osteoporosis, 333
    for vision problems, 221
Magnetic resonance imaging (MRI),
    45–46, 318
Maitake mushroom extract, 72
Mammograms
    abnormal test results, next steps, 47–48
Mandarin Medallions recipe, 258
Massage, to relieve cancer symptoms, 85
Measles vaccines
    and multiple myeloma, 77
Meat, red. *See also* Beef
    and breast cancer risk, 48–49
    and chronic pain, 282–283
    and diabetes risk, 99
    and kidney stones, 160
    linked to gout, 286
Medical bills, 294
Medical care
    inpatient doctors, 307–309
    traveling, to reduce cost of, 287–289
Medical insurance, after serious illness,
    303–304
Medicare, 303–304
Medicines. *See* Drugs; *specific conditions*
Meditation
    lowering of pain response, 279–280
    for stress relief, 125
Mediterranean diet
    and Alzheimer's risk, 8–9
    and cancer prevention, 64
    and coronary artery disease, 188
    for quality longevity, 21–22
Melanoma, and sun exposure, 219–220
Melatonin
    depletion of, by beta-blockers, 106–107
    for tinnitus, 108
Memory
    and Alzheimer's disease, 2–3
    exercise to improve, 138
    and folic acid, 217
    and intake of fruits and vegetables, 1–2
    and low-dose aspirin, 3–4
    and uric acid testing, 4
Men
    advanced age fatherhood, 18–19
    and breast cancer, 51–52
    communicating with, tips for women,
    130–131
    elderly, and testosterone levels, 17
    and shopping addiction, 146–147
Meningitis, misdiagnosis of, 149
Menopausal symptoms
    hot flashes, 324
    and HRT, 59–60
Mental health professionals, 309
Metabolism, pills to increase, 104–105
Methicillin-resistant *Staphylococcus
    aureus* (MRSA), 152–154